Concepts in Clinical

Pharmacokinetics

Fourth Edition

Concepts in Clinical
Pharmacokinetics

Fourth Edition

Joseph T. DiPiro, Pharm.D.

Professor and Executive Dean, South Carolina College of Pharmacy, The University of South Carolina, Columbia, Medical University of South Carolina, Charleston, South Carolina

William J. Spruill, Pharm.D., FASHP

Professor, Department of Clinical and Administrative Pharmacy at the University of Georgia College of Pharmacy, Athens, Georgia

William E. Wade, Pharm.D., FASHP

Professor, Department of Clinical and Administrative Pharmacy at the University of Georgia College of Pharmacy, Athens, Georgia

Robert A. Blouin, Pharm.D.

Professor and Dean, School of Pharmacy, University of North Carolina at Chapel Hill, Chapel Hill, North Carolina

Jane M. Pruemer, Pharm.D., BCOP

Associate Professor of Clinical Pharmacy Practice, University of Cincinnati College of Pharmacy, Cincinnati, Ohio

American Society of Health-System Pharmacists®

Any correspondence regarding this publication should be sent to the publisher, American Society of Health-System Pharmacists, 7272 Wisconsin Avenue, Bethesda, MD 20814, attn: Special Publishing. Produced in conjunction with the ASHP Publications Production Center.

The information presented herein reflects the opinions of the contributors and reviewers. It should not be interpreted as an official policy of ASHP or as an endorsement of any product.

Drug information and its applications are constantly evolving because of ongoing research and clinical experience and are often subject to professional judgment and interpretation by the practitioner and to the uniqueness of a clinical situation. The editors, authors, and ASHP have made every effort to ensure the accuracy and completeness of the information presented in this book. However, the reader is advised that the publisher, author, contributors, editors, and reviewers cannot be responsible for the continued currency or accuracy of the information, for any errors or omissions, and/or for any consequences arising from the use of the information in the clinical setting.

The reader is cautioned that ASHP makes no representation, guarantee, or warranty, express or implied, that the use of the information contained in this book will prevent problems with insurers and will bear no responsibility or liability for the results or consequences of its use.

Acquisition Editor: Hal Pollard
Managing/Development Editor: Dana Battaglia
Production: Silverchair Science + Communications, Inc.

Library of Congress Cataloging-in-Publication Data
    Concepts in clinical pharmacokinetics / Joseph T. DiPiro ... [et al.]. – 4th ed.
       p. ; cm. --
    Includes bibliographical references and index.
    ISBN 1-58528-124-7
   1. Pharmacokinetics.
   [DNLM: 1. Pharmacokinetics—Programmed Instruction. 2. Pharmaceutical Preparations--administration & dosage—Programmed Instruction. QV 18.2 C744 2005] I. Title: Clinical pharmacokinetics. II. DiPiro, Joseph T. III. American Society of Health-System Pharmacists

   RM301.5.C66 2005
   615'.7--dc22

                         2005011225

Contents

Lessons and Practice Sets

Acknowledgments

The authors are indebted to George Francisco, Kim Brouwer, Stan Greene, Cecily DiPiro, William H. Asbury, Maureen S. Boro, W. Greg Leader, Daniel Maddix, Gary R. Matzke, Page H. Pigg, Carl Possidente, and John R. Reynolds for their review and suggestions during the preparation of the first and second editions. The third and fourth editions reflect the suggestions of many individuals who used the manual and recommended improvements. The rigorous effort and valuable suggestions provided by Dana Battaglia for this edition are greatly appreciated.

Preface to the Third Edition

This programmed manual presents basic pharmacokinetic concepts and procedures that are useful in pharmacy, medicine, and other health professions. Most of the material relates to individualization of drug dosing regimens. Although this text is not intended to create a practitioner fully competent in clinical pharmacokinetics, it will provide an orientation to the concepts involved.

After completing this text, the reader should be prepared to begin learning the pharmacokinetic techniques for clinical situations. The reader should participate in structured educational settings, such as a formal clinical pharmacokinetics course or a clerkship under an experienced clinical practitioner, to develop clinical skills related to pharmacokinetics. Readers who want in-depth understanding of the derivations of pharmacokinetic equations should consult an appropriate text.

In this third edition, the manual is divided into 15 lessons to allow progression on a typical semester schedule of 15 weeks. The first 11 lessons include pharmacokinetic and pharmacodynamic principles as well as an overview of biopharmaceutic principles. Each of these lessons begins with a list of educational objectives and concludes with a series of questions. Answers and feedback for incorrect responses have been provided for the short-answer questions. Discussion questions have been added. Lessons 12 through 15 present brief patient case studies with aminoglycosides, theophylline, vancomycin, digoxin, and phenytoin so the reader can practice the use of pharmacokinetic equations.

This edition will be accompanied by a Web-based version that will provide lessons to parallel each of the lessons in the print version. The Web-based version will include dynamic figures and simulators, calculators for applying pharmacokinetic equations, links to important Web pages, and interactive capability for discussion questions. Although the print version may be used independently, we believe that concurrent use of both versions will enhance learning.

Joseph T. DiPiro
William J. Spruill
Robert A. Blouin
Jane M. Pruemer

January 2002

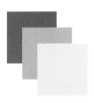

Preface to the Fourth Edition

Although the fourth edition of *Concepts in Clinical Pharmacokinetics* continues to provide basic pharmacokinetic concepts and procedures that are useful in pharmacy, medicine, and other health professions, this new edition has been revised to be, we anticipate, even more instructive and user-friendly for the reader.

All of the chapters are revised, with many new clinical correlates and some new figures. All similar equations are cross-referenced throughout the book to allow the student to compare the various equations. All cases are revised and new ones added. A new appendix, Basic and Drug-Specific Pharmacokinetic Equations, summarizes and lists all equations needed to dose selected drugs (aminoglycoside, vancomycin, theophylline, digoxin, and phenytoin). In addition, more in-depth answers and feedback for incorrect responses are provided for the short-answer questions.

Overall, this edition looks different as well. Figures are larger and equations clearer. All features are designated with specific design elements for easy navigation throughout the chapters. Our goal is to provide the student with an optimum learning experience. We hope this new design and the other enhancements help to achieve that goal.

Joseph T. DiPiro
William J. Spruill
William E. Wade
Robert A. Blouin
Jane M. Pruemer

March 2005

Abbreviations

α: distribution rate constant for two-compartment model

AUC: area under plasma drug concentration versus time curve

AUMC: area under the (drug concentration $\times$ time) versus time (moment) curve

β: terminal elimination rate constant

C: concentration

$\bar{C}$: average steady-state concentration

C_0, C_1, C_2: initial (just after infusion), first, second concentrations

C_{in}: concentration in blood on entering organ

C_{last}: last measured concentration

C_{max}: maximum concentration

C_{max1}, C_{max2}: first, second maximum concentrations

$C_{max(steady\ state)}$: steady-state maximum concentration

$C_{min(steady\ state)}$: steady-state minimum concentration

C_{min}: minimum concentration

C_{out}: concentration in blood on leaving organ

C_{peak}: peak concentration

C_{ss}: steady-state concentration

C_t: concentration at time t

C_{trough}: trough concentration

Cl: clearance

Cl_b: biliary clearance

Cl_h: hepatic (liver) clearance

Cl_i: intrinsic clearance

Cl_m: clearance by metabolism (mainly liver)

$Cl_{other\ organs}$: clearance by other organs

$Cl_{P \to mX}$: formation clearance for a given metabolite X

$Cl_{P \to m1}$: fractional clearance of parent drug (P) to form metabolite 1 (m_1)

Cl_r: renal clearance

Cl_t: total body clearance

conc: concentration

Δ: change in

E: extraction ratio

e: base of natural logarithm

F: fraction of drug absorbed that reaches systemic circulation (bioavailability)

F_p: fraction of unbound drug in plasma

F_t: fraction of unbound drug in tissue

F_{m1}: fraction of metabolite m_1 formed from a single dose of the parent drug

GFR: glomerular filtration rate

GI: gastrointestinal

K: elimination rate constant

K_0: rate of drug infusion

K_{12}: rate constant for transfer of drug from compartment 1 to compartment 2

K_{21}: rate constant for transfer of drug from compartment 2 to compartment 1

K_a: absorption rate constant

K_m: Michaelis–Menten constant (drug concentration at which elimination rate = $\frac{1}{2} V_{max}$)

λ: terminal elimination rate constant

m_1, m_2, m_3: metabolites 1, 2, and 3

$m_{1,u}, m_{2,u}, m_{3,u}$: amount of m_1, m_2, or m_3 excreted in the urine

MRT: mean residence time

n: number of doses

Q: blood flow

Q_h: hepatic blood flow

S: salt form of drug

SST: serum separator tube

τ: dosing interval

t: time (after dose)

t': time after end of infusion ($t' = \tau - t$ for trough concentration)

t'': time (duration) of loading infusion

t_0: time zero

$T^{1/2}$: half-life

$t_{90\%}$: time required to reach 90% of steady-state concentration

V: volume; volume of distribution

   V_{area}: volume of distribution by area

   V_c: volume of central compartment

   V_{extrap}: extrapolated volume of distribution

   V_p: plasma volume

   V_{ss}: steady-state volume of distribution

V_t: tissue volume

V_{max}: maximum rate of the elimination process

X: amount of drug

   X_0: dose (or initial dose) of drug

   X_1, X_2: amount of drug at different times

   X_c: amount of drug in central compartment

   X_d: daily dose of drug

   X_p: amount of drug in peripheral compartment

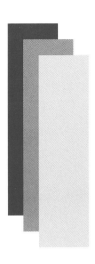

Pharmacy Continuing Education Program

HOW TO EARN CONTINUING EDUCATION

The continuing pharmacy education (CE) test for *Concepts in Clinical Pharmacokinetics*, fourth edition (Accreditation Council for Pharmacy Education Program [ACPE] Number: 204-000-05-083-H01) can only be taken online at the American Society of Health-System Pharmacists (ASHP) CE Testing Center at http://ce.ashp.org. If you score 70% or better on the test, you will be able to immediately print your own CE statement. You will have two opportunities to pass the CE test, and you can start and return to the test at any time before submitting your final answers.

Use your eight-digit ASHP member ID or Customer ID to log on (be sure to include any leading zeroes). Your member ID can be found on your membership card or on the mailing label of your copy of AJHP. To log on, click on "Enter the CE Testing Center" and type your ID number and password on the left-navigation column of the page. Follow the instructions below to purchase a CE Exam Processing Fee and to select the CE test for *Concepts in Clinical Pharmacokinetics*, fourth edition.

If you are not an ASHP member or do not have a Customer ID, you can click on the link to obtain an ASHP Customer ID or connect to the ASHP shopping cart to purchase the CE Exam Processing Fee. The system will automatically create a Customer ID and password when you purchase an item online.

Program Title: *Concepts in Clinical Pharmacokinetics*, fourth edition
ACPE Program #: 204-000-05-083-H01
CE credit: 20 hours (2.0 CEUs)

CE Exam Processing Fee

There is a nominal fee to access the test on the CE testing center. The fee for ASHP members is $20.95, and it is $30.95 for non-ASHP members.

Go the ASHP Shopping Cart (www.ashp.org/products-services), select "Browse Online Catalog," select "Products" in the navigation bar, and select "Continuing Education." Click on the "Add to Cart" icon, and check out. You can access the CE Testing Center immediately after your purchase to begin to take the CE test.

Cannot Remember Your Password?

Click on the "forgot password" link at http://www.ashp.org/ce/homepage.cfm

Questions

Call the ASHP Customer Service Center toll free at (866) 279-0681.

 The American Society of Health-System Pharmacists is accredited by the Accreditation Council for Pharmacy Education as a provider for continuing pharmacy education.

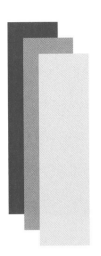

LESSON

1

Introduction to Pharmacokinetics and Pharmacodynamics

 OBJECTIVES

After completing Lesson 1, you should be able to:

1. Define and differentiate between *pharmacokinetics* and *clinical pharmacokinetics*.

2. Define *pharmacodynamics* and relate it to pharmacokinetics.

3. Describe the concept of the therapeutic concentration range.

4. Identify factors that cause interpatient variability in drug disposition and drug response.

5. Describe situations in which routine clinical pharmacokinetic monitoring would be advantageous.

6. Use both *one-* and *two-compartment models* and list the assumptions made about drug distribution patterns in each.

7. Represent graphically the typical natural log of plasma drug concentration versus time curve for a one-compartment model after an intravenous dose.

Pharmacokinetics is currently defined as the study of the time course of drug absorption, distribution, metabolism, and excretion. *Clinical pharmacokinetics* is the application of pharmacokinetic principles to the safe and effective therapeutic management of drugs in an individual patient.

Primary goals of clinical pharmacokinetics include enhancing efficacy and decreasing toxicity of a patient's drug therapy. The development of strong correlations between drug concentrations and their pharmacologic responses has enabled clinicians to apply pharmacokinetic principles to actual patient situations.

A drug's effect is often related to its concentration at the site of action, so it would be useful to monitor this concentration. Receptor sites of drugs are generally inaccessible to our observations or are widely distributed in the body, and therefore direct measurement of drug concentrations at these sites is not practical. For example, the receptor sites for digoxin are believed to be within the myocardium, and we cannot directly sample drug concentration in this tissue. However, we can measure drug concentration in the blood or plasma, urine, saliva, and other easily sampled fluids (Figure 1-1). *Kinetic homogeneity* describes the predictable relationship between plasma drug concentration and concentration at the receptor site (Figure 1-2). Changes in the plasma drug concentration reflect changes in drug concentrations in other tissues. As the concentration of drug in plasma increases, the concentration of drug in most tissues will increase proportionally.

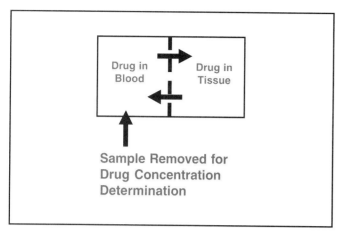

FIGURE 1-1.
Blood is the fluid most often sampled for drug concentration determination.

Similarly, if the plasma concentration of a drug is decreasing, the concentration in tissues will also decrease. Figure 1-3 is a simplified plot of the drug concentration versus time profile after an intravenous drug dose and illustrates the property of kinetic homogeneity.

The property of kinetic homogeneity is important for the assumptions made in clinical pharmacokinetics. It is the foundation on which all therapeutic and toxic plasma drug concentrations are established. That is, when studying concentrations of a drug in plasma, we assume that these plasma concentrations directly relate to concentrations in tissues where the disease process is to be modified by the drug (e.g., the central nervous system in Parkinson's disease or bone in osteomyelitis). This assumption, however, may not be true for all drugs.

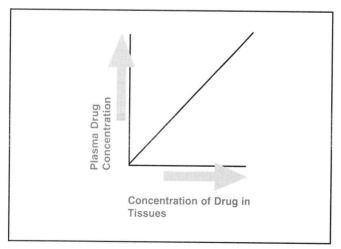

FIGURE 1-2.
Relationship of plasma to tissue drug concentrations.

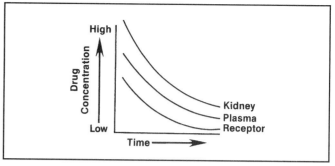

FIGURE 1-3.
Drug concentration versus time.

▮ CLINICAL CORRELATE

Drugs concentrate in some tissues because of physical or chemical properties. Examples include digoxin, which concentrates in the myocardium, and lipid-soluble drugs, such as benzodiazepines, which concentrate in fat.

BASIC PHARMACODYNAMIC CONCEPTS

Pharmacodynamics refers to the relationship between drug concentration at the site of action and the resulting effect, including the time course and intensity of therapeutic and adverse effects. The effect of a drug present at the site of action is determined by that drug's binding with a receptor. Receptors may be present on neurons in the central nervous system to depress pain sensation, on cardiac muscle to affect the intensity of contraction, or even within bacteria to disrupt maintenance of the bacterial cell wall.

For most drugs, the concentration at the site of the receptor determines the intensity of a drug's effect (Figure 1-4). However, other factors affect drug response as well. The drug's effect may ultimately be determined by the density of receptors on the cell surface, the mechanism by which a signal is transmitted into the cell by second messengers (substances within the cell), or regulatory factors that control gene translation and protein production. This multilevel regulation of drug effect results in variation of sensitivity to drug effect from one individual to another and also determines enhancement of or tolerance to drug effects.

In the simplest examples of drug effect, there is a relationship between the concentration of drug at the receptor site and the pharmacologic effect. If enough concentrations are tested, a maximum effect (E_{max}) can be determined (Figure 1-5). When the logarithm of concentration is plotted versus effect (Figure 1-5), one can see that there is a concentration below which no effect is observed and a concentration above which no greater effect is achieved.

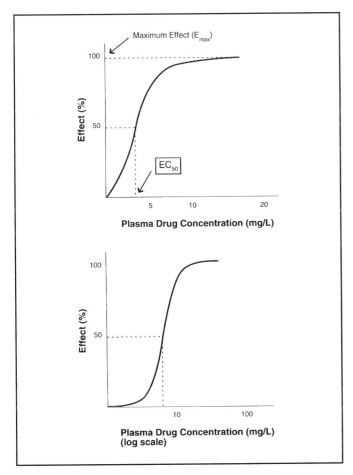

FIGURE 1-4.
Relationship of drug concentration to drug effect at the receptor site.

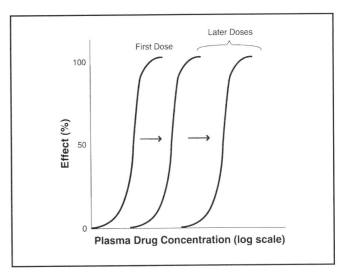

FIGURE 1-6.
Demonstration of tolerance to drug effect with repeated dosing.

One way of comparing **drug potency** is by the concentration at which 50% of the maximum effect is achieved. This is referred to as the *50% effective concentration* or *EC₅₀*. When two drugs are tested in the same individual, the drug with a lower EC_{50} would be considered more potent. This means that a lesser amount of a more potent drug is needed to achieve the same effect as a less potent drug.

The EC_{50} does not, however, indicate other important determinants of drug response, such as the duration of effect. Duration of effect is determined by a complex set of factors, including the time that a drug is engaged on the receptor as well as intracellular signaling and gene regulation.

For some drugs, the effectiveness can decrease with continued use. This is referred to as *tolerance*. Tolerance may be caused by pharmacokinetic factors, such as increased drug metabolism, that decrease the concentrations achieved with a dose. There can also be pharmacodynamic tolerance, which occurs when the same concentration at the receptor site results in a reduced effect with repeated exposure. Tolerance can be described in terms of the dose–response curve, as shown in Figure 1-6.

To assess the effect that a drug regimen is likely to have, the clinician should consider pharmacokinetic and pharmacodynamic factors. Both are important in determining a drug's effect.

▌ CLINICAL CORRELATE

Tolerance can occur with many commonly used drugs. One example is the hemodynamic tolerance that occurs with continued use of organic nitrates, such as nitroglycerin. For this drug, tolerance can be reversed by interspersing drug-free intervals with chronic drug use.

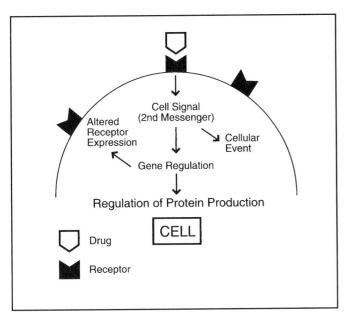

FIGURE 1-5.
Relationship of drug concentration at the receptor site to effect (as a percentage of maximal effect).

For some patients with diabetes mellitus there is a reduction in the number of insulin receptors on the surface of cells using glucose. These patients then become relatively insensitive to insulin and require higher doses. Therefore, the pharmacologic response for one person can be quite different from another, even with the same insulin concentrations at the receptor site.

◼ CLINICAL CORRELATE

One way to compare potency of two drugs that are in the same pharmacologic class is to compare EC_{50}. The drug with a lower EC_{50} is considered more potent.

THERAPEUTIC DRUG MONITORING

The usefulness of plasma drug concentration data is based on the concept that pharmacologic response is closely related to drug concentration at the site of action. For certain drugs, studies in patients have provided information on the plasma concentration range that is safe and effective in treating specific diseases—the therapeutic range (Figure 1-7). Within this therapeutic range, the desired effects of the drug are seen. Below it, there is greater probability that the therapeutic benefits are not realized; above it, toxic effects may occur.

No absolute boundaries divide subtherapeutic, therapeutic, and toxic drug concentrations. A gray area usually exists for most drugs in which these concentrations overlap due to variability in individual patient response. Both pharmacodynamic and pharmacokinetic factors contribute to this variability in patient response.

Although this course focuses on pharmacokinetics, it is important to remember the fundamental relationship between drug pharmacokinetics and pharmacologic response. The pharmacokinetics of a drug determine the blood concentration achieved from a prescribed dosing regimen. It is generally assumed that after continued drug dosing, the blood concentration will mirror the drug concentration at the receptor site; and it is the receptor site concentration that should principally determine the intensity of a drug's effect. Consequently, both the pharmacokinetics and pharmacologic response characteristics of a drug and the relationship between them must be understood before predicting a patient's response to a drug regimen.

Theophylline is an excellent example of a drug whose pharmacokinetics and pharmacodynamics are fairly well understood. When theophylline is administered at a fixed dosage to numerous patients, the blood concentrations achieved vary greatly. That is, wide interpatient variability exists in the pharmacokinetics of theophylline. This is important for theophylline because subtle changes in the blood concentration may result in significant changes in drug response.

Figure 1-8 shows the relationship between theophylline concentration (x-axis, on a logarithmic scale) and its pharmacologic effect, (changes in pulmonary function [y-axis]). Figure 1-8 illustrates that as the concentration of theophylline increases, so does the intensity of the response for some patients. Wide interpatient variability is also shown.

Theophylline concentrations below 5 mg/L are generally considered inadequate for a desired therapeutic effect, and side effects (tachycardia, nausea and vomiting, and nervousness) are more likely to occur at concentrations above 20 mg/L. Drugs like theophylline possess a narrow therapeutic index because the concentrations that may produce toxic effects are close to those required for therapeutic effects. The importance of considering both pharmacokinetics and pharmacodynamics is clear. Examples of therapeutic ranges for commonly used drugs are shown in Table 1-1.

As can be seen in this table, most drug concentrations are expressed as a unit of mass per volume (e.g., mg/L or mcg/mL, which are equivalent).

Many pharmacokinetic factors cause variability in the plasma drug concentration and, consequently, the pharmacologic response of a drug. Among these factors are:

- Differences in an individual's ability to metabolize and eliminate the drug (e.g., genetics)
- Variations in drug absorption

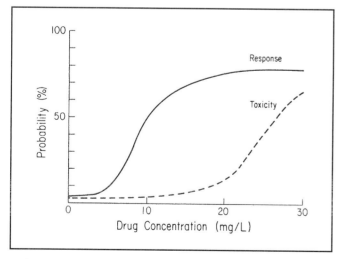

FIGURE 1-7.
Relationship between drug concentration and drug effects for a hypothetical drug. **Source:** Adapted with permission from Evans WE, editor. General principles of applied pharmacokinetics. In: *Applied Pharmacokinetics*, 3rd ed. Vancouver, WA: Applied Therapeutics; 1992. p.1–3.

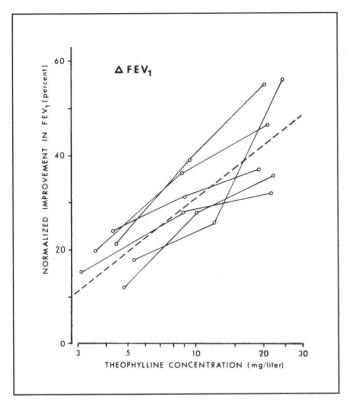

FIGURE 1-8.
Relationship between plasma theophylline concentration and change in forced expiratory volume (FEV) in asthmatic patients. **Source:** Reproduced with permission from Mitenko PA, Ogilvie RI. Rational intravenous doses of theophylline. *N Engl J Med* 1973; 289:600–3. Copyright 1973, Massachusetts Medical Society.

TABLE 1-1.
Therapeutic Ranges for Commonly Used Drugs

Drug	Range
Digoxin	0.5–2.0 ng/mL
Lidocaine	1.5–5.0 mg/L
Lithium	0.6–1.4 mEq/L
Phenobarbital	15–40 mg/L
Phenytoin	10–20 mg/L
Quinidine	2–5 mg/L
Theophylline	5–15 mg/L

Source: Adapted with permission from Bauer LA. Clinical pharmacokinetics and pharmacodynamics. In: DiPiro JT, Talbert RL, Yee GC, et al., editors. *Pharmacotherapy: a Pathophysiologic Approach.* 5th ed. New York: McGraw-Hill; 2002. p. 34.

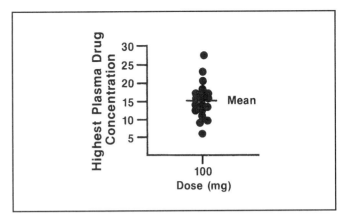

FIGURE 1-9.
Example of variability in plasma drug concentration among subjects given the same drug dose.

- Disease states or physiologic states (e.g., extremes of age) that alter drug absorption, distribution, or elimination
- Drug interactions

We could study a large group of patients by measuring the highest plasma drug concentrations resulting after administration of the same drug dose to each patient. For most drugs, the intersubject variability is likely to result in differing plasma drug concentrations (Figure 1-9). This variability is primarily attributed to factors influencing drug absorption, distribution, metabolism, or excretion. Disease states (e.g., renal or hepatic failure) and other conditions (e.g., obesity and aging) that may alter these processes must be considered for the individualization of drug dosage regimens (dose and frequency of dosing).

Therapeutic drug monitoring is defined as the use of assay procedures for determination of drug concentrations in plasma, and the interpretation and application of the resulting concentration data to develop safe and effective drug regimens. If performed properly, this process allows for the achievement of therapeutic concentrations of a drug more rapidly and safely than can be attained with empiric dose changes. Together with observations of the drug's clinical effects, it should provide the safest approach to optimal drug therapy.

The major potential advantages of therapeutic drug monitoring include maximization of therapeutic drug benefits as well as minimization of toxic drug effects. Therapeutic drug monitoring may be used in designing safe and effective drug therapy regimens. (Figure 1-10).

Recall the definition of pharmacodynamics as the relationship between drug concentration at the site of action and pharmacologic response. As demonstrated in Figure 1-10, pharmacodynamics and pharmacokinetics are closely interrelated (Figure 1-11).

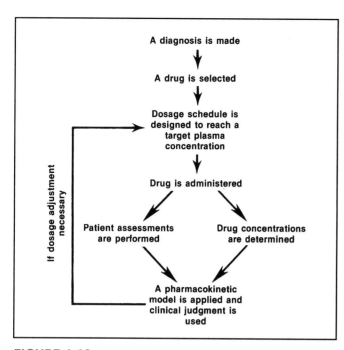

FIGURE 1-10.
Process for reaching dosage decisions with therapeutic drug monitoring.

TABLE 1-2.
Drugs for Which Plasma Levels May Be Monitored

Aminoglycosides

Cyclosporine

Digoxin

Lidocaine

Lithium

Methotrexate

Phenobarbital

Phenytoin

Procainamide

Theophylline

Quinidine

Valproic acid

Vancomycin

Carbamazepine

Some drugs lend themselves to clinical pharmacokinetic monitoring because their concentrations in plasma correlate well with pharmacologic response; for other drugs, this approach is not valuable. For example, it is advantageous to know the plasma theophylline concentration in a patient receiving this drug for the management of asthma. Because plasma theophylline concentration is related to pharmacologic effect, knowing that the plasma concentration is below the therapeutic range could justify increasing the dose. However, it is of little value to determine the plasma concentration of an antihypertensive agent, as it may not correlate well with pharmacologic effects and the end-point of treatment, blood pressure, is much easier to measure than the plasma concentration. Plasma levels are often monitored for the drugs listed in Table 1-2.

Therapeutic monitoring using drug concentration data is valuable when:

1. A good correlation exists between the pharmacologic response and plasma concentration. Over at least a limited concentration range, the intensity of pharmacologic effects should increase with plasma concentration. This relationship allows us to predict pharmacologic effects with changing plasma drug concentrations (Figure 1-12).
2. Wide intersubject variation in plasma drug concentrations results from a given dose.
3. The drug has a narrow therapeutic index (i.e., the therapeutic concentration is close to the toxic concentration).

FIGURE 1-11.
Relationship of pharmacokinetics and pharmacodynamics and factors that affect each.

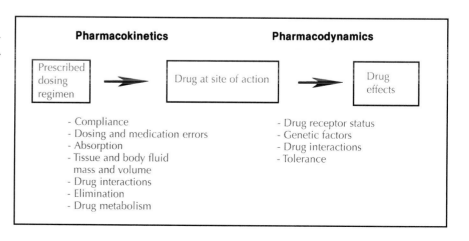

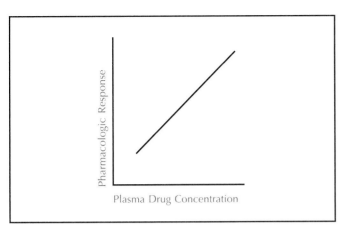

FIGURE 1-12.
When pharmacologic effects relate to plasma drug concentrations, the latter can be used to predict the former.

4. The drug's desired pharmacologic effects cannot be assessed readily by other simple means (e.g., blood pressure measurement for antihypertensives).

The value of therapeutic drug monitoring is limited in situations in which:

1. There is no well-defined therapeutic plasma concentration range.
2. The formation of pharmacologically active metabolites of a drug complicates the application of plasma drug concentration data to clinical effect unless metabolite concentrations are also considered.
3. Toxic effects may occur at unexpectedly low drug concentrations as well as at high concentrations.
4. There are no significant consequences associated with too high or too low levels.

◼ CLINICAL CORRELATE

A drug's effect may also be determined by the amount of time that the drug is present at the site of action. An example is with beta-lactam antimicrobials. The rate of bacterial killing by beta-lactams (the bacterial cell would be considered the site of action) is usually determined by the length of time that the drug concentration remains above the minimal concentration that inhibits bacterial growth.

PHARMACOKINETIC MODELS

The handling of a drug by the body can be very complex, as several processes (such as absorption, distribution, metabolism, and elimination) work to alter drug concentrations in tissues and fluids. Simplifications of body processes are necessary to predict a drug's behavior in the

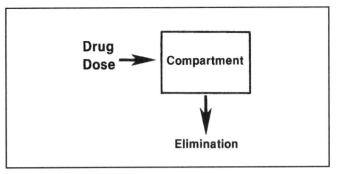

FIGURE 1-13.
Simple compartmental model.

body. One way to make these simplifications is to apply mathematical principles to the various processes.

To apply mathematical principles, a model of the body must be selected. A basic type of model used in pharmacokinetics is the compartmental model. Compartmental models are categorized by the number of compartments needed to describe the drug's behavior in the body. There are one-compartment, two-compartment, and multicompartment models. The compartments do not represent a specific tissue or fluid but may represent a group of similar tissues or fluids. These models can be used to predict the time course of drug concentrations in the body (Figure 1-13).

Compartmental models are termed *deterministic* because the observed drug concentrations determine the type of compartmental model required to describe the pharmacokinetics of the drug. This concept will become evident when we examine one- and two-compartment models.

To construct a compartmental model as a representation of the body, simplifications of body structures are made. Organs and tissues in which drug distribution is similar are grouped into one compartment. For example, distribution into adipose tissue differs from distribution into renal tissue for most drugs. Therefore, these tissues may be in different compartments. The highly perfused organs (e.g., heart, liver, and kidneys) often have similar drug distribution patterns, so these areas may be considered as one compartment. The compartment that includes blood (plasma), heart, lungs, liver, and kidneys is usually referred to as the *central compartment* or the *highly blood-perfused compartment* (Figure 1-14). The other compartment that includes the fat tissue, muscle tissue, and cerebrospinal fluid is the peripheral compartment, which is less well perfused than the central compartment.

Another simplification of body processes concerns the expression of changes in the amount of drug in the body over time. These changes with time are known as *rates*. The elimination rate describes the change in the amount of drug in the body due to drug elimination over

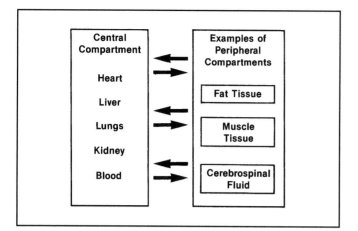

FIGURE 1-14.
Typical organ groups for central and peripheral compartments.

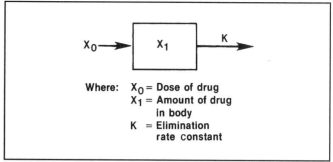

FIGURE 1-15.
One-compartment model.

time. Most pharmacokinetic models assume that elimination does not change over time.

The value of any model is determined by how well it predicts drug concentrations in fluids and tissues. Generally, it is best to use the simplest model that accurately predicts changes in drug concentrations over time. If a one-compartment model is sufficient to predict plasma drug concentrations (and those concentrations are of most interest to us), then a more complex (two-compartment or more) model is not needed. However, more complex models are often required to predict tissue drug concentrations.

◼ CLINICAL CORRELATE

Drugs that do not extensively distribute into extra-vascular tissues, such as aminoglycosides, are generally well described by one-compartment models. Extent of distribution is partly determined by the chemistry of the agents. Aminoglycosides are polar molecules, so their distribution is limited primarily to extracellular water. Drugs extensively distributed in tissue (such as lipophilic drugs like the benzodiazepines) or those that have extensive intracellular uptake may be better described by the more complex models.

COMPARTMENTAL MODELS

The one-compartment model is the most frequently used model in clinical practice. In structuring the model, a visual representation is helpful. The compartment is represented by an enclosed square or rectangle, and rates of drug transfer are represented by straight arrows (Figure 1-15). The arrow pointing into the box simply indicates that drug is put into that compartment. And the arrow

pointing out of the box indicates that drug is leaving the compartment.

This model is the simplest because there is only one compartment. All body tissues and fluids are considered a part of this compartment. Furthermore, it is assumed that after a dose of drug is administered, it distributes instantaneously to all body areas. Common abbreviations are shown in Figure 1-15.

Some drugs do not distribute instantaneously to all parts of the body, however, even after intravenous bolus administration. *Intravenous bolus dosing* means administering a dose of drug over a very short time period. A common distribution pattern is for the drug to distribute rapidly in the bloodstream and to the highly perfused organs, such as the liver and kidneys. Then, at a slower rate, the drug distributes to other body tissues. This pattern of drug distribution may be represented by a two-compartment model. The rapidly distributing tissues are called the *central compartment*, and the slowly distributing tissues are called the *peripheral compartment*. Drug moves back and forth between these tissues to maintain equilibrium (Figure 1-16).

Figure 1-17 simplifies the difference between one- and two-compartment models. Again, the one-compartment model assumes that the drug is distributed to tissues very rapidly after intravenous administration.

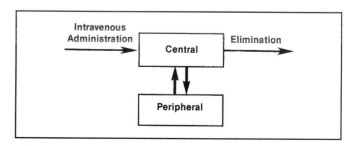

FIGURE 1-16.
Compartmental model representing transfer of drug to and from central and peripheral compartments.

FIGURE 1-17.
Drug distribution in one- and two-compartment models.

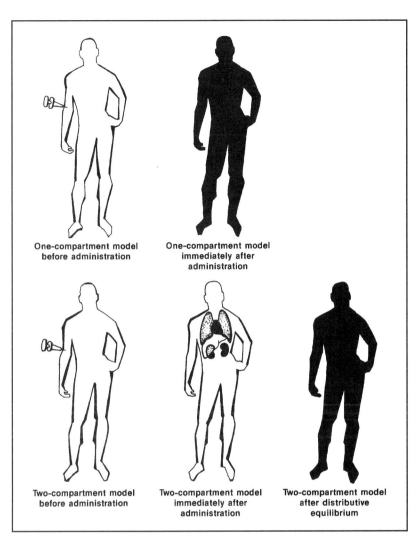

One-compartment model before administration

One-compartment model immediately after administration

Two-compartment model before administration

Two-compartment model immediately after administration

Two-compartment model after distributive equilibrium

The two-compartment model can be represented as in Figure 1-18, where:

X_0 = dose of drug
X_1 = amount of drug in central compartment
X_2 = amount of drug in peripheral compartment
K = elimination rate constant of drug from central compartment to outside the body
K_{12} = elimination rate constant of drug from central compartment to peripheral compartment
K_{21} = elimination rate constant of drug from peripheral compartment to central compartment

in tissue and plasma, plasma concentrations decline less rapidly (Figure 1-19). The plasma would be the central compartment, and muscle tissue would be the peripheral compartment.

Until now, we have spoken of the amount of drug (X) in a compartment. If we also consider the volume of the compartment, we can describe the concept of drug concentra-

■ CLINICAL CORRELATE

Digoxin, particularly when given intravenously, is an example of a drug that is well described by two-compartment pharmacokinetics. After an intravenous dose is administered, plasma concentrations rise and then rapidly decline as drug distributes out of plasma and into muscle tissue. After equilibration between drug

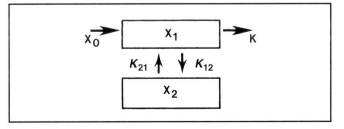

FIGURE 1-18.
Two-compartment model.

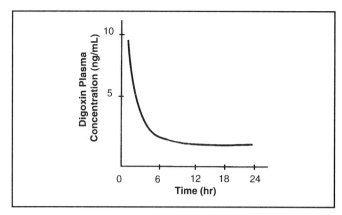

FIGURE 1-19.
Plasma concentrations of digoxin after an intravenous dose.

tion. *Drug concentration* in the compartment is defined as the amount of drug in a given volume, such as mg/L:

⚠ 1-1

$$\text{concentration of drug} = \frac{\text{amount of drug}}{\begin{array}{c}\text{volume in which}\\\text{drug is distributed}\end{array}}$$

Volume of distribution (*V*) is an important indicator of the extent of drug distribution into body fluids and tissues. *V* relates the amount of drug in the body (*X*) to the measured concentration in the plasma (*C*). Thus, *V* is the volume required to account for all of the drug in the body if the concentrations in all tissues are the same as the plasma concentration:

$$\text{volume of distribution} = \frac{\text{amount of drug}}{\text{concentration}}$$

A large volume of distribution usually indicates that the drug distributes extensively into body tissues and fluids. Conversely, a small volume of distribution often indicates limited drug distribution.

Volume of distribution indicates the extent of distribution but not the tissues or fluids into which the drug is distributing. Two drugs can have the same volume of distribution, but one may distribute primarily into muscle tissues, whereas the other may concentrate in adipose tissues. Approximate volumes of distribution for some commonly used drugs are shown in Table 1-3.

When *V* is many times the volume of the body, the drug concentrations in some tissues should be much greater than those in plasma. The smallest volume in which a drug may distribute is the plasma volume.

To illustrate the concept of volume of distribution, let us first imagine the body as a tank filled with fluid, as the body is primarily composed of water. To calculate the volume of the tank, we can place a known quantity of substance into it and then measure its concentration in the fluid (Figure 1-20). If the amount of substance (*X*) and the resulting concentration (*C*) is known, then the

TABLE 1-3.

Approximate Volumes of Distribution of Commonly Used Drugs

Drug	Volume of Distribution (L)
Nortriptyline	1300
Digoxin	440
Propranolol	270
Lidocaine	77
Phenytoin	45
Theophylline	35
Gentamicin	18

Source: Shargel L, Yu ABC. *Applied Biopharmaceutics and Pharmacokinetics.* 4th ed. New York: McGraw-Hill; 1999. pp. 732–6.

volume of distribution (*V*) can be calculated using the simplified equations:

$$X = VC \qquad \text{or} \qquad C = \frac{X}{V} \qquad \text{or} \qquad V = \frac{X}{C}$$

V = volume of distribution
X = amount of drug in body
C = concentration in the plasma

As with other pharmacokinetic parameters, volume of distribution can vary considerably from one person to another because of differences in physiology or disease states. Something to note: the dose of a drug (X_0) and the amount of drug in the body (X) are essentially the same thing because all of the dose goes into the body.

In this example, important assumptions have been made: that instantaneous distribution occurs and that it occurs equally throughout the tank. In the closed tank, there is no elimination. This example is analogous to a one-compartment model of the body after intravenous

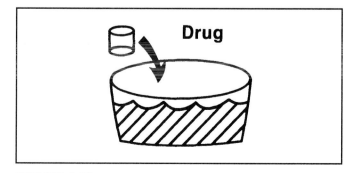

FIGURE 1-20.
The volume of a tank can be determined from the amount of substance added and the resulting concentration.

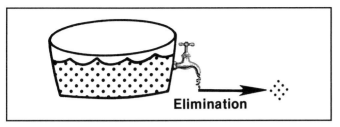

FIGURE 1-21.
Drug elimination complicates the determination of the "volume" of the body from drug concentrations.

bolus administration. However, there is one complicating factor—during the entire time that the drug is in the body, elimination is taking place. So, if we consider the body as a tank with an open outlet valve, the concentration used to calculate the volume of the tank would be constantly changing (Figure 1-21).

We can use the relationship given in **Equation 1-1** for volume, amount of drug administered, and resulting concentration to estimate a drug's volume of distribution in a patient. If we give a known dose of a drug and determine the concentration of that drug achieved in the plasma, we can calculate a volume of distribution. However, the concentration used for this estimation must take into account changes resulting from drug elimination, as discussed in Lessons 3 and 9.

For example:
If 100 mg of drug X is administered intravenously and the plasma concentration is determined to be 5 mg/L just after the dose is given, then:

$$\text{volume of distribution } (V) = \frac{\text{dose}}{\text{resulting concentration}} = \frac{X_0}{C} = \frac{100 \text{ mg}}{5 \text{ mg/L}} = 2$$

 CLINICAL CORRELATE

The volume of distribution is easily approximated for many drugs. For example, if the first 80-mg dose of gentamicin is administered intravenously and results in a peak plasma concentration of 8 mg/L, volume of distribution would be calculated as follows:

$$\text{volume of distribution } (V) = \frac{\text{dose}}{\text{resulting concentration}} = \frac{X_0}{C} = \frac{80 \text{ mg}}{8 \text{ mg/L}} = 10 \text{ L}$$

CLINICAL CORRELATE

Drugs that have extensive distribution outside of plasma appear to have a large volume of distribution.

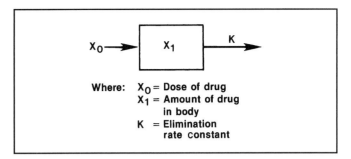

FIGURE 1-22.
One-compartment model.

Examples include chloroquine, digoxin, diltiazem, dirithromycin, imipramine, labetalol, metoprolol, meperidine, and nortriptyline.

PLASMA DRUG CONCENTRATION VERSUS TIME CURVES

With the one-compartment model (Figure 1-22), if we continuously measure the concentration of a drug in the plasma after an intravenous bolus dose and then plot these plasma drug concentrations against the times they are obtained, the curve shown in Figure 1-23 would result. Note that this plot is a curve and that the plasma concentration is highest just after the dose is administered, at time zero (t_0).

Because of cost limitations and patient convenience in clinical situations, only a small number of plasma samples can usually be obtained for measuring drug concentrations (Figure 1-24). From these known values, we are able to predict the plasma drug concentrations for the times when we have no samples (Figure 1-25). In clinical situations, it is rare to collect more than two samples after a dose.

The prediction of drug concentrations based on known concentrations can be subject to multiple sources of error. However, if we realize the assumptions

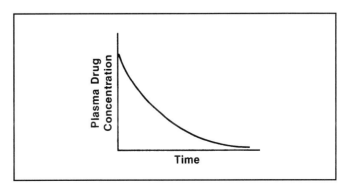

FIGURE 1-23.
Typical plasma drug concentration versus time curve for a one-compartment model.

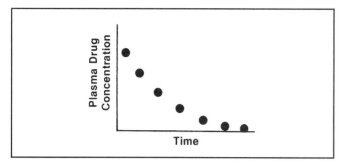

FIGURE 1-24.
Plasma drug concentrations determined at specific time points.

used to make the predictions, some errors can be avoided. These assumptions are pointed out as we review the one-compartment system.

From a mathematical standpoint, the prediction of plasma concentrations is easier if we know that the concentrations are all on a straight line rather than a curve. This conversion can be accomplished for most drugs by plotting the natural logarithm (ln) of the plasma drug concentration versus time. The plot of a curve (Figure 1-25) is, in effect, converted to a straight line by using the natural log of the plasma drug concentration (Figure 1-26).

A straight line is obtained from the natural log of plasma drug concentration versus time plot only for drugs that follow first-order elimination processes and exhibit one-compartment distribution. First-order elimination occurs when the amount of drug eliminated from the body in a specific time is dependent on the amount of drug in the body at that time. This concept is explained further in Lesson 2.

An alternative to calculating the natural log values is to plot the actual concentration and time values on semilogarithmic (or semilog) paper (Figure 1-27), a special graph paper that automatically adjusts for the logarithmic relationship by altering the distance between lines on the *y*-axis. The lines on the *y*-axis are not evenly spaced but

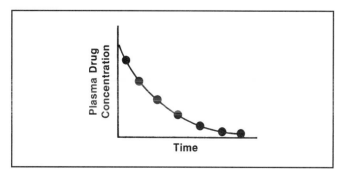

FIGURE 1-25.
Plasma drug concentrations can be predicted for times when they were not determined. Concentrations on the line drawn through the measured concentrations are predicted concentrations.

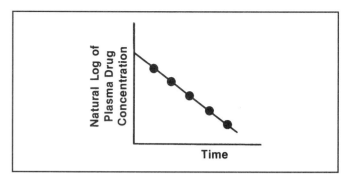

FIGURE 1-26.
With a simple one-compartment, intravenous bolus model, a plot of the natural log of plasma concentration versus time results in a straight line.

rather are logarithmically related within each log cycle (or multiple of 10). So when the actual values of plasma drug concentrations are plotted against the time values, a straight line results. The *x*-axis has evenly spaced lines; there is no conversion to the log of those values. (The term *semilogarithmic* indicates that only one axis is converted.) The numbers on the *y*-axis may be used to represent 0.1 through 1, 1 through 10, 10 through 100, or any series with a 10-fold difference in the range of values.

If a series of plasma concentration versus time points are known and plotted on semilog paper, a straight line can be drawn through the points by visual inspection or, more accurately, by linear regression techniques. Linear regression is a mathematical method used to determine the line that best represents a set of plotted points. From this line,

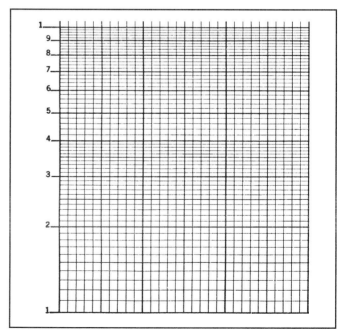

FIGURE 1-27.
Paper with one log-scale axis is called *semilog paper*.

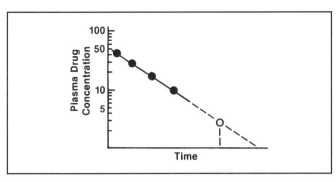

FIGURE 1-28.

When plasma concentration versus time points fall on a straight line, concentrations at various times can be predicted simply by picking a time point and matching concentration on the line at that time.

we can predict plasma drug concentrations at times for which no measurements are available (Figure 1-28).

■ CLINICAL CORRELATE

For a typical patient, plasma concentrations resulting from an 80-mg dose of gentamicin may be as shown in Table 1-4. The plasma concentrations plotted on linear and semilogarithmic graph paper are shown in Figure 1-29. With the semilog paper, it is easier to predict what the gentamicin plasma concentration would be 10 hours after the dose is administered.

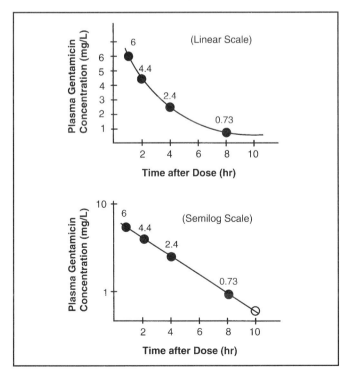

FIGURE 1-29.

Predicting plasma drug concentrations with semilog scale.

TABLE 1-4.

Time Course of Plasma Gentamicin Concentration

Concentration (mg/L)	Time after Dose (hours)
6	1
4.4	2
2.4	4
0.73	8

LOGARITHM PRIMER

The log of a number is the power to which a given base number must be raised to equal that number. With natural logarithms, the base is 2.718. For example, the natural logarithm of 8.0 is x, where $2.718^x = 8.0$ and x = 2.08. Natural logarithms are used because they relate to natural processes such as drug elimination, radioactive decay, and bacterial growth. Instead of 2.718 to indicate the base of the natural log function, the abbreviation "e" is used. Also, instead of writing "natural logarithm of 8.0," we shall use the abbreviation ln 8.0.

Natural logarithms can be related to common logarithms (base 10 logarithms) as follows:

$$\text{log base } 10 = \frac{\text{log base e}}{2.303}$$

USING THE CALCULATOR WITH NATURAL LOG AND EXPONENTIAL KEYS

There are two major keys that will be used to calculate pharmacokinetic values from either known or estimated data. These are the "ln" key and the "e^x" key. Certain calculators do not have the "e^x" key. Instead, they will have an "ln" key and an "INV" key. Pressing the "INV" key and then the "ln" key will give "e^x" values.

▌ Review Questions _____

1-1. The study of the time course of drug absorption, distribution, metabolism, and excretion is called:

A. pharmacodynamics.

B. drug concentration.

C. pharmacokinetics.

D. kinetic homogeneity.

1-2. The application of pharmacokinetic principles to the safe and effective therapeutic management of drugs in an individual patient is known as:

A. pharmacodynamics.

B. clinical pharmacokinetics.

1-3. Since we cannot practically measure drug concentration in specific tissues, we measure it in the plasma and assume that this concentration is the same as that in tissue.

A. True

B. False

1-4. *Pharmacodynamics* refers to the relationship of drug:

A. dose to drug concentration in plasma.

B. dose to drug concentration at the receptor site.

C. concentrations to drug effect.

D. dose to drug effect.

1-5. Drug pharmacodynamics are affected by the drug concentration at the site of the receptor, density of receptors on the target cell surface, mechanism by which a signal is transmitted into the cell by second messengers, and regulatory factors that control gene translation and protein production.

A. True

B. False

1-6. The EC_{50} refers to the drug concentration at which:

A. one-half the maximum response is achieved.

B. the maximal effect is achieved.

C. tolerance is likely to be observed.

1-7. The therapeutic range is the range of plasma drug concentrations that clearly defines optimal drug therapy and where toxic effects cannot occur.

A. True

B. False

1-8. Therapeutic drug concentration monitoring with plasma drug concentration data assumes that pharmacologic response is related to the drug concentration in plasma.

A. True

B. False

1-9. Factors that cause variability in plasma drug concentrations after the same drug dose is given to different patients include variations in the:

A. drug absorption.

B. EC_{50} of the drug.

1-10. An example of a situation that would not support therapeutic drug concentration monitoring with plasma drug concentrations would be one in which:

A. a wide variation in plasma drug concentrations is achieved in different patients given a standard drug dose.

B. the toxic plasma concentration is many times the therapeutic concentration range.

C. correlation between a drug's plasma concentration and therapeutic response is good.

1-11. For a drug with a narrow therapeutic index, the plasma concentration required for therapeutic effects is near the concentration that produces toxic effects.

A. True

B. False

1-12. In pharmacokinetics, the term *rate* refers to a change in which of the following measurements over time.

A. drug dose

B. drug elimination

C. concentration of drug in plasma

1-13. The most commonly used model in clinical pharmacokinetic situations is the:

A. one-compartment model.

B. two-compartment model.

C. multicompartment model.

1-14. Highly perfused organs and blood make up what is usually known as the peripheral compartment.

A. True

B. False

1-15. Instantaneous distribution to most body tissues and fluids is assumed in which of the following models?

A. one-compartment model

B. two-compartment model

C. multi-compartment model

1-16. The amount of drug per unit of volume is defined as the:

A. volume of distribution.

B. concentration.

C. rate.

1-17. If 3 g of a drug are added and distributed throughout a tank and the resulting concentration is 0.15 g/L, calculate the volume of the tank.

A. 10 L

B. 20 L

C. 30 L

D. 200 L

1-18. For a drug that has first-order elimination and follows a one-compartment model, which of the following plots would result in a curved line?

A. plasma concentration versus time

B. natural log of plasma concentration versus time

1-19. A drug that follows a one-compartment model is given as an intravenous injection, and the following plasma concentrations are determined at the times indicated:

Plasma Concentration (mg/L)	Time after Dose (hours)
81	1
67	2
55	3

Using semilog graph paper, determine the approximate concentration in plasma at 6 hours after the dose.

A. 18 mg/L

B. 30 mg/L

C. <1 mg/L

▋ Answers

1-1. A. Incorrect answer. Pharmacodynamics deals with the relationship between the drug concentration at the site of action and the resulting effect.

B. Incorrect answer. Drug concentrations in plasma and tissues are what results from pharmacokinetic processes.

C. CORRECT ANSWER

D. Incorrect answer. Kinetic homogeneity describes the relationship between plasma drug concentration and concentration at a receptor or site of action.

1-2. A. Incorrect answer. Pharmacodynamics alone is not sufficient for effective therapeutic management as it does not account for absorption, distribution, metabolism, and excretion.

B. CORRECT ANSWER

1-3. A. Incorrect answer. The plasma drug concentration is not the same as that in the tissue but rather is related to the tissue concentration by the volume of distribution (V). Plasma drug concentrations are commonly used because blood, being

readily accessible via venipuncture, is the body fluid most often collected for drug measurement.

B. CORRECT ANSWER

1-4. A, B. Incorrect answers. These statements are definitions of pharmacokinetics.

C. CORRECT ANSWER

D. Incorrect answer. This statement refers to the effect of pharmacokinetic and pharmacodynamic processes.

1-5. A. CORRECT ANSWER

B. Incorrect answer

1-6. A. CORRECT ANSWER

B. Incorrect answer. The "50" in "EC_{50}" refers to 50% of the maximal effect.

C. Incorrect answer. The term EC_{50} refers to pharmacologic effect and not to tolerance.

1-7. A. Incorrect answer. Although the therapeutic range of a drug describes a range of plasma drug concentrations generally considered safe and effective in a patient population, no absolute boundaries divide subtherapeutic, therapeutic, and toxic drug concentrations for an individual patient. Both pharmacodynamic and pharmacokinetic factors influence a patient's response.

B. CORRECT ANSWER

1-8. A. CORRECT ANSWER

B. Incorrect answer. This statement is the basic assumption underlying the use of plasma drug concentrations.

1-9. A. CORRECT ANSWER

B. Incorrect answer. The EC_{50}, 50% effective concentration, is a way of comparing drug potency. The EC_{50} is the concentration at which 50% of the maximum effect of the drug is achieved.

1-10. A. Incorrect answer. A wide variation in plasma drug concentrations would be a good justification for therapeutic drug level monitoring.

B. CORRECT ANSWER. When the toxic plasma concentration is much greater than the therapeutic concentration range, then there is less need for drug level monitoring.

C. Incorrect answer. A good correlation between concentration and response makes therapeutic drug level monitoring more useful.

1-11. For a drug with a narrow therapeutic index, the plasma concentration required for therapeutic effects is near the concentration that produces toxic effects. The dosage of such a drug must be chosen carefully.

1-12. A. Incorrect answer. The dose is the amount of drug given at one time or in divided amounts within a given period.

B. Incorrect answer. Most pharmacokinetic models assume that elimination does not change over time.

C. CORRECT ANSWER

1-13. A. CORRECT ANSWER

B. Incorrect answer. Although a two-compartment model is often used, it is not used as commonly as a one-compartment model.

C. Incorrect answer. Multicompartment models are used occasionally for research purposes but are not normally used in clinical pharmacokinetics.

1-14. A. Incorrect answer. The peripheral compartment is generally made up of less-well-perfused tissues, such as muscle and fat.

B. CORRECT ANSWER

1-15. A. CORRECT ANSWER

B. Incorrect answer. In a two-compartment model, it is assumed that drug distribution to some tissues proceeds at a lower rate than for other tissues.

C. Incorrect answer. In a multicompartment model, it is also assumed that drug distribution to some tissues proceeds at a lower rate than for other tissues.

1-16. A. Incorrect answer. The volume of distribution refers to the dose over the resulting concentration.

B. CORRECT ANSWER

C. Incorrect answer. The amount per unit of volume is a static value and would not change over time; therefore, it would not be considered a rate.

1-17. A, C, D. Incorrect answers. A math error must have been made. The answer can be found by dividing 3 g by 0.15 g/L.

B. CORRECT ANSWER

1-18. A. CORRECT ANSWER

B. Incorrect answer. This plot would be a straight line (see Figure 1-29).

1-19. A, C. Incorrect answers. These results might have been determined if linear graph paper was used or if the points were plotted incorrectly.

B. CORRECT ANSWER

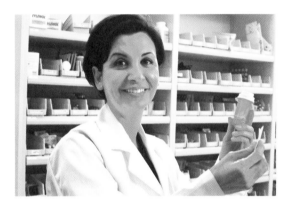

Discussion Points

D-1. An H_2-receptor antagonist is given to control gastric pH and prevent stress bleeding. The following gastric pHs were observed when steady-state concentrations of the drug were achieved. What are the E_{max} and EC_{50} of this drug?

Plasma Concentration (mg/L)	Resulting pH
0.25	1.0
0.5	1.0
1	1.4
2	2.6
3	3.8
4	4.8
5	4.8

D-2. The relationship shown in Figure 1-30 is observed from a clinical study. What are some of the likely reasons for this result?

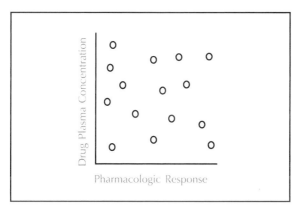

FIGURE 1-30.
Pharmacologic response versus drug plasma concentration.

(continued)

D-3.   The models shown in Figure 1-31 both well represent actual plasma concentrations of a drug after a dose. Which one should be preferred to predict plasma levels? Provide a justification for your answer.

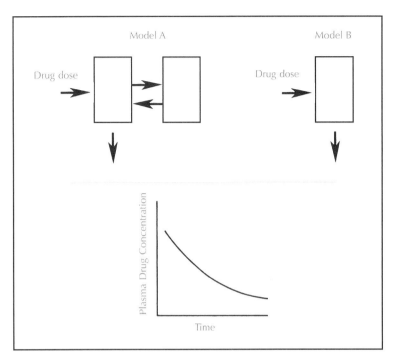

FIGURE 1-31.
Models for predicting plasma drug concentrations over time.

D-4.   Would you expect that a large drug molecule that does not cross physiologic membranes very well and is not lipid soluble to have a relatively high or low volume of distribution? Explain your answer.

D-5.   When plotting plasma drug concentration (y-axis) versus time (x-axis), what are the advantages of using a natural log scale for the y-axis rather than a linear scale?

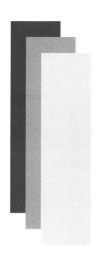

LESSON

2

Basic Pharmacokinetics

 OBJECTIVES

After completing Lesson 2, you should be able to:

1. Calculate the volume of distribution.
2. Identify the components of body fluids that make up extracellular and intracellular fluids and know the percentage of each component.
3. Describe the difference between whole blood, plasma, and serum.
4. Define drug clearance and show how it is related to organ blood flow.
5. Describe the difference between first- and zero-order elimination and how each appear graphically.

To examine the concept of volume of distribution (volume of distribution may be represented by "V" or "Vd") further, let's return to our example of the body as a tank described in Lesson 1. We assumed that no drug was being removed from the tank while we were determining volume. In reality, drug concentration in the body is constantly changing, primarily due to elimination. This flux makes it more difficult to calculate the apparent volume in which a drug distributes.

One way to calculate the apparent volume of drug distribution in the body is to measure the plasma concentration immediately after intravenous administration before elimination has had a significant effect. The concentration just after intravenous administration (at time zero, t_0) is abbreviated as C_0 (Figure 2-1). The volume of distribution can be calculated using the equation:

$$\text{volume of distribution} = \frac{\text{amount of drug administered (dose)}}{\text{initial drug concentration}} \text{ or } V_d(L) = \frac{X_0 \text{ (mg)}}{C_0 \text{ (mg/L)}}$$

(See **Equation 1-1**.)

C_0 can be determined from a direct measurement or estimated by back-extrapolation from concentrations determined at any time after the dose. If two concentrations have been determined, a line containing the two values and extending through the y-axis can be drawn on semilog paper. The point where that line crosses the y-axis gives an estimate of C_0. Both the direct measurement and back-extrapolation approaches assume that the drug distributes instantaneously into a single homogeneous compartment.

The volume of distribution is an important parameter for determining proper drug dosing regimens. Often referred to as the *apparent* volume of distribution, it does not have an exact physiologic significance, but it can indicate the extent of drug distribution and aid in determination of dosage requirements. Generally, dosing is proportional to the volume of distribution. For example: the larger the volume of distribution, the larger a dose must be to achieve a desired target concentration.

To understand how distribution occurs, you must have a basic understanding of body fluids and tissues (Figure 2-2). The fluid portion (water) in an adult makes up approximately 60% of total body weight and is composed of intracellular fluid (35%) and extracellular fluid (25%). Extracellular fluid is made up of plasma (4%) and interstitial fluid (21%). Interstitial fluid surrounds

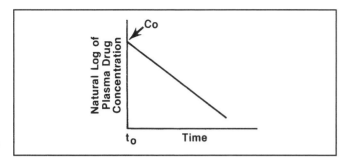

FIGURE 2-1.
Concentration resulting immediately after an intravenous injection of a drug is referred to as C_0.

cells outside the vascular system. These percentages vary somewhat in a child.

If a drug has a volume of distribution of approximately 15–18 L in a 70-kg person, we might assume that its distribution is limited to extracellular fluid, as that is the approximate volume of extracellular fluid in the body. If a drug has a volume of distribution of about 40 L, the drug may be distributing into all body water, because a 70-kg person has approximately 40 L of body water (70 kg × 60%). If the volume of distribution is much greater than 40–50 L, the drug probably is being concentrated in tissue outside the plasma and interstitial fluid.

If a drug distributes extensively into tissues, the volume of distribution calculated from plasma concentrations could be much higher than the actual physiologic volume in which it distributes. For example, by measuring plasma concentrations, it appears that digoxin distributes in approximately 440 L in an adult. Because digoxin binds extensively to muscle tissue, plasma levels are fairly low relative to concentrations in muscle tissue. For other drugs, tissue concentrations may not be as high as the plasma concentration, so it may appear that these drugs distribute into a relatively small volume.

It is also important to distinguish among blood, plasma, and serum. *Blood* refers to the fluid portion in combina-

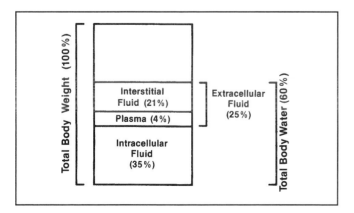

FIGURE 2-2.
Fluid distribution in an adult.

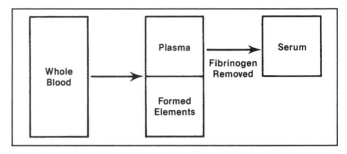

FIGURE 2-3.
Relationship of whole blood, plasma, and serum.

tion with formed elements (white cells, red cells, and platelets). *Plasma* refers only to the fluid portion of blood (including soluble proteins but not formed elements). When the soluble protein fibrinogen is removed from plasma, the remaining product is *serum* (Figure 2-3).

These differences in biologic fluids must be recognized when considering reported drug concentrations. The plasma concentration of a drug may be much less than the whole blood concentration if the drug is preferentially sequestered by red blood cells.

☐ CLINICAL CORRELATE

Most drug concentrations are measured using plasma or serum that usually generate similar values. It is more relevant to use plasma or serum than whole blood measurements to estimate drug concentrations at the site of effect. However, some drugs such as antimalarials are extensively taken up by red blood cells. In these situations, whole blood concentrations would be more relevant, although they are not commonly used in clinical practice.

CLEARANCE

Another important parameter in pharmacokinetics is *clearance*. Clearance is a measure of the removal of drug from the body. Plasma drug concentrations are affected by the rate at which drug is administered, the volume in which it distributes, and its clearance. A drug's clearance and the volume of distribution determine its half-life. The concept of half-life and its relevant equations are discussed in Lesson 3.

Clearance (expressed as volume/time) describes the removal of drug from a volume of plasma in a given unit of time (drug loss from the body). Clearance does not indicate the amount of drug being removed. It indicates the volume of plasma (or blood) from which the drug is completely removed, or cleared, in a given time period. Figures 2-4 and 2-5 represent two ways of thinking about drug clearance. In Figure 2-4, the amount of drug (the

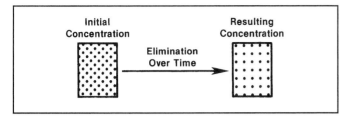

FIGURE 2-4.
Decrease in drug concentration due to drug clearance.

number of dots) decreases but fills the same volume, resulting in a lower concentration. Another way of viewing the same decrease would be to calculate the volume that would be drug-free if the concentration were held constant.

Drugs can be cleared from the body by many different mechanisms, pathways, or organs, including hepatic biotransformation and renal and biliary excretion. Total body clearance of a drug is the sum of all the clearances by various mechanisms.

$$Cl_t = Cl_r + Cl_m + Cl_b + Cl_{other}$$

2-1

where

Cl_t = total body clearance (from all mechanisms, where t refers to total);

Cl_r = renal clearance (through renal excretion);

Cl_m = clearance by liver metabolism or biotransformation;

Cl_b = biliary clearance (through biliary excretion); and

Cl_{other} = clearance by all other routes (gastrointestinal tract, pulmonary, etc.).

For an agent removed primarily by the kidneys, renal clearance (Cl_r) makes up most of the total body clearance. For a drug primarily metabolized by the liver, hepatic clearance (Cl_m) is most important.

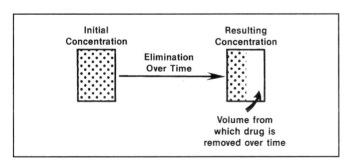

FIGURE 2-5.
Clearance may be viewed as the volume of plasma from which drug is totally removed over a specified period.

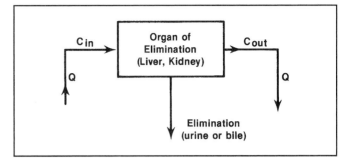

FIGURE 2-6.
Model for organ clearance of a drug.

A good way to understand clearance is to consider a single well-perfused organ that eliminates drug. Blood flow through the organ is referred to as Q (mL/minute) as seen in Figure 2-6, where C_{in} is the drug concentration in the blood entering the organ and C_{out} is the drug concentration in the exiting blood. If the organ eliminates some of the drug, C_{in} is greater than C_{out}.

We can measure an organ's ability to remove a drug by relating C_{in} and C_{out}. This extraction ratio (E) is:

$$E = \frac{C_{in} - C_{out}}{C_{in}}$$

This ratio must be a fraction between zero and one. Organs that are very efficient at eliminating a drug will have an extraction ratio approaching one (i.e., 100% extraction). Table 2-1 is used as a general guide.

The drug clearance of any organ is determined by blood flow and the extraction ratio:

organ clearance = blood flow × extraction ratio

or:

$$Cl_{organ} = Q \times \frac{C_{in} - C_{out}}{C_{in}} \quad \text{or} \quad Cl_{organ} = QE$$

2-2

If an organ is very efficient in removing drug (i.e., extraction ratio near one) but blood flow is low, clearance will also be low. Also, if an organ is inefficient in

TABLE 2-1.
Rating of Extraction Ratios

Extraction Ratio (E)	Rating
> 0.7	High
0.3–0.7	Intermediate
< 0.3	Low

TABLE 2-2.
Effect on Clearance

Extraction Ratio (E)	Blood Flow (Q) (L/hour)	Clearance (Cl) (L/hour)
High (0.7–1.0)	Low	Low
Low (< 0.3)	High	Low
High (0.7–1.0)	High	High
Low (< 0.3)	Low	Low

TABLE 2-3.
Average Clearances of Common Drugs

Aspirin	650 mL/minute
Cephalexin	300 mL/minute
Digoxin	130 mL/minute
Gentamicin	90 mL/minute
Lovastatin	4–18 mL/minute
Ranitidine	730 mL/minute
Vancomycin	98 mL/minute
Zidovudine	26 mL/minute

Source: Shargel L, Yu ABC. *Applied Biopharmaceutics and Pharmacokinetics.* 4th ed. New York: McGraw-Hill; 1999. pp. 732–6.

removing drug (i.e., extraction ratio close to zero) even if blood flow is high, clearance would again be low. See Table 2-2.

The equations noted previously are not used routinely in clinical drug monitoring, but they describe the concept of drug clearance. Examination of a single well-perfused organ to understand clearance is a noncompartmental approach; no assumptions about the number of compartments have to be made. Therefore, *clearance* is said to be a model-independent parameter. Clearance also can be related to the model-dependent parameters volume of distribution and elimination rate (discussed in Lesson 3).

Clearance can also be a useful parameter for constructing dosage recommendations in clinical situations. It is an index of the capacity for drug removal by the body organs.

 CLINICAL CORRELATE

Blood flow and the extraction ratio will determine a drug's clearance. Propranolol is a drug that is eliminated exclusively by hepatic metabolism. The extraction ratio for propranolol is greater than 0.9, so most of the drug presented to the liver is removed by one pass through the liver. Therefore, clearance is approximately equal to liver blood flow (Cl = Q × E: when E ~ 1.0, Cl ~ Q). One indication of the high extraction ratio is the relatively high oral dose of propranolol compared with the intravenous dose; an oral dose is 10–20 times the equivalent intravenous dose. The difference reflects the amount of drug removed by first-pass metabolism after absorption from the gastrointestinal tract and before entry into the general circulation.

The average clearances of some commonly used drugs are shown in Table 2-3. These values can vary considerably between individuals and may be altered by disease.

FIRST-ORDER AND ZERO-ORDER ELIMINATION

The simplest example of drug elimination in a one-compartment model is a single intravenous bolus dose of a drug. It is first assumed that:

1. Distribution and equilibration to all tissues and fluids occurs instantaneously, so a one-compartment model applies.
2. Elimination is first order.

Most drugs are eliminated by a first-order process, and the concept of first-order elimination must be understood. With first-order elimination, the amount of drug eliminated in a set amount of time is directly proportional to the amount of drug in the body. The amount of drug eliminated over a certain time period increases as the amount of drug in the body increases; likewise, the amount of drug eliminated per unit of time decreases as the amount of drug in the body decreases. This concept is different from zero-order elimination, in which the amount of drug eliminated for each time interval is constant, regardless of the amount of drug in the body.

With the first-order elimination process, although the amount of drug eliminated may change with the amount of drug in the body, the fraction of a drug in the body eliminated over a given time remains constant. In practical terms, the fraction or percentage of drug being removed is the same with either high or low drug concentrations. For example, if 1000 mg of a drug is administered and the drug follows first-order elimination, we might observe the patterns in Table 2-4.

TABLE 2-4.
First-Order Elimination

Time after Drug Administration (hours)	Amount of Drug in Body (mg)	Amount of Drug Eliminated Over Preceding Hour (mg)	Fraction of Drug Eliminated Over Preceding Hour
0	1000	—	—
1	850	150	0.15
2	723	127	0.15
3	614	109	0.15
4	522	92	0.15
5	444	78	0.15
6	377	67	0.15

The actual amount of drug eliminated is different for each fixed time period, depending on the initial amount in the body, but the fraction removed is the same, so this elimination is first order. Because the elimination of this drug (like most drugs) occurs by a first-order process, the amount of drug eliminated decreases as the concentration in plasma decreases. The actual fraction of drug eliminated over any given time (in this case 15%) depends on the drug itself and the individual patient's capacity to eliminate the drug.

On the other hand, with zero-order elimination, the amount of drug eliminated does not change with the amount or concentration of drug in the body, but the fraction removed varies (Figure 2-7). For example, if 1000 mg of a drug is administered and the drug follows zero-order elimination, we might observe the patterns in Table 2-5.

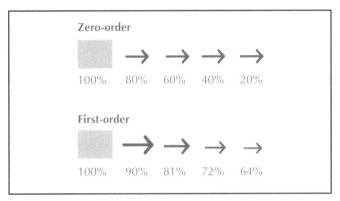

FIGURE 2-7.
Zero- versus first-order elimination. The size of the arrow represents the amount of drug eliminated over a unit of time. Percentages are the fraction of the initial drug amount remaining in the body.

TABLE 2-5.
Zero-Order Elimination

Time after Drug Administration (hours)	Amount of Drug in Body (mg)	Amount of Drug Eliminated Over Preceding Hour (mg)	Fraction of Drug Eliminated Over Preceding Hour
0	1000	—	—
1	850	150	0.15
2	700	150	0.18
3	550	150	0.21
4	400	150	0.27
5	250	150	0.38

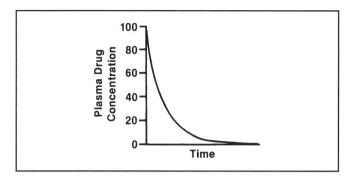

FIGURE 2-8.
Plasma drug concentration versus time after an intravenous (bolus) drug dose, assuming a one-compartment model with first-order elimination (linear y-scale).

Now that we have examined zero- and first-order elimination, let's return to our simple one-compartment, intravenous bolus situation. If the plasma drug concentration is continuously measured and plotted against time after administration of an intravenous dose of a drug with first-order elimination, the plasma concentration curve shown in Figure 2-8 would result. To predict concentrations at times when we did not collect samples, we must linearize the plot by using semilog paper (Figure 2-9).

For a drug with first-order elimination, the natural log of plasma concentration versus time plot is a straight line. Conversely, plots with zero-order elimination would be as shown in Figure 2-10. Note that for a drug with zero-order elimination, the plot of the plasma concentration versus time is linear (plot A in Figure 2-10), whereas on semilog paper (representing the natural log of plasma concentration versus time) it is a curve (bottom plot in Figure 2-10).

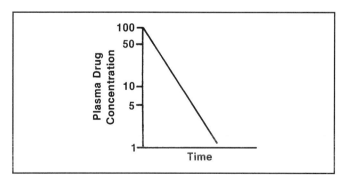

FIGURE 2-9.
As in Figure 2-8, but with a log scale y-axis.

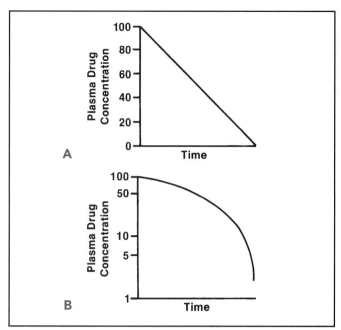

FIGURE 2-10.
Plasma drug concentrations versus time after an intravenous (bolus) drug dose, assuming a one-compartment model with zero-order elimination (**A**, linear plot; **B**, log plot).

If the natural log of a plasma drug concentration versus time plot is linear, it generally can be assumed that the drug follows first-order elimination.

▮ CLINICAL CORRELATE

Most antimicrobial agents (e.g., aminoglycosides, cephalosporins, and vancomycin) display first-order elimination when administered in usual doses. The pharmacokinetic parameters for these drugs are not affected by the size of the dose given. As the dose and drug concentrations increase, the amount of drug eliminated per hour increases while the fraction of drug removed remains the same.

Some drugs (e.g., phenytoin), when given in high doses, display zero-order elimination. Zero-order elimination occurs when the body's ability to eliminate a drug has reached its maximum capability (i.e., all transporters are being used). As the dose and drug concentration increase, the amount of drug eliminated per hour does not increase, and the fraction of drug removed declines.

Review Questions

2-1. The volume of distribution equals the dose divided by:

A. clearance

B. initial drug concentration

C. half-life

D. final concentration

2-2. A dose of 1000 mg of a drug is administered to a patient, and the following concentrations result at the indicated times below. Assume a one-compartment model.

Plasma Concentration (mg/L)	Time after Dose (hours)
100	2
67	4
45	6

An estimate of the volume of distribution would be:

A. 10 L.

B. 22.2 L.

C. 6.7 L.

D. 5 L.

2-3. If a drug is extensively distributed to tissues, its apparent volume of distribution is probably very:

A. large.

B. small.

2-4. For the body fluid compartments below, rank them from the lowest volume to the highest, in a typical 70-kg person.

A. Plasma < extracellular fluid < intracellular fluid < total body water

B. Extracellular fluid < intracellular fluid < plasma < total body water

C. Intracellular fluid < extracellular fluid < plasma < total body water

D. Total body water < plasma < intracellular fluid < extracellular fluid

2-5. *Plasma* refers only to the fluid portion of blood, including soluble proteins but not formed elements.

A. True

B. False

2-6. Clearance describes the removal of drug from the body over:

A. concentration.

B. dose.

C. one half-life.

D. time.

2-7. Total body clearance is the sum of clearance by the kidneys, liver, and other routes of elimination.

A. True

B. False

2-8. To determine drug clearance, we must first determine whether a drug best fits a one- or two-compartment model.

A. True

B. False

2-9. With a drug that follows first-order elimination, the amount of drug eliminated per unit time:

A. remains constant while the fraction of drug eliminated decreases.

B. decreases while the fraction of drug eliminated remains constant.

Answers

2-1. A, C, D. Incorrect answers

B. CORRECT ANSWER. You can determine the correct answer from the units in the numerator and denominator. They should cancel to yield a volume unit. "Grams" divided by "grams per liter" would leave you with "liter" as the unit. The volume is therefore determined from the dose, or amount of drug given, and the resulting initial concentration.

2-2. A. Incorrect answer. You may have used 100 mg/L as the initial concentration.

B. Incorrect answer. You may have used an incorrect initial concentration.

C. CORRECT ANSWER. To find the initial concentration, plot the given plasma concentration and time values on semilog paper, connect the points, and read the value of the y-axis (concentration) when x (time) = 0. This should be 150 mg/L. You can then determine the volume of distribution using the equation volume of distribution = dose/initial concentration.

D. Incorrect answer. You may have used an incorrect initial concentration, or you may have used linear graph paper instead of semilog paper.

2-3.   A. CORRECT ANSWER. Drug concentrations are generally measured in plasma. When drug distributes extensively into tissues, the plasma level will be reduced. This will make it seem as if the drug distributes over a very large volume. Examining the equation volume of distribution = dose/initial concentration, as the initial concentration decreases, the volume will increase.

B. Incorrect answer

2-4.   A. CORRECT ANSWER. See Figure 2-2. Plasma would be 2.8 L, extracellular fluid would be 18 L, intracellular fluid would be 25 L, and total body water would be 42 L.

B, C, D. Incorrect answers

2-5.   A. CORRECT ANSWER

B. Incorrect answer

2-6.   A, B, C. Incorrect answers. (Although half-life is a unit of time, clearance is usually expressed per minute or per hour.)

D. CORRECT ANSWER. The units for clearance are volume/time.

2-7.   A. CORRECT ANSWER. Total body clearance can be determined as the sum of individual clearances from all organs or routes of elimination.

B. Incorrect answer

2-8.   A. Incorrect answer

B. CORRECT ANSWER. It is not necessary to specify a model to determine drug clearance.

2-9.   A. Incorrect answer

B. CORRECT ANSWER. With first-order elimination, the amount of drug eliminated in any time period is determined by the amount of drug present at the start. Although the amount of drug eliminated in successive time periods may decrease, the fraction of the initial drug that is eliminated remains constant.

Discussion Points

D-1. Explain how a person who weighs 70 kg can have a volume of distribution for a drug of 700 L.

D-2. For drug X, individual organ clearances have been determined as follows:

Renal clearance   180 mL/minute
Hepatic clearance   22 mL/minute
Pulmonary clearance   5.2 mL/minute

How would you describe the clearance of drug X?

D-3. Drug Y is given by an intravenous injection and plasma concentrations are then determined as follows:

Time after Injection (hours)	Concentration (mg/L)
0	12
1	9.8
2	7.9
3	6.4
4	5.2
5	4.2
6	3.4
7	2.8
8	2.2

Is this drug eliminated by a first- or zero-order process? Defend your answer.

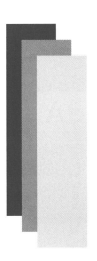

LESSON

3

Half-Life, Elimination Rate, and AUC

 OBJECTIVES

After completing Lesson 3, you should be able to:

1. Calculate the elimination rate constant given a natural log of plasma drug concentration versus time curve.

2. Define *half-life*.

3. Calculate a drug's half-life given a natural log of plasma drug concentration versus time curve.

4. Define the relationship between half-life and elimination rate constant.

5. Calculate a drug's half-life given its elimination rate constant.

6. Define *drug clearance* and relate it to the area under the plasma drug concentration curve and drug dose.

7. Calculate a drug's volume of distribution, concentration at time zero, and area under the plasma concentration versus time curve, given plasma concentration data after an intravenous bolus drug dose.

In Lesson 2, we learned that for most drugs (those following first-order elimination) a straight line can describe the change in natural log of plasma concentration over time. Recognizing this relationship, we can now develop mathematical methods to predict drug concentrations.

Whenever you have a straight line such as that in Figure 3-1, the line is defined by the equation:

$$Y = mX + b$$

where m is the slope of the line and b is the intercept of the y-axis. If you know the slope and the y-intercept, you can find the value of Y for any given X value.

As the value for the y-intercept may be obtained easily by visual inspection, the only part of the equation that must be calculated is the slope of the line. A slope is calculated from the change in the y-axis (the vertical change) divided by the change in the x-axis (the horizontal change), as in Figure 3-2:

$$\text{slope} = \frac{\Delta Y}{\Delta X} \quad \text{or} \quad \text{slope} = \frac{Y_2 - Y_1}{X_2 - X_1}$$

where Δ means "change in."

The slope is obtained by selecting two different points on the line and calculating the differences between their values: We can apply these same mathematical principles to the natural log of plasma concentration versus time plot (Figure 3-3). The slope is the change in the natural log of plasma concentrations divided by the change in time between the concentrations:

$$\text{slope} = \frac{\Delta \ln \text{conc}}{\Delta \text{time}} \quad \text{or} \quad \text{slope} = \frac{\ln C_1 - \ln C_0}{t_1 - t_0}$$

If, for example, 10 mg/L is the first concentration (C_0) drawn immediately after administration ($t_0 = 0$ hour) and 1 mg/L is the second concentration (C_1) drawn 2.5 hours after administration ($t_1 = 2.5$ hours):

$$\begin{aligned} \text{slope} &= \frac{\ln C_1 - \ln C_0}{t_1 - t_0} \\ &= \frac{\ln 1 - \ln 10}{2.5 \text{ hr} - 0 \text{ hr}} = \frac{0 - 2.303}{2.5 \text{ hr}} \\ &= -0.92 \text{ hr}^{-1} \end{aligned}$$

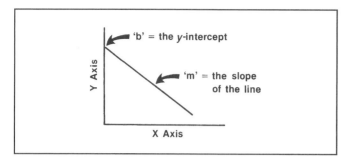

FIGURE 3-1.
Straight-line plot showing slope and *y*-intercept.

Note that the slope is calculated using $\ln C_1 - \ln C_0$ or $\ln(C_1/C_0)$ and not $\ln(C_1 - C_0)$. The latter would give an incorrect result. A negative slope indicates that the natural log of concentration declines with increasing time.

When the natural log of drug concentration is plotted versus time and a straight line results, as in the previous example, the slope of that line indicates the rate of drug elimination. A steeper slope (Figure 3-4, top graph) indicates a faster rate of elimination than does a flatter slope (Figure 3-4, bottom graph). For first-order processes, the rate of elimination (expressed as the fraction of drug in the body removed over a unit of time) is the same at high or low concentrations and is therefore called an *elimination rate constant*.

In fact, when drug elimination is first order, the negative slope of the natural log of drug concentration versus time plot equals the drug's elimination rate constant:

slope = –elimination rate constant

or:

–slope = elimination rate constant

Remember that the elimination rate constant is the fraction of drug removed over a unit of time. If the elim-

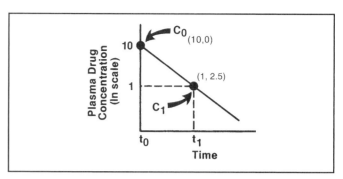

FIGURE 3-3.
The slope of the natural log of plasma concentration versus time curve can be determined if two plasma concentrations and their corresponding times are known.

ination rate constant is 0.25 hr^{-1}, then 25% of the drug remaining in the body is removed each hour.

Because we know that a plot of the natural log of drug concentration over time is a straight line for a drug following first-order elimination, we can predict drug concentrations for any time after the dose if we know the equation for this line. Remember that all straight lines can be defined by:

$$Y = mX + b$$

As shown in Figure 3-3:

Y axis = natural log of drug concentration in plasma
X axis = time after dose

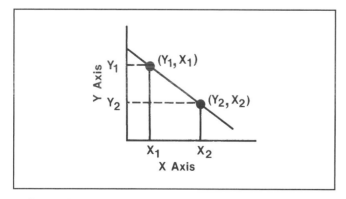

FIGURE 3-2.
The slope of a straight line can be determined from any two points on the line.

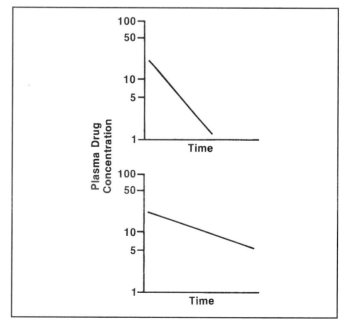

FIGURE 3-4.
A steeper slope (*top*) indicates a faster rate of elimination.

m = slope of line, "or negative elimination rate constant"

b = intercept on natural log of plasma drug concentration axis (y-intercept)

Now, when we convert to our new terms:

ln drug concentration = (–elimination rate constant × time) + ln concentration at y-intercept

If we know the slope of the line and the intercept of the y-axis, we can predict the natural log of drug concentration at any time after a dose.

Drug concentrations can be predicted using these mathematical methods instead of the previously described graphical methods. With mathematical methods, our predictions of drug concentrations over time are more accurate. So, if the negative slope of the natural log of drug concentration versus time plot equals the elimination rate constant, our equation for the line:

$$Y = mX + b$$

becomes:

ln (drug concentration) = (–elimination rate constant × time) + ln y-intercept

To simplify our terminology here, let:

ln C = natural log of drug concentration,
K = elimination rate constant, and
t = time after dose.

Also, we shall call the y-intercept "ln C_0," the drug concentration immediately after a dose is administered (at time zero, or t_0). Therefore, our equation becomes:

$$\ln C = (-K \times t) + \ln C_0 \text{ or } -K = \frac{\ln C - \ln C_0}{t}$$

This last equation is valuable in therapeutic drug monitoring. If two plasma drug concentrations and the time between them are known, then the elimination rate can be calculated. If one plasma drug concentration and the elimination rate are known, then the plasma concentration at any later time can be calculated.

■ CLINICAL CORRELATE

The concepts presented in this lesson can be used to predict plasma concentrations in some situations. For example, if a patient with renal dysfunction received a dose of vancomycin and plasma concentrations were determined 24 and 48 hours after the dose, then two plasma concentrations could be plotted on semilog

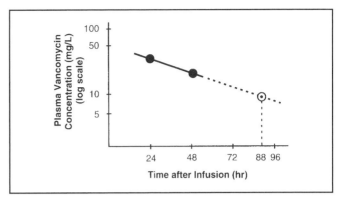

FIGURE 3-5.
Predicting plasma drug concentrations.

paper to determine when the concentration would reach 10 mg/L (Figure 3-5). This would be approximately 88 hours after the infusion. This information can be used to determine when the next dose should be given.

ELIMINATION RATE CONSTANT

As stated in the previous section, the elimination rate constant (K) represents the fraction of drug removed per unit of time and has units of reciprocal time (e.g., minute^{-1}, hour^{-1}, and day^{-1}). These units are evident from examination of the calculation of K. For example, in Figure 3-6, C_0 is the first plasma drug concentration, measured just after the dose is given, and C_1 is the second plasma drug concentration, measured at a later time (t_1). From our previous discussion, we know that the equation for this line ($y = mX + b$) is:

$$\ln C_1 = -Kt + \ln C_0$$

Furthermore, we know that the slope of the line equals $-K$, and we can calculate this slope:

⚠ 3-1 $$\text{slope} = -K = \frac{\ln C_1 - \ln C_0}{t_1 - t_0}$$

It is a property of logarithms that:

$$\ln C_1 - \ln C_0 = \ln \frac{C_1}{C_0}$$

Then, using numbers from Figure 3-6:

$$-K = \frac{\ln \frac{C_1}{C_0}}{t_1 - t_0} = \frac{\ln \left(\frac{5 \text{ mg/L}}{12.3 \text{ mg/L}} \right)}{6 \text{ hr} - 0 \text{ hr}}$$

So, $-K = -0.15$ hr^{-1}, or $K = 0.15$ hr^{-1}.

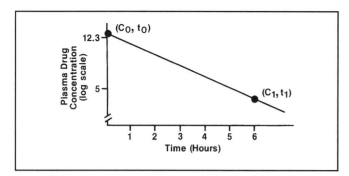

FIGURE 3-6.
Determination of a line (log scale) from two known plasma drug concentrations.

In this case, the elimination rate constant is 0.15 hr^{-1}. This means that 15% of the drug remaining in the body is removed each hour, so an initial plasma concentration of 10 mg/L will decrease 15% ($0.15 \times 10 \text{ mg/L} = 1.5$ mg/L) to 8.5 mg/L by the end of the first hour. By the end of the second hour, the concentration will be 7.2 mg/L, a 15% reduction from 8.5 mg/L ($0.15 \times 8.5 \text{ mg/L} = 1.3$).

The equation $\ln C = -Kt + \ln C_0$ is important because it allows the estimation of the concentration at any given time. Remember that it is in the form of an equation for a line, $Y = mX + b$. Remembering the rule of logarithms, that $\ln X^p = P \ln X$, if we take the antilog of each part of this equation, we get:

⚠️
3-2
$$C = C_0 e^{-Kt}$$

where:
   C = plasma drug concentration at time = t,
   C_0 = plasma drug concentration at time = 0,
   K = elimination rate constant,
   t = time after dose, and
   e = base of the natural log (approximately 2.718).
   e^{-Kt} = percent or fraction remaining after time (t)

To determine the e^{-Kt} portion on a calculator, enter the value for $-Kt$ and then the function for e^x, or inverse natural log, or raise 2.718 to the power of the value of $-Kt$. The antilog of a number is equal to e (or 2.718) raised to a power equal to that number. The preceding equation can also be used to predict the concentration at any time, given an initial concentration of C_0 and an elimination rate of K.

Through these mathematical manipulations, simple equations have been derived to aid in predicting drug plasma concentration after a given dose. The equation $C = C_0 e^{-Kt}$ is also helpful in clinical situations. It is essentially the same as the equation for the straight line

($\ln C_1 = -Kt + \ln C_0$), and either equation can be used to predict drug concentrations.

HALF-LIFE

Another important parameter that relates to the rate of drug elimination is half-life ($T\frac{1}{2}$). The half-life is the time necessary for the concentration of drug in the plasma to decrease by half. A drug's half-life is often related to its duration of action and also may indicate when another dose should be given.

One way to estimate the half-life is to visually examine the natural log of plasma drug concentration versus time plot and note the time required for the plasma concentration to decrease by half. For example, in Figure 3-7, the decrease from 10 to 5 mg/L takes approximately 1.5 hours. It also takes 1.5 hours for the concentration to decrease from 5.0 to 2.5 mg/L, from 7.0 to 3.5 mg/L, etc. At any point, the decrease in concentration by half takes approximately 1.5 hours, even when the decrease is from a concentration as low as 0.05 to 0.025 mg/L. Thus, the half-life can be estimated to be 1.5 hours.

There is another way to estimate the half-life from two known concentrations. Because the half-life is the time for a concentration to decrease by half, $T\frac{1}{2}$ can be estimated by halving the initial concentration, then taking half of that concentration to get a second concentration, and so on until the final concentration is reached. The number of halves required to reach the final concentration, divided into the time between

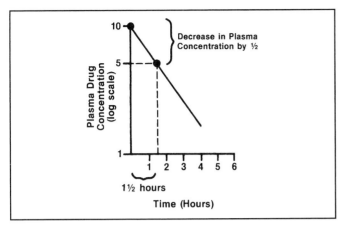

FIGURE 3-7.
Half-life can be determined from the natural log of plasma concentration versus time plot.

TABLE 3-1.
Example of Half-Life

Time after Peak Concentration (hours)	Plasma Concentration (mg/L)
0	100
2	50
4	25
6	12.5
7	6.25
8	3.125

the two concentrations, is the estimated half-life. For example, the following two concentrations were determined at the times stated after a dose was administered:

C (mg/L)	8.0	4.0
t (hour)	0	6

Because the concentration drops from 8.0 to 4.0 mg/L in 6 hours, the half-life is 6 hours. Consider a case in which concentrations and times were as follows:

C (mg/L)	12.0	3.0
t (hour)	8	12

The concentration drops from 12 mg/L to 3 mg/L in 4 hours. To get from 12 to 3 requires a halving of 12 to 6 and a halving of 6 to 3, representing two half-lives in 4 hours, or one half-life of 2 hours.

The half-life and the elimination rate constant express the same idea. They indicate how quickly a drug is removed from the plasma and, therefore, how often a dose has to be administered.

If the half-life and peak plasma concentration of a drug are known, then the plasma drug concentration at any time can be estimated. For example, if the peak plasma concentration is 100 mg/L after an intravenous dose of a drug with a 2-hour half-life, then the concentration will be 50 mg/L 2 hours after the peak concentration (a decrease by half). At 4 hours after the peak concentration, it will have decreased by half again, to 25 mg/L, and so on as shown in Table 3-1.

Half-life may be mathematically calculated with the following equation:

$$\text{⚠}\quad T\tfrac{1}{2} = \frac{0.693}{K}$$

3-3

The equation represents the important relationship between the half-life and the elimination rate constant shown by mathematical manipulation. We already know that:

$$\ln C = \ln C_0 - Kt$$

By definition, the concentration (C) at the time (t) equal to the half-life ($T\tfrac{1}{2}$) is half the original concentration (C_0). Therefore, at one half-life, the concentration is half of what it was initially. So we can say that at $t = T\tfrac{1}{2}$, $C = \tfrac{1}{2}C_0$. For simplicity, let's assume that $C_0 = 1$. Therefore:

$$\ln 0.5C_0 = \ln C_0 - K(T\tfrac{1}{2})$$

$$\ln 0.5 = \ln 1 - K(T\tfrac{1}{2})$$

Transforming this equation algebraically gives:

$$K(T\tfrac{1}{2}) = \ln 1 - \ln \tfrac{1}{2}$$
$$T\tfrac{1}{2} = \frac{0 - (-0.693)}{K}$$
$$T\tfrac{1}{2} = \frac{0.693}{K}$$

and

$$K = \frac{0.693}{T\tfrac{1}{2}}$$

Therefore, the half-life can be determined if we know the elimination rate constant and, conversely, the elimination rate constant can be determined if we know the half-life. This relationship between the half-life and elimination rate constant is important in determining drug dosages and dosing intervals.

CLINICAL CORRELATE

Half-life can be calculated from two plasma concentrations after a dose is given. First the elimination rate constant (K) is calculated as shown previously. For example, if a dose of gentamicin is administered and a peak plasma concentration is 6 mg/L after the infusion is completed and is 1.5 mg/L 4 hours later, the elimination rate constant is calculated as follows:

$$K = -\frac{\ln C_1 - \ln C_0}{t_1 - t_0}$$

$$= -\frac{\ln 1.5 - \ln 6}{4\ \text{hr} - 0\ \text{hr}}$$

$$= -\frac{-1.39}{4\ \text{hr}}$$

$$= 0.348\ \text{hr}^{-1}$$

Then:

$$T\tfrac{1}{2} = \frac{0.693}{K} = 2.0\ \text{hr}$$

CLINICAL CORRELATE

The average plasma half-lives of some commonly used drugs are shown in Table 3-2. These may vary considerably between individuals and may be altered by disease. Note that drug effects may persist for a period of time longer than would be predicted by a drug's half-life. The greater the value of the half-life, the longer the drug stays in the body. As an example from Table 3-2, half of a dose of vancomycin takes approximately 5.6 hours to be eliminated from the body (no matter the size of the dose). Also, half of a dose of cephalexin is eliminated in approximately 0.9 hour after administration, and so on.

RELATIONSHIPS AMONG PHARMACOKINETIC PARAMETERS

In previous lessons, we discussed elimination rate, volume of distribution, and clearance. These important parameters aid in calculating a drug dosage regimen. All three relate to how fast a drug effect will terminate. There are significant relationships among these parameters, the drug dose, and plasma drug concentrations. In

TABLE 3-2.
Half-Lives of Common Drugs

Drug	Half-Life (hours)
Aspirin	0.3
Cephalexin	0.9
Digoxin	39
Gentamicin	2–3
Lovastatin	1.1–1.7
Ranitidine	2.1
Vancomycin	5.6
Zidovudine	1.1

Source: Shargel L, YU ABC. *Applied Biopharmaceutics and Pharmacokinetics.* 4th ed. New York: McGraw-Hill; 1999. pp. 732–6.

this lesson, we begin to explore these relationships so that we can better predict plasma drug concentrations achieved with drug doses.

Although clearance is a model-independent pharmacokinetic parameter, and is not physiologically dependent only on elimination rate, it is sometimes useful to relate it to such parameters as the elimination rate constant (K) and the volume of distribution (V). Mathematically, systemic clearance (Cl_t) is related to V and K by:

$$Cl_t/V = K$$

or:

3-4

$$Cl_t = V \times K$$

Clearance and volume are independent factors that together determine K (and $T\tfrac{1}{2}$). Because V has units of volume (milliliters or liters) and clearance has units of volume/time (usually milliliters per minute), K has units of reciprocal time (minute^{-1}, hour^{-1}, or day^{-1}). It is important to understand that the elimination rate constant and plasma drug concentration versus time curve are determined by drug clearance and volume of distribution.

Clearance can be related to drug dose by first evaluating the plasma drug concentration versus time curve after a dose. In examining this curve (Figure 3-8), we see that there is a definite area under the curve, referred to as the *area under the plasma drug concentration versus time curve* or *AUC.*

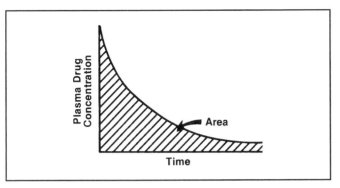

FIGURE 3-8.
Area under the plasma drug concentration versus time curve.

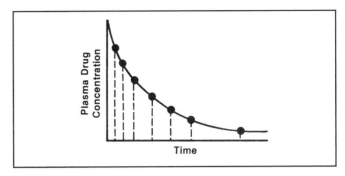

FIGURE 3-9.
A plasma drug concentration versus time curve can be divided into a series of trapezoids.

The AUC is determined by drug clearance and the dose given:

> ⚠
> 3-5

$$AUC = \frac{\text{dose administered}}{\text{drug clearance}}$$

When clearance remains constant, the AUC is directly proportional to the dose administered. If the dose doubled, the AUC would also double. Another way to think about this concept is that clearance is the parameter relating the AUC to the drug dose.

We usually know the dose of drug being administered and can determine plasma drug concentrations over time. From the plasma concentrations, the AUC can be estimated and drug clearance can be determined easily by rearranging the previous equation to:

$$\text{drug clearance} = \frac{\text{dose administered}}{AUC}$$

With a one-compartment model, first-order elimination, and intravenous drug administration, the AUC can be calculated easily:

$$AUC = \frac{\text{initial concentration } (C_0)}{\text{elimination rate constant } (K)}$$

C_0 has units of concentration, usually milligrams per liter ($\frac{mg}{L}$), and K is expressed as reciprocal time (usually hour^{-1}), so the AUC is expressed as milligrams per liter times hours ($\frac{mg \times hr}{L}$). These units make sense graphically as well, because when we multiply length times width to measure area, the product of the axes (concentration, in milligrams per liter, and time, in hours) would be expressed as milligrams per liter times hours.

AUC can be calculated by computer modeling of the above AUC equation, or by applying the "trapezoidal rule". The trapezoidal rule method is rarely used, but provides visual means to understand AUC. If a line is

drawn vertically to the *x*-axis from each measured concentration, a number of smaller areas is described (Figure 3-9). Because we are using the determined concentrations rather than their natural logs, the plasma drug concentration versus time plot is curved. The tops of the resulting shapes are curved as well, which makes their areas difficult to calculate. The area of each shape can be estimated, however, by drawing a straight line between adjacent concentrations and calculating the area of the resulting trapezoid (Figure 3-10).

If the time between measurements (and hence the width of the trapezoid) is small, only a slight error results. These smaller areas can be summed to estimate the AUC, as shown in the following equation.

$$AUC = [(\frac{C_2 + C_1}{2})(t_2 - t_1)] + [(\frac{C_3 + C_2}{2})(t3 - t2)]...etc$$

To calculate drug clearance, however, we need the AUC from time zero to infinity, and the preceding method only estimates the AUC to the final measured drug concentration. The terminal part of the AUC is estimated by dividing the last measured plasma concentration by the elimination rate constant (Figure 3-11):

$$\text{terminal area} = \frac{C_{last}}{K}$$

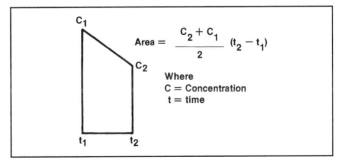

FIGURE 3-10.
Calculation of the area of a trapezoid.

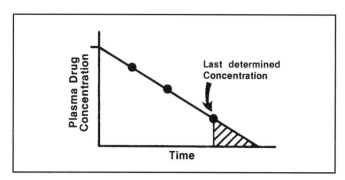

FIGURE 3-11.
Terminal area.

Add the terminal area to the value of AUC from the preceding equation to find the value of AUC from zero to infinity.

To calculate drug clearance, divide drug dose by AUC. By knowing how to calculate clearance by the area method, it is not necessary to decide first which model (i.e., one, two, or more compartments) best fits the observed plasma levels.

CLINICAL CORRELATE

The AUC can be used to determine a drug's clearance. For an individual patient, when the same drug dose is given over a period of time and the volume of distribution remains constant, changes in clearance can be assessed by changes in the AUC. For example, a doubling of the AUC would result if clearance decreased by half. For orally administered drugs, this would only be true if the fraction of drug absorbed from the gastrointestinal tract remained constant. AUC is only rarely used in clinical situations to determine clearance. It is used more frequently in clinical research.

■ Review Questions

3-1. Which of the following is the equation for a straight line?

A. $X = mY + b$

B. $b = mY + X$

C. $Y = mX + b$

D. $mX + Y = b$

3-2. Which of the following would be the slope of the straight line in Figure 3-12?

A. $\ln (C_0 - C_1)$

B. $t_0 - t_1$

C. $C_0 - t_0$

D. $(\ln C_1 - \ln C_0)/(t_1 - t_0)$

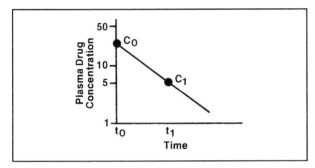

FIGURE 3-12.
Plasma drug concentration versus time.

3-3. Which of the following is the elimination rate constant for Figure 3-13?

A. −0.173

B. 0.52

C. 0.231

D. 0.173

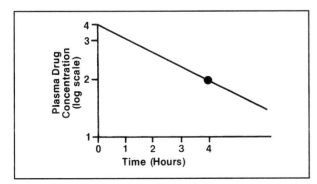

FIGURE 3-13.
Plasma drug concentration versus time.

3-4. If two patients receive the same drug and the plots in Figure 3-14 result, which patient has the larger elimination rate constant (faster elimination)?

A. Patient A

B. Patient B

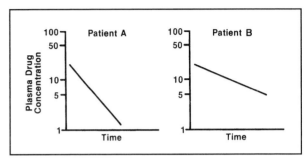

FIGURE 3-14.
Plasma drug concentration versus time.

3-5. A patient with renal dysfunction received a dose of vancomycin. Plasma concentrations were 22 and 15 mg/L at 24 and 48 hours after infusion, respectively. Plot these two plasma concentrations on semilog paper and determine when the concentration would reach 10 mg/L.

A. 54 hours

B. 72 hours

C. 96 hours

D. 128 hours

3-6. Using the equation $C = C_0 e^{-Kt}$, determine the plasma concentration of a drug 24 hours after a peak level of 10 mg/L is observed if the elimination rate constant is 0.05 hr^{-1}.

A. 3.01 mg/L

B. 33.2 mg/L

C. 18.1 mg/L

3-7. Which of the following is a proper unit for the elimination rate constant?

A. minutes

B. mg/minute

C. hr^{-1}

D. mg/L

3-8. If the elimination rate constant is 0.2 hr⁻¹ the percent of drug removed per hour is:

A. 20%.

B. 1%.

C. 0.1%.

D. 10%.

3-9. If the plasma concentration just after a gentamicin dose is 10 mg/L and the patient's elimination rate constant is 0.15 hr⁻¹, predict what the plasma concentration will be 8 hours later.

A. 6.0 mg/L

B. 3.0 mg/L

C. 1.5 mg/L

D. 1.0 mg/L

3-10. For a drug that has an initial plasma concentration of 120 mg/L and a half-life of 3 hours, what would the plasma concentration be 12 hours after the initial concentration?

A. 15 mg/L

B. 112.5

C. 7.5 mg/L

D. 60

3-11. From Figure 3-15, the approximate $T\frac{1}{2}$ is:

A. 5 hours.

B. 10 hours.

C. 20 hours.

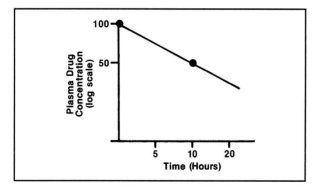

FIGURE 3-15.
Plasma drug concentration versus time.

3-12. If a drug has an elimination rate constant of 0.564 hr⁻¹, what is the half-life?

A. 1.23 hours

B. 0.81 hour

C. 1.77 hours

3-13. To calculate drug clearance by the area method, it is necessary to first determine whether the drug best fits a one- or two-compartment model.

A. True

B. False

3-14. In the trapezoid shown in Figure 3-16, what is the area?

A. 150 (mg/L) × hour

B. 300 (mg/L) × hour

C. 100 (mg/L) × hour

D. 25 (mg/L) × hour

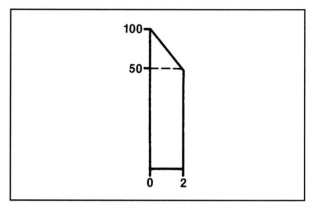

FIGURE 3-16.
Trapezoid.

3-15. If the dose (X_0) and AUC are known, the clearance (area method) is calculated by:

A. AUC/dose.

B. dose/AUC.

C. plasma concentration/AUC.

D. K/AUC.

3-16. Using Figure 3-17 and knowing that a 500-mg dose was given intravenously, calculate clearance by the area method.

A. 42 L/hour

B. 8.4 L/hour

C. 3 L/hour

D. 4.2 L/hour

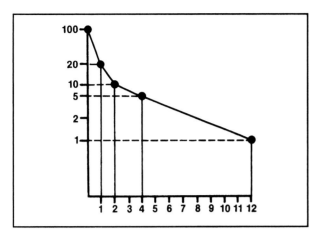

FIGURE 3-17.
Plasma drug concentration versus time.

▌ Answers

3-1. A, B, D. Incorrect answers

C. CORRECT ANSWER. The slope is m, and b is the y-intercept.

3-2. A. Incorrect answer. This value should be $(\ln C_1 - \ln C_0)$ and should be divided by the change in time $(t_1 - t_0)$.

B. Incorrect answer. The numerator $[(\ln C_1 - \ln C_0)]$ hasn't been included.

C. Incorrect answer

D. CORRECT ANSWER. The slope is the natural log of change in concentration divided by the change in time: $(\ln C_1 - \ln C_0)/(t_1 - t_0)$.

3-3. A. Incorrect answer. The elimination rate constant would not have a negative value; this is merely the slope of the line.

B. Incorrect answer. You may have added ln 2 and ln 4 rather than subtracted ln 4 from ln 2.

C. Incorrect answer. You may have used 3 hours in the denominator rather than 4 hours for change in time.

D. CORRECT ANSWER

3-4. A. CORRECT ANSWER. The larger the slope of the line is (i.e., the steeper the line is), the larger the elimination rate constant will be.

B. Incorrect answer. Note that the slope of the line is smaller (i.e., the line is less steep).

3-5. A, C, D. Incorrect answers. Be sure your points are plotted on paper that has a log scale for y (concen-

tration) values. Double-check the placement of your points.

B. CORRECT ANSWER

3-6. A. CORRECT ANSWER

B. Incorrect answer. You may have used Kt and not $-Kt$.

C. Incorrect answer. Check the $-Kt$ term, which should be -0.1 hr^{-1} × 24 hours (or -2.4).

3-7. A. Incorrect answer. A rate constant is a unit change per time expressed as reciprocal time units (e.g., minute^{-1}).

B. Incorrect answer. The elimination rate constant does not include mass units.

C. CORRECT ANSWER

D. Incorrect answer. These are the proper units for concentration.

3-8. A. CORRECT ANSWER

B, C, D. Incorrect Answer. The elimination rate constant is 0.2 hr^{-1}, meaning one fifth (or 20% per hour.

3-9. A, C, D. Incorrect answers

B. CORRECT ANSWER. $C_{8\ hr} = C_0 e^{-Kt}$, where $C_0 = 10$ mg/L, $K = 0.1$ hr^{-1}, and $t = 8$ hours.

3-10. A, B, D. Incorrect answers

C. CORRECT ANSWER. $C_{12\ hr} = C_0 e^{-Kt}$, where $C_0 = 120$ mg/L, $K = 0.231$ hr^{-1}, and $t = 12$ hours. K is calculated from half-life ($K = 0.693/T\frac{1}{2}$). Also, 12 hours represents four half-lives. We would expect the concentration to decrease from 120 mg/L to 60 mg/L, then to 30 mg/L, 15 mg/L, and finally, to 7.5 mg/L.

3-11. A, C. Incorrect answers

B. CORRECT ANSWER. To find the $T\frac{1}{2}$ of 10 hours, find the interval of time necessary for the concentration to decrease from 100 to 50.

3-12. A. CORRECT ANSWER

B. Incorrect answer. You may have used $T\frac{1}{2} = K/0.693$ rather than $T\frac{1}{2} = 0.693/K$.

C. Incorrect answer. You may have used $T\frac{1}{2} = 1/0.564$ rather than $T\frac{1}{2} = 0.693/K$.

3-13. A. Incorrect answer

B. CORRECT ANSWER. When using the area method, it does not matter if the drug best fits any particular model.

3-14. A. CORRECT ANSWER

B. Incorrect answer. You may have neglected to divide the sum of 100 plus 50 by 2 before then multiplying by the width of 2.

C, D. Incorrect answers. Be sure you calculated the height correctly as the average of 50 and 100.

3-15. A, C, D. Incorrect answers

B. CORRECT ANSWER. Remember, clearance has units of volume/time, so the units in the equation must result in volume/time. Dose/AUC has units of mg/(mg/L) × hour, which reduces to L/hour.

3-16. A, B, C. Incorrect answers

D. CORRECT ANSWER. To calculate clearance, the AUC from time zero to infinity must be used. The AUC from time zero to 12 hours can be calculated, and to this area is added the estimated area from 12 hours to infinity. This area is estimated by dividing the drug concentration at 12 hours, 1 mg/L, by the elimination rate constant, 0.20 hr^{-1} (estimated by the slope of the line between the last two points), thereby obtaining an area of 5 (mg/L) × hour from 12 hours to infinity. Clearance = dose/AUC. Dose is 500 mg. AUC is 119 mg/L, which is the sum of 114 mg/L (from 0 to 12 hours) and 5 mg/L (from 12 hours to infinity).

Discussion Points

D-1. Drug X is given by intravenous administration to two patients. Two plasma concentrations are then determined, and the slope of the plasma concentration versus time curve is calculated. Determine which patient (A or B) has the greater elimination rate constant.

	Patient A	Patient B
Slope of plasma concentration versus time curve	−0.55	−0.23

D-2. Drug X is given to two patients, and two plasma drug concentrations are then determined for each patient. Determine which patient has the greater elimination rate constant.

Time after Dose (hours)	Plasma Concentration (mg/L)	
	Patient A	Patient B
8	22	30
16	5	8

D-3. Why is the half-life of most drugs the same at high and low plasma concentrations?

D-4. The plasma concentration versus time curves for two different drugs are exactly parallel; however, one of the drugs has much higher plasma concentrations. What can you say about the two drug half-lives?

D-5. For drug X, the AUC determines the intensity of drug effect. Explain why a reduction of drug clearance by 50% would result in the same intensity of effect as doubling the dose.

Practice Set 1

The following problems are for your review. Definitions of symbols and key equations are provided here:

X_0 = dose administered
K = elimination rate constant
V = volume of distribution
$T\frac{1}{2}$ = half-life
t_0 = time immediately after drug administration
C_0 = concentration of drug in plasma at t_0
$C_t = C_0 e^{-Kt}$ = concentration of drug in plasma at any time (t) after drug administration
AUC = area under plasma concentration versus time curve
Cl_t = total drug clearance from body = dose/AUC

$$K = \frac{\ln C_0 - \ln C}{t_1 - t_0}$$

The following applies to questions PS1-1 to PS1-3. A 1-g dose of drug X is administered by intravenous injection, and the following plasma concentrations result (a one-compartment model is assumed):

Time after Dose (hours)	Plasma Concentration (mg/L)
2	15
4	9.5
6	6

QUESTIONS

PS1-1. The plasma concentration at 9 hours after the dose estimated from a plot of the points on semi-log graph paper is:

　A. < 0.1 mg/L.

　B. 0.7 mg/L.

　C. 3.1 mg/L.

　D. 4.8 mg/L.

PS1-2. An estimate for the volume of distribution would be:

　A. 67 L.

　B. 43 L.

　C. 53 L.

PS1-3. For this same example, the half-life would be:

　A. 1.3 hours.

　B. 1.5 hours.

　C. 3.1 hours.

　D. 4.6 hours.

The following applies to questions PS1-4 to PS1-6. An 80-mg dose of drug Y is administered as an intravenous bolus, and the following plasma concentrations result:

Time after Dose (hours)	Plasma Concentration (mg/L)
0	6.7
0.5	6.0
1	5.3
2	4.2
4	2.6
8	1.0

PS1-4. Using the plasma concentrations at 4 and 8 hours, K is:

　A. 0.118 hr^{-1}.

　B. 0.239 hr^{-1}.

　C. 0.478 hr^{-1}.

　D. 0.960 hr^{-1}.

PS1-5. Using the trapezoidal rule, calculate the area under the curve from 0 to 8 hours (AUC$_{0-8}$). Then calculate it from 0 hours to infinity (∞). *Remember*: AUC$_{0\to8}$ equals AUC$_{0-8}$ plus the area under the curve after 8 hours. This terminal area is calculated by taking the final concentration (at 8 hours) and dividing by K above.

　A. 4.2 (mg/L) × hour

　B. 24.8 (mg/L) × hour

　C. 28.9 (mg/L) × hour

　D. 53.7 (mg/L) × hour

PS1-6. For this same example, the clearance calculated by the area method would be:

A. 0.36 L/hour.

B. 0.78 L/hour.

C. 1.52 L/hour.

D. 2.76 L/hour.

ANSWERS

PS1-1. A, B. Incorrect answers. You may have used linear graph paper rather than semilog paper.

C. CORRECT ANSWER

D. Incorrect answer. Be sure your x-scale for time is correct and that you extrapolated the concentration for 9 hours.

PS1-2. A, C. Incorrect answers

B. CORRECT ANSWER. First, estimate C_0 by drawing a line back to time = 0 (t_0) using the three plotted points. This should equal 23 mg/L. Then, V = dose/C_0 = 1000 mg/23 mg/L = 43 L.

PS1-3. A. Incorrect answer. You may have calculated the numerator incorrectly.

B, D. Incorrect answers. You may have used the wrong time interval.

C. CORRECT ANSWER. Half life = 0.693/K, where: K = (ln 6 – ln 15)/(6 hours – 2 hours) = 0.23 hr^{-1}. So, half-life = 0.693/0.23 = 3.1 hours.

PS1-4. A, C, D. Incorrect answers

B. CORRECT ANSWER.

$$K = \frac{\ln 1 - \ln 2.6}{8 \text{ hr} - 4 \text{ hr}} = \frac{0 - 0.96}{4 \text{ hr}}$$
$$= 0.239 \text{ hr}^{-1}$$

PS1-5. A. Incorrect answer. You may have included just the area from 8 hours to infinity.

B. Incorrect answer. You may not have included the area from 8 hours to infinity.

C. CORRECT ANSWER.

For AUC from 0 to 8 hours:

$$\frac{6.7 + 6.0}{2}(0.5) = 3.18$$

$$\frac{6.0 + 5.3}{2}(0.5) = 2.82$$

$$\frac{5.3 + 4.2}{2}(1) = 4.75$$

$$\frac{4.2 + 2.6}{2}(2) = 6.80$$

$$\frac{2.6 + 1.0}{2}(4) = 7.20$$

$$3.18 + 2.82 + 4.75 + 6.80 + 7.20 = 24.8 \text{ (mg/L)} \times \text{hr}$$

For AUC from 8 hours to infinity:

$$C_{8 \text{ hr}} = \frac{1.0 \text{ mg/L}}{0.239 \text{ hr}^{-1}} = 4.18 \text{ (mg/L)} \times \text{hr}$$

Therefore, the AUC from time zero to infinity equals:

$$24.8 \text{ (mg/L)} \times \text{hr} + 4.18 \text{ (mg/L)} \times \text{hr} = 28.93 \text{ (mg/L)} \times \text{hr}$$

D. Incorrect answer. You may not have multiplied by ½ when calculating the area from 8 hours to infinity.

PS1-6. A. Incorrect answer. You may have inverted the formula.

B, C. Incorrect answers

D. CORRECT ANSWER.

$$\text{clearance} = \frac{\text{dose}}{\text{AUC}} = \frac{80 \text{ mg}}{28.93 \text{ (mg/L)} \times \text{hr}}$$
$$= 2.76 \text{L/hr}$$

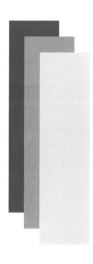

LESSON
4

Intravenous Bolus Administration, Multiple Drug Administration, and Steady-State Average Concentrations

 OBJECTIVES

After completing Lesson 4, you should be able to:

1. Describe the principle of superposition and how it applies to multiple drug dosing.
2. Define *steady state* and describe how it relates to a drug's half-life.
3. Calculate the estimated peak plasma concentration after multiple drug dosing (at steady state).
4. Calculate the estimated trough plasma concentration after multiple drug dosing (at steady state).
5. Understand the equation for accumulation factor at steady state.

In clinical practice, most pharmacokinetic dosing is performed with one-compartment, intermittent infusion models at steady state. Using these models, we can obtain an elimination rate constant (K) and then calculate volume of distribution (V) and dosing interval (τ) based on this K value. So far, our discussion has been limited to a single intravenous (IV) bolus dose of drug. Most clinical situations, however, require a therapeutic effect for time periods extending beyond the effect of one dose. In these situations, **multiple doses** of drug are given. The goal is to maintain a therapeutic effect by keeping the amount of drug in the body, as well as the concentration of drug in the plasma, within a fairly constant range (the therapeutic range). In this lesson, we construct equations for predicting drug concentrations after multiple IV doses. Although intermediate equations are used, only the final equation is important to remember.

INTRAVENOUS BOLUS DOSE MODEL

Although not used often clinically, the simplest example of multiple dosing is the administration of rapid IV doses (IV boluses) of drug at constant time intervals, in which the drug is represented by a one-compartment model with first-order elimination.

 CLINICAL CORRELATE

This lesson describes a one-compartment, first-order, IV bolus pharmacokinetic model. It is used only to illustrate certain math concepts that will be further explored with the more commonly used IV intermittent infusion (i.e., IV piggyback) models described in Lesson 5. Consequently, only read this IV bolus section for general conceptual understanding, knowing that it is seldom applied clinically.

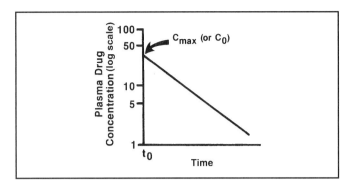

FIGURE 4-1.
Plasma drug concentrations after a first dose.

The first dose produces a plasma drug concentration versus time curve like the one in Figure 4-1. C_0 is now referred to as C_{max}, meaning maximum concentration, to group it with the other peak concentrations that occur with multiple dosing.

If a second bolus dose is administered before the first dose is completely eliminated, the maximum concentration after the second dose (C_{max2}) will be higher than that after the first dose (C_{max1}) (Figure 4-2). The second part of the curve will be very similar to the first curve but will be higher (have a greater concentration) because some drug remains from the first dose when the second dose is administered.

The time between administration of doses is the **dosing interval**. The dosing interval, symbolized by the Greek letter tau (τ), is determined by a drug's half-life. Rapidly eliminated drugs (i.e., those having a short half-life) generally have to be given more frequently (shorter τ), than drugs with a longer half-life.

If a drug follows first-order elimination (i.e., the fraction of drug eliminated per unit of time is constant), then plasma drug concentrations after **multiple dosing** can be predicted from concentrations after a single dose. This method uses the **principle of superposition**, a simple overlay technique. If the early doses of drug do not affect

the pharmacokinetics (e.g., absorption and clearance) of subsequent doses, then plasma drug concentration versus time curves after each dose will look the same; they will be superimposable. The only difference is that the actual concentrations may be higher at later doses, because drug has accumulated.

Recall that the y-intercept is called C_0 and the slope of the line is $-K$. Furthermore, the drug concentration at any time (C_t) after the first IV bolus dose is given by:

$$\ln C_t = \ln C_0 - Kt \quad \text{(See **Equation 3-2**.)}$$

or

$$C_t = C_0 e^{-Kt}$$

A second IV bolus dose is administered after the dosing interval (τ), but before the first dose is completely eliminated. Because $C_t = C_0 e^{-Kt}$ at any time (t) after the first dose, it follows that:

$$C_{min1} = C_{max1} e^{-K\tau}$$

where C_{min1} is the concentration just before the next dose is given and τ, the dosing interval, is the time from C_{max} to C_{min}.

C_{max2} is the sum of C_{min1} and C_{max1} (Figure 4-3), as the same dose is given again:

$$C_{max2} = C_{max1} + C_{min1}$$

We showed that:

$$C_{min1} = C_{max1} e^{-K\tau}$$

so:

$$C_{max2} = C_{max1} + C_{max1} e^{-K\tau}$$

By rearranging, we get:

$$C_{max2} = C_{max1}(1 + e^{-K\tau})$$

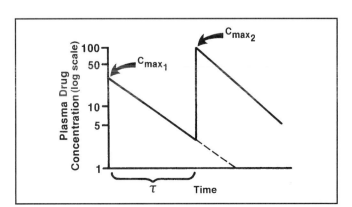

FIGURE 4-2.
Plasma drug concentrations resulting from a second dose.

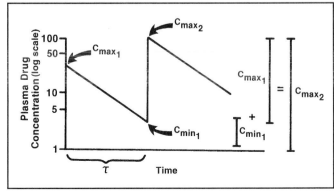

FIGURE 4-3.
C_{max2} calculation.

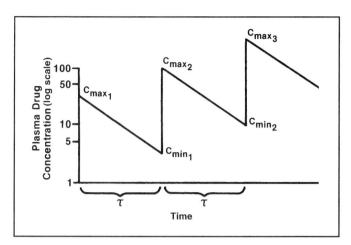

FIGURE 4-4.
Increase in C_{max}.

A third IV bolus dose can be administered after the same dosing interval (τ). The plasma drug concentration versus time profile reveals a further increase in the maximum concentration immediately after the third dose, as shown in Figure 4-4. Just as after the first dose:

$$C_{min2} = C_{max2}e^{-K\tau}$$

which, by substitution for C_{max2}, equals $C_{max1}(1 + e^{-K\tau})e^{-K\tau}$. Moreover:

$$C_{max3} = C_{min2} + C_{max1}$$

which, substituting for C_{min2}, equals $C_{max1}(1 + e^{-K\tau})e^{-K\tau} + C_{max1}$. This simplifies as follows:

$$C_{max3} = C_{max1}[(1 + e^{-K\tau})(e^{-K\tau}) + 1]$$

$$= C_{max1}[e^{-K\tau} + e^{-2K\tau} + 1]$$

$$= C_{max1}[1 + e^{-K\tau} + e^{-2K\tau}]$$

As we can see, a pattern emerges—after any number of dosing intervals, the maximum concentration will be:

$$C_{maxn} = C_{max1}[1 + e^{-K\tau} + e^{-2K\tau} + \ldots + e^{-(n-1)K\tau}]$$

where n is the number of doses given. This equation can be simplified by mathematical procedures to a more useful form:

$$C_{maxn} = C_{max1}\frac{(1-e^{-nK\tau})}{(1-e^{-K\tau})}$$

where C_{maxn} is the concentration just after n number of doses are given. So, if we know C_{max1}, the elimination rate, and the dosing interval, we can predict the maximum plasma concentration after any number (n) of doses.

We also know that C_{minn} (concentration just before a dose is given) equals $C_{maxn}e^{-K\tau}$. Therefore:

$$C_{minn} = C_{max1}\frac{(1-e^{-nK\tau})}{(1-e^{-K\tau})}e^{-K\tau}$$

and because $C_{max1} = X_0/V$ (i.e., dose divided by volume of distribution):

$$C_{minn} = \frac{X_0}{V}\frac{(1-e^{-nK\tau})}{(1-e^{-K\tau})}e^{-K\tau}$$

This latter change allows us to calculate C_{min} if we know the dose and volume of distribution, a likely situation in clinical practice.

In each of the preceding equations, the term $(1 - e^{-nK\tau})/(1 - e^{-K\tau})$ appears. It is called the *accumulation factor* because it relates drug concentration after a single dose to drug concentration after n doses with multiple dosing. This factor is a number greater than 1, which indicates how much higher the concentration will be after n doses compared with the first dose For example, if 100 doses of a certain drug are given to a patient, where $K = 0.05$ hr^{-1} and $\tau = 8$ hours, the accumulation factor is calculated as follows:

$$\frac{(1-e^{-nK\tau})}{(1-e^{-K\tau})} = \frac{(1-e^{-100(0.05\text{ hr}^{-1})8\text{ hr}})}{(1-e^{-(0.05\text{ hr}^{-1})8\text{ hr}})} = 3.03$$

This means that the peak (or trough) concentration after 100 doses will be 3.03 times the peak (or trough) concentration after the first dose.

The accumulation factor for two or three doses can also be calculated to predict concentrations before achievement of steady-state. Remember:

⚠️ 4-1 $\text{accumulation factor} = \dfrac{(1-e^{-nK\tau})}{(1-e^{-K\tau})}$

So for the second IV bolus dose:

$$\begin{aligned}\text{accumulation factor (two doses)} &= \frac{(1-e^{-2(0.05\text{ hr}^{-1})8\text{ hr}})}{(1-e^{-(0.05\text{ hr}^{-1})8\text{ hr}})} \\ &= \frac{(1-0.449)}{(1-0.670)} \\ &= 1.67\end{aligned}$$

For the third IV bolus dose:

$$\begin{aligned}\text{accumulation factor (three doses)} &= \frac{(1-e^{-3(0.05\text{ hr}^{-1})8\text{ hr}})}{(1-e^{-(0.05\text{ hr}^{-1})8\text{ hr}})} \\ &= \frac{(1-0.301)}{(1-0.670)} \\ &= 2.12\end{aligned}$$

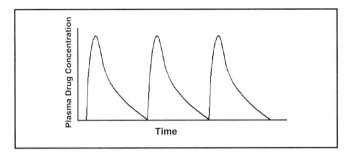

FIGURE 4-5.
Plasma drug concentration versus time.

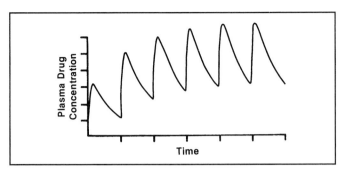

FIGURE 4-6.
Multiple-dose drug administration.

Therefore, after two or three doses, the observed peak drug concentration will be 1.67 or 2.12 times the peak concentration after the first dose, respectively. The concept of accumulation factor is discussed in more detail in the section Accumulation Factor later in this lesson.

These equations will be used later to predict drug concentrations for given dosage regimens. For certain drugs (e.g., aminoglycosides), it is important to predict peak (C_{max}) and trough (C_{min}) concentrations in various clinical situations.

> ### ▮ CLINICAL CORRELATE
>
> If a drug has a very short half-life (much less than the dosing interval) then the plasma concentrations resulting from each dose will be the same and accumulation of drug will not occur (as shown in Figure 4-5). An example would be a drug such as gentamicin given every 8 hr intravenously to a patient whose excellent renal function results in a drug half-life of 1.0–1.5 hours.

INTRAVENOUS BOLUS EQUATIONS AT STEADY STATE

As successive doses of a drug are administered, the drug begins to accumulate in the body. With first-order elimination, the amount of drug eliminated per unit of time is proportional to the amount of drug in the body. Accumulation continues until the rate of elimination approaches the rate of administration:

rate of drug going in = rate of drug going out

As the rate of drug elimination increases and then approaches that of drug administration, the maximum (peak) and minimum (trough) concentrations increase until an equilibrium is reached. After that point, there will be no additional accumulation; the maximum and minimum concentrations will remain constant with each subsequent dose of drug (Figure 4-6).

When this equilibrium occurs, the maximum (and minimum) drug concentrations are the same for each additional dose given (assuming the same dose and dosing interval are used). When the maximum (and minimum) drug concentrations for successive doses are the same, the amount of drug eliminated over the dosing interval (rate out) equals the dose administered (rate in) and the condition of "steady state" is reached.

Steady state will always be reached after repeated drug administration at the same dosing interval if the drug follows first-order elimination. However, the time required to reach steady state varies from drug to drug, depending on the elimination rate constant. With a higher elimination rate constant (a shorter half-life), steady state is reached sooner than with a lower one (a longer half-life) (Figure 4-7).

Steady state is the point at which the amount of drug administered over a dosing interval equals the amount of drug being eliminated over that same period and is totally dependent on the elimination rate constant. Therefore, when the elimination rate is higher, a greater amount of drug is eliminated over a given time interval; it then takes a shorter time for the amount of drug eliminated and the amount of drug administered to become equivalent (and, therefore, achieve steady state). If the half-life of a drug is known, the time to reach steady state can be determined. If repeated doses of drug are

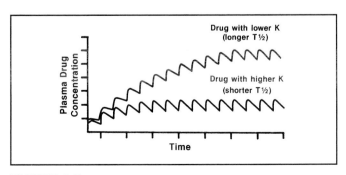

FIGURE 4-7.
Steady state is reached sooner with a drug having a shorter half-life.

TABLE 4-1.
Percentage of Steady-State Concentration Reached

Duration of Drug Administration (half-lives)	Steady-State Concentration Reached (%)
1	50
2	75
3	87.5
4	93.75
5	96.875
6	98.4735
7	99.25

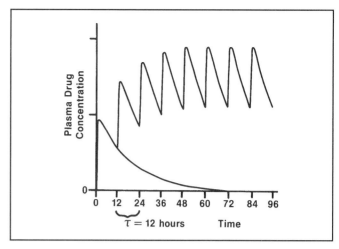

FIGURE 4-8.
At steady state, the time required to eliminate one dose of drug is one dosing interval.

given at a fixed interval, then in one half-life the plasma concentrations will reach 50% of those at steady state. By the end of the second half-life, the concentrations will be 75% of steady state, and so on as shown in Table 4-1. The plasma concentrations will increase by progressively smaller increments. *For all practical purposes, steady state will be reached after approximately four or five half-lives;* the concentrations at steady state may be abbreviated as C_{ss}.

For a drug such as gentamicin, with a 1- to 4-hour half-life in patients with normal renal function, steady-state concentration is achieved within 10–20 hours. For agents such as digoxin and phenobarbital, however, a week or longer may be needed to reach steady state.

With multiple drug doses (Figure 4-8), steady state is reached when the drug from the first dose is almost entirely eliminated from the body. At this point, the amount of drug remaining from the first dose does not contribute significantly to the total amount of drug in the body. After a single dose, approximately four or five half-lives are required for the body to eliminate the amount of drug equivalent to the one dose. However, at steady state, the amount of drug equivalent to one dose is eliminated over one dosing interval. This apparently faster elimination is a result of accumulation of drug in the body. Although the same percentage of drug is eliminated per hour, the greater amount of drug in the body at steady state causes a greater amount to be eliminated over the same time period.

The average times to reach steady-state for some commonly used drugs are shown in Table 4-2. These values may vary considerably between individuals and may be altered by disease. For some drugs (e.g., aspirin, ranitidine, and gentamicin), the therapeutic effects will begin before steady-state plasma concentrations are reached. For others (e.g., zidovudine or lovastatin), a much longer time period than that

needed to reach steady state is necessary for full therapeutic benefits.

■ CLINICAL CORRELATE

Time to achieve steady state is a physiologic function based solely on the drug's K or half-life, and the amount of time it takes to "get to" steady state cannot be increased or decreased. However, administration of a loading dose for drugs that take many hours to reach steady state is commonly used to achieve a concentration approximately equal to the eventual actual steady-state concentration.

TABLE 4-2.
Time to Reach Steady State for Commonly Used Drugs[a]

Drug	Time to Reach Steady State (hours)
Aspirin	1.3
Cephalexin	4.5
Digoxin	120–148
Gentamicin	10–15
Lovastatin	5.5–8.5
Ranitidine	10.5
Vancomycin	25–30
Zidovudine	5.5

[a]Calculated from average drug half-lives.

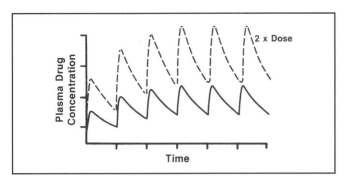

FIGURE 4-9.
Dose increase with no change in dosing interval to achieve higher concentrations.

The time to reach steady state is determined by the drug's elimination rate constant (K), but what determines the actual plasma drug concentrations achieved? At steady state, the levels achieved depend on the drug's clearance, volume of distribution, dose, and dosing interval (τ). When equivalent doses are given, a drug with a low elimination rate constant and small volume of distribution should achieve higher steady-state plasma concentrations than an otherwise similar agent with a high elimination rate constant and large volume of distribution. In the remainder of this lesson, we examine some aspects of multiple drug dosing.

Steady-state concentrations are commonly increased in two ways:

- Method 1—Increase the drug dose but maintain the same dosing interval (τ), as shown in Figure 4-9, which results in wider fluctuations between the maximum (peak) and minimum (trough) concentrations after each dose.
- Method 2—Keep the same dose but give it more frequently, as shown in Figure 4-10, which reduces the differences between the peak and trough concentrations.

Note that the time to achieve steady state is the same in both figures.

CLINICAL CORRELATE

You may wish to change a patient's steady-state drug concentrations. For example, the patient is not receiving maximal benefits because the steady-state concentrations are relatively low or the steady-state levels are high, causing the patient to experience toxic effects. Remember from earlier in this lesson that repeated doses of drug require approximately four or five half-lives to reach steady state. Clinically, this means that each time a dose or dosing interval is changed, four or five half-lives are needed to reach a new steady state. Of course, a drug with a long half-life will require a longer time to achieve the new steady state than a drug with a relatively short half-life. For example, Drug A has a half-life of 6 hours therefore if the dose or dosing interval is changed, steady state will not be reached for 24–30 hours after the change. If Drug B has a half-life of 3 hours, steady state will be reached only after 12–15 hours after a change in the dose or dosing interval.

In deciding on a specific dosing regimen for a patient, the goal is to achieve a certain plasma concentration of drug at steady state. Ideally, peak and trough concentrations will both be within the therapeutic range (Figure 4-11).

ACCUMULATION FACTOR

Equations can describe the plasma concentrations and pharmacokinetics of a drug at steady state. Remember, steady state will be reached only after four or five half-lives.

Recall that with an IV bolus injection of a drug fitting a one-compartment model and first-order elimination,

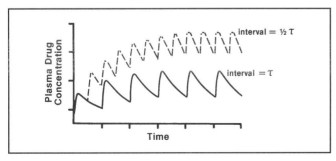

FIGURE 4-10.
Dosing interval decrease with no change in dose to achieve higher concentrations.

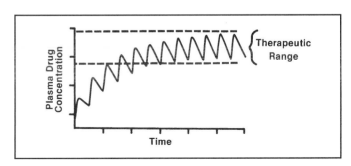

FIGURE 4-11.
Maintenance of plasma drug concentrations within the therapeutic range.

the drug concentration at any time (t) after any number of doses (n), **not necessarily at steady state**, can be described by:

$$C_{n(t)} = \frac{X_0}{V} \frac{(1-e^{-nK\tau})}{(1-e^{-K\tau})} e^{-Kt}$$

To predict the plasma concentration of a drug at any time t after n number of doses, we therefore need to know four values:

- drug dose (X_0),
- volume of distribution (V),
- elimination rate constant (K), and
- dosing interval (τ).

As multiple drug doses are administered, n increases and approaches infinity (abbreviated as $n \to \infty$). The preceding equation can then be simplified. As n becomes a large number, $e^{-nK\tau}$ approaches $e^{-\infty}$, which approaches zero, so $1 - e^{-nK\tau}$ approaches 1. As $1 - e^{-nK\tau}$ approaches 1, the value of this numerator becomes 1 and the resultant numerator/denominator combination is termed the *accumulation factor at steady state*:

⚠️
4-2
$$\frac{1}{(1-e^{-K\tau})}$$

Consequently, the equation above can now be re-written to described the C_{pmax} concentration at steady state:

$$C_{pmax} = \frac{X_0}{V} \frac{(1-e^{-K\tau})}{(1-e^{-K\tau})} e^{-Kt}$$

If we wish to predict the steady-state peak concentration immediately after an IV bolus dose, where $t = 0$ and $e^{-0} = 1$, the equation above for $C_{n(t)}$ becomes:

$$C_{peak(n)} = \frac{X_0}{V} \frac{(1-e^{-nK\tau})}{(1-e^{-K\tau})}$$

because time after the dose equals zero ($t = 0$, and $e^{-0} = 1$). When n (the number of doses given) is sufficiently large (>4 or 5 doses), the equation above simplifies to:

$$C_{peak(steady\ state)} = \frac{X_0}{V} \left[\frac{1}{(1-e^{-K\tau})} \right]$$

We can estimate the minimum or trough concentration at steady state. The trough concentration occurs just before the administration of the next dose (at $t = \tau$). In this situation, the general equation for the equation for $C_{n(t)}$ becomes:

$$C_{trough(steady\ state)} = \frac{X_0}{V} \left[\frac{1}{(1-e^{-K\tau})} \right] e^{-K\tau}$$

CLINICAL CORRELATE

In most clinical situations it is preferable to wait until a drug concentration is at steady state before obtaining serum drug concentrations. Use of steady-state concentrations are more accurate and make the numerous required calculations easier.

Note the similarity between the equations for $C_{peak(steady\ state)}$ and $C_{trough(steady\ state)}$. The expression for $C_{trough(steady\ state)}$ simplifies to $C_{peak(steady\ state)}$ times e^{-Kt}. An almost identical equation (below) can be used to calculate the concentration at any time after the peak. The only difference is that t is replaced by the time elapsed since the peak level. Therefore:

$$C_{(t)} = C_{peak(steady\ state)} e^{-Kt}$$

where t is the time after the peak.

This last relationship is very useful in clinical pharmacokinetics. It is really the same as an equation presented earlier. (See **Equation 3-2**.):

$$C_t = C_0 e^{-Kt}$$

The preceding equation, stated in words, means "a concentration at any time (C_t) is equal to some previous concentration (C_0) multiplied by the fraction (or percent) of that previous concentration (i.e., e^{-Kt}) remaining after it has been allowed to be eliminated from the body for a number of hours represented by t.

If two drug concentrations and the time between them are known, K can be calculated. If one concentration after a dose (e.g., a peak concentration) and K are known, then other concentrations at any time after a dose (before the next dose) can be estimated.

AVERAGE STEADY-STATE CONCENTRATION WITH INTRAVENOUS BOLUS DOSING

We now have examined both the maximum and minimum concentrations that occur at steady state. Another useful parameter in multiple IV dosing situations is the average concentration of drug in the plasma at steady state ($\bar{C}$) (Figure 4-12). Because $\bar{C}$ is independent of any pharmacokinetic model, it is helpful to the practicing clinician (model assumptions do not have to be made). $\bar{C}$ is not an arithmetic or geometric mean.

Several mathematical methods may be used to calculate the average drug concentration, but only one is presented here. A plasma drug concentration versus time curve, after steady state has been achieved with IV dos-

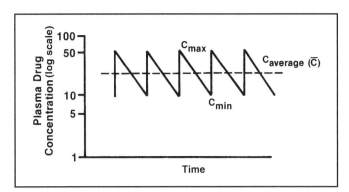

FIGURE 4-12.
Average plasma drug concentration at steady state.

ing, is illustrated in Figure 4-13. By knowing the dose given (X_0) and the dosing interval (τ), we can determine the average concentration if we also know the area under the plasma drug concentration versus time curve (AUC) over τ. Therefore:

$$\bar{C} = \frac{AUC}{\tau}$$

and since:

$$AUC = \frac{dose}{drug\ clearance}$$

$$\bar{C} = \frac{dose}{drug\ clearance \times \tau}$$

The equation:

⚠
4-3

$$\bar{C} = \frac{dose}{Cl_t \times \tau}$$

is very useful, particularly with drugs having a long half-life, in which the difference between peak and trough steady-state levels may not be large.

It is important to recognize from the equations that $\bar{C}$ at steady state is determined by the clearance and

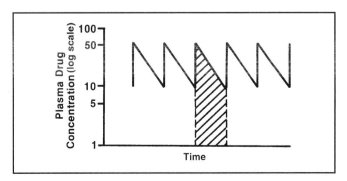

FIGURE 4-13.
AUC for one dosing interval.

drug dose (dose/τ). If the dose remains the same [n = a time period such as a day (e.g., 80 mg every 8 hours [80 × 3] or 120 mg every 12 hours [120 × 2])] while τ is changed, $\bar{C}$ would remain the same. Also, changes in V or K that are not related to a change in clearance would not alter $\bar{C}$. With multiple drug dosing at steady state, changes in τ, K, or V (with no change in clearance) would alter the observed peak and trough drug concentrations but not $\bar{C}$.

In dealing with such equations, it is helpful to remember that the units of measure on both sides must be the same. For example, in the equation above, $\bar{C}$ should be in micrograms per milliliter, milligrams per liter, or similar concentration units. Therefore, the right side of the equation must have the same units, as is the case when:

- dose is in a consistent mass unit, such as milligrams,
- clearance is in liters per hour or milliliters per minute, and
- dosing interval is in hours.

So dose/(Cl × τ) has the following units:

$$\frac{amount}{(volume/time) \times time}$$

Then, as both hour terms cancel out, we see that amount per volume (concentration) is left.

PREDICTING STEADY-STATE CONCENTRATION

The equation for $C_{peak(steady\ state)}$ derived above (and shown below) is valuable because it allows us to predict the peak plasma concentration achieved when a drug is given in a specified dose (X_0) at a consistent and repeated interval (τ). To predict peak concentration at steady state, however, we also must have an estimate of the elimination rate (K) and the volume of distribution (V); therefore, the following equation is only used for IV bolus dosing:

$$C_{peak(steady\ state)} = \frac{X_0}{V}\left[\frac{1}{\left(1 - e^{-K\tau}\right)}\right]$$

It is possible to estimate a patient's K and V from published reports of similar patients. For example, most patients with normal renal function will have a gentamicin V of 0.20–0.30 L/kg and a K of 0.035–0.2 hr^{-1}. In a clinical setting, where a drug is administered and plasma concentrations are then determined, it is possible to calculate a patient's actual K and V using plasma concentrations and the above equation. Such calculations can be performed as follows.

Example 1

A patient receives 500 mg of drug X intravenously every 6 hours until steady state is reached. Just after the dose is injected, a blood sample is drawn to determine a peak plasma concentration. Then, 5 hours later, a second plasma concentration is determined. Using the two plasma concentrations, we first calculate K, as described previously:

$$K = \frac{\ln C_{peak} - \ln C_{5\,hr}}{5\,hr}$$

Then we insert the known C_{peak}, K, X_0, and τ values in the equation for C_{peak}. By rearranging the equation to isolate the only remaining unknown variable, we can then use it to calculate V:

$$V = \frac{X_0}{C_{peak(steady\,state)}}\left[\frac{1}{\left(1 - e^{-K\tau}\right)}\right]$$

Now we know the values of all the variables in the equation (V, K, C_{peak}, X_0, and τ) and can use this information to calculate a new C_{peak} if we change the dose (e.g., if the previous C_{peak} is too high or too low). For example, if we want the peak level to be higher and wish to calculate the required dose to reach this new peak level, we can rearrange our equation:

$$X_0 = V \times C_{peak(steady\,state)}(1 - e^{-K\tau})$$

and substitute our calculated V and K and the desired C_{peak}. Or we can choose a new dose (X_0) and calculate the resulting C_{peak} by inserting the calculated K and V with τ into the original equation:

$$C_{peak(steady\,state)} = \frac{X_0}{V}\left[\frac{1}{\left(1 - e^{-K\tau}\right)}\right]$$

Remember that each time we calculate a peak plasma level (C_{peak}), the trough plasma level also can be calculated if we know K and τ:

$$C_{trough} = C_{peak}e^{-K\tau}$$

If the dosing interval is not changed, new doses and concentrations are directly proportional if nothing else changes (i.e., K or V).

So,

$$X_{0\,(new)} = \frac{C_{peak(steady\,state)new}}{C_{peak(steady\,state)old}} \times X_{0\,(old)}$$

And,

$$C_{peak(steady\,state)new} = \frac{X_{0\,(new)}}{X_{0\,(old)}} \times C_{steady\,state(old)}$$

■ Review Questions

Note: Refer to Figure 4-14 when answering questions 4-1 through 4-3.

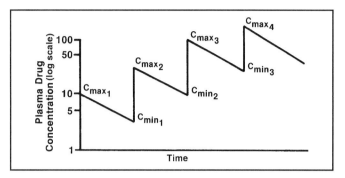

FIGURE 4-14.
Plasma drug concentration versus time.

4-1.   If C_{max1}, K, and τ are 100 mg/L, 0.40 hr^{-1}, and 6 hours, respectively, what is the value of C_{max2}?

A. 109.1 mg/L

B. 9.1 mg/L

C. 100 mg/L

D. 110 mg/L

4-2.   For the example given in the previous question, what is the value of C_{min2}?

A. 9.1 mg/L

B. 43.6 mg/L

C. 85.3 mg/L

D. 9.9 mg/L

4-3.   What is the maximum concentration after 15 doses if the dose (X_0) is 800 mg and the volume of distribution (V) is 20 L? Assume that τ equals 6 hours and K equals 0.50 hr^{-1}.

A. 42.1 mg/L

B. 66.7 mg/L

C. 52.9 mg/L

D. 156.8 mg/L

4-4.   When multiple drug doses are given and steady state is reached, the amount of drug eliminated during one dosing interval (τ) is equal to the drug dose.

A. True

B. False

4-5.   A drug with a relatively small K (long $T\frac{1}{2}$) takes a longer time to reach steady state than a drug with a large K.

A. True

B. False

4-6.   If a drug with a $T\frac{1}{2}$ of 12 hours is given every 6 hours and a peak concentration at steady state is 10 mg/L, what will be the approximate peak concentration just after the fifth dose is administered?

A. 5 mg/L

B. 7.5 mg/L

C. 10 mg/L

4-7.   A 100-mg dose of drug X is given to two different patients every 8 hours. Which patient (A or B) is likely to achieve higher steady-state plasma concentrations?

Patient	Elimination Rate (hr^{-1})	Volume of Distribution (L)
A	0.2	10
B	0.4	20

A. Patient A

B. Patient B

4-8.   Decreasing the dosing interval while keeping the dose constant will result in lower steady-state concentrations.

A. True

B. False

4-9.   Which of the following dosage techniques results in the greatest difference between maximum (peak) and minimum (trough) concentrations after a dose?

A. Small doses given at a short dosing interval

B. Large doses given at a long dosing interval

4-10. What is the peak drug X concentration attained at steady state if 100 mg is given by intravenous injection every 6 hours, the patient's K = 0.35 hr^{-1}, and V = 20 L? Assume one-compartment distribution.

A. 3.4 mg/L

B. 5.7 mg/L

C. 16.3 mg/L

D. 41 mg/L

4-11. What would be the trough level for the example in problem 4-10?

A. 0.41 mg/L

B. 0.7 mg/L

C. 2 mg/L

D. 5 mg/L

4-12. A 500-mg dose of drug X is given every 6 hours until steady-state levels are reached. At steady state, the AUC for one dosing interval is 42 (mg/L) × hour. What is the average concentration over that dosing interval?

A. 3.1 mg/L

B. 7 mg/L

C. 12.5 mg/L

D. 22 mg/L

4-13. A patient receives an antimicrobial dose of 400 mg intravenously every 8 hours. After steady state is reached, a peak level of 15 mg/L is determined; the level 4 hours after the peak is 4.5 mg/L. What dose is required to attain a peak plasma level of 35 mg/L? (Assume IV bolus drug administration.)

A. 400 mg

B. 800 mg

C. 933 mg

D. 3108 mg

4-14. For the example given in the last question, when the peak plasma level is 35 mg/L, what will the trough plasma level be?

A. 2.3 mg/L

B. 3.2 mg/L

C. 4.8 mg/L

D. 32 mg/L

Answers

4-1. A. CORRECT ANSWER

B. Incorrect answer. This value is the minimum concentration after the first dose. Remember to add the value of C_{max1}, which was 100 mg/L.

C. Incorrect answer. This is the value of C_{max1}. C_{max2} is calculated as the sum of C_{max1} and C_{min1}.

D. Incorrect answer. This is close to the C_{max2} but is actually the steady-state C_{max}. C_{max2} is calculated as the sum of C_{max1} and C_{min1}.

4-2. A. Incorrect answer. This is C_{min1}.

B, C. Incorrect answers

D. CORRECT ANSWER. C_{min2} can be found from C_{max2} as follows: $C_{min2} = C_{max2} (e^{-Kt})$, so $C_{min2} = $ 109.1 mg/L$(e^{-0.4/hr \times 6\ hr}) = 109.1 \times 0.091 = 9.9$ mg/L.

4-3 A. CORRECT ANSWER.

$$C_{maxn} = C_{max1} \frac{\left(1 - e^{-nK\tau}\right)}{1 - e^{-K\tau}}$$

$$C_{max1} = \frac{X_0}{V} = \frac{800\ mg}{20\ L}$$

then

$$C_{max15} = \left(\frac{800\ mg}{20\ L}\right)\left[\frac{\left(1 - e^{-15\left(0.5\ hr^{-1}\right)6\ hr}\right)}{\left(1 - e^{-\left(0.5\ hr^{-1}\right)6\ hr}\right)}\right]$$

$$C_{max15} = 42.1\ mg/L$$

B, C, D. Incorrect answers

4-4. A. CORRECT ANSWER. When steady state is reached, the amount of drug eliminated over one dosing interval is equal to the dose.

B. Incorrect answer

4-5. A. CORRECT ANSWER. The half-life directly relates to the time required to reach steady state. Approximately five half-lives are required to reach steady state. A longer half-life (lower K) will mean that more time is required to reach steady state.

B. Incorrect answer

4-6. A, C. Incorrect answers

B. CORRECT ANSWER. Administration of five doses would take 24 hours, which is two drug half-lives. After one half-life, the peak concentration would be 50% of steady-state concentration; at two half-lives, it would be 75%. So the peak concentration just after the fifth dose would be approximately 7.5 mg/L.

4-7. A. CORRECT ANSWER. Higher concentrations would result with a lower K and V.

B. Incorrect answer

4-8. A. Incorrect answer

B. CORRECT ANSWER. By decreasing the dosing interval the amount of drug administered per unit of time will increase and steady state concentrations will increase.

4-9. A. Incorrect answer. A small dose given very frequently results in less of a change from peak to trough concentrations.

B. CORRECT ANSWER

4-10. A, C, D. Incorrect answers

B. CORRECT ANSWER. The peak concentration is calculated as follows:

$$C_{peak} = X_0/V(1/[1 - e^{-K\tau}])$$

$$= 100 \text{ mg}/20 \text{ L}(1/[1 - e^{-0.35 \text{ hr}^{-1} \times 6 \text{ hr}}])$$

$$= 5.7 \text{ mg/L}$$

4-11. A, C, D. Incorrect answers

B. CORRECT ANSWER. The trough concentration is calculated as follows:

$$C_{trough} = C_{peak} \times e^{-K\tau}$$

$$= 5.7 \text{ mg/L} \times e^{-0.35 \text{ hr}^{-1} \times 6 \text{ hr}}$$

$$= 0.7 \text{ mg/L}$$

In this case, the elapsed time t is equal to τ.

4-12. A, C, D. Incorrect answers

B. CORRECT ANSWER. The average plasma concentration is determined as follows:

$$C = AUC/\tau$$

$$= 42 \text{ (mg/L)} \times \text{hr} / 6 \text{ hr}$$

$$= 7 \text{ mg/L}$$

4-13. A. Incorrect answer. Giving the same dose would result in the same peak concentration of 15 mg/L.

B. Incorrect answer. Doubling the dose would result in a doubling of the steady-state peak concentration to 30 mg/L.

C. CORRECT ANSWER

D. Incorrect answer. This dose would result in a steady-state peak concentration of 117 mg/L.

4-14. A, C, D. Incorrect answers

B. CORRECT ANSWER. To answer this question, K must first be calculated:

$$K = (\ln C_{4 \text{ hr}} - \ln C_{peak}) / 4 = 0.3 \text{ hr}^{-1}$$

Then, use the following to calculate the trough plasma concentration:

$$C_{trough} = C_{peak} \times e^{-K\tau} = 35 \text{ mg/L} \times e^{-0.30 \text{ hr}^{-1} \times 8 \text{ hr}}$$

$$= 35 \text{ mg/L} \times 0.091 = 3.2 \text{ mg/L}$$

Discussion Points

D-1. Explain why, for most drugs, the increase in drug plasma concentrations resulting from a single dose will be the same magnitude whether it is the first or tenth dose.

D-2. Explain why the plasma concentrations (maximum or minimum) remain the same for each dose after steady state is reached.

D-3. Explain why changing the dose or the dosing interval does not affect the time to reach steady state.

D-4. The peak plasma concentration achieved after the first intravenous dose of drug X is 25 mg/L. The drug's half-life is 3.5 hours, and it is administered every 12 hours. What will the peak plasma concentration at steady state be?

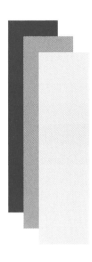

Relationships of Pharmacokinetic Parameters and Intravenous Intermittent and Continuous Infusions

OBJECTIVES

After completing Lesson 5, you should be able to:

1. Explain the relationships of pharmacokinetic parameters and how changes in each parameter affect the others.

2. Describe the relationship between the rate of continuous intravenous (IV) drug infusion, drug clearance, and steady-state plasma concentration.

3. Calculate plasma drug concentrations during and after continuous IV infusion.

4. Calculate an appropriate loading dose to achieve therapeutic range at onset of infusion.

5. Calculate peak and trough concentrations at steady state after intermittent IV infusions.

RELATIONSHIPS OF PHARMACOKINETIC PARAMETERS

Understanding the relationships of pharmacokinetic parameters is important to determine what will occur to the plasma concentration versus time curve when changes in any of the parameters arise. If we administer multiple IV doses of a drug that exhibits one-compartment, first-order elimination kinetics, we might find a plasma drug concentration versus time curve that resembles Figure 5-1.

Changes in Elimination Rate Constant

If the dose, the volume of distribution, and the dosing interval (τ) all remain the same but the elimination rate constant (K) **decreases** (as with decreasing renal or hepatic function), the curve should change as shown in Figure 5-2. With a lower K, we would see that:

1. Peak and trough concentrations at steady state are higher than before.

2. The difference between peak and trough levels at steady state is smaller because the elimination rate is lower.

Because K is decreased in this situation, the half-life ($T^{1/2}$) is increased and, therefore, the time to reach steady state ($5 \times T^{1/2}$) is also lengthened. This concept is important in designing dosing regimens for patients with progressing diseases of the primary organs of drug elimination (kidneys and liver).

Changes in Dosing Interval

For another example, suppose everything, including the elimination rate, remains constant but the dosing interval (τ) is decreased. The resulting plasma drug concentration versus time curve would be similar to that in Figure 5-3.

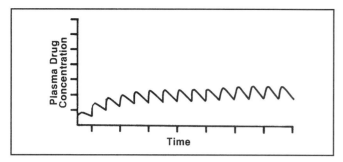

FIGURE 5-1.
Plasma drug concentrations after multiple intravenous doses.

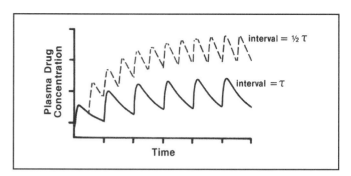

FIGURE 5-3.
Effect of decreased τ on plasma drug concentrations.

The peak and trough concentrations at steady state are increased. Also, the difference between peak and trough plasma concentrations at steady state is smaller (only because the body is allowed less time to eliminate drug before receiving the next dose). Because K (and therefore $T^{1/2}$) is the same, the **time** to reach steady state remains **unchanged**.

Changes in Dose

Now, suppose that K, V, and τ remain constant but the dose (X_0) is increased. The plasma concentration versus time curve shown in Figure 5-4 would result. The drug concentrations at steady state are higher, but there is no difference in the time required to reach steady state, as it is dependent only on $T^{1/2}$.

With some drugs, it is preferable to give a smaller dose at more frequent intervals; with other drugs, the reverse is true. The disadvantage of larger, less frequent dosing is that the fluctuation from peak to trough concentrations is greater. Thus, the possibility of being in a toxic range just after a dose is given and in a subtherapeutic range before the next dose is given is also greater. The problem with smaller, more frequent doses is that such administration may not be practical, even though plasma concentrations may be within the therapeutic range for a greater portion of the dosing interval.

Changes in Clearance and Volume of Distribution

A drug's half-life and elimination rate constant are determined by its clearance and volume of distribution (discussed in Lessons 2 and 3). These last two pharmacokinetic parameters determine the plasma drug concentrations that result from a dosing regimen, so changes in clearance or volume of distribution result in changes in steady-state plasma drug concentrations.

Volume of distribution and clearance may change independently. However, some disease states may alter both the clearance and the volume of distribution. An example is the effect of renal failure on aminoglycoside concentrations. The renal clearance of aminoglycosides decreases in patients with renal failure, and the volume of distribution may increase because of the fluid accumulation that occurs with oliguric renal failure.

There are a number of conditions that may increase or decrease volume of distribution. The volume of distribution of drugs that distribute primarily in body water increase in patients with conditions that cause fluid accumulation (e.g., renal failure, heart failure, liver failure with ascites, and inflammatory processes such as sepsis). As one would expect, dehydration results in a decreased volume of distribution for drugs of this type. Drugs that are highly bound to plasma protein (such as phenytoin) have a greater volume of distribution when

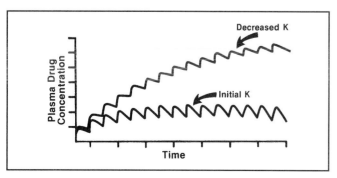

FIGURE 5-2.
Effect of decreased K (and therefore increased $T^{1/2}$) on plasma drug concentrations.

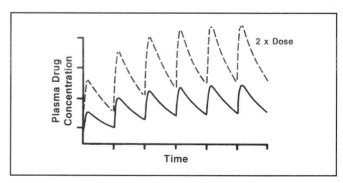

FIGURE 5-4.
Effect of increased dose on plasma drug concentrations.

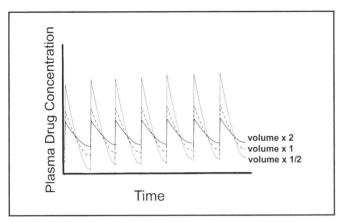

FIGURE 5-5.
Effect of changes in volume of distribution on plasma drug concentrations.

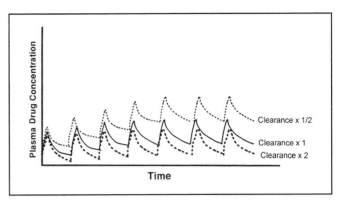

FIGURE 5-6.
Effect of changes in clearance on plasma drug concentrations.

protein binding is decreased by hypoalbuminemia or phenytoin-displacing agents. If less proteins are available for binding, then to maintain equilibrium with the tissues, free drug moves from the plasma to the tissues, thus increasing the "apparent" volume of distribution.

Changes in the volume of distribution directly affect steady-state plasma drug concentrations. In general, if the drug dose, dosing interval (τ), and drug clearance are all unchanged but the volume of distribution decreases, there will be greater fluctuation of plasma concentrations with higher peak concentrations. Conversely, if the volume of distribution increases, there will be less fluctuation of plasma concentrations with a lower peak (Figure 5-5).

The effect of volume of distribution changes on plasma drug concentrations can be easily estimated for most drugs. When the volume of distribution increases, assuming there are no other changes, peak steady-state plasma drug concentrations decrease. Conversely, if the volume of distribution decreases, the peak steady-state plasma drug concentrations increase. This can also be demonstrated by the following equation:

$$C_{ss} = K_0/KV$$

where K_0 = the rate of drug infusion (or administration). (Note: This equation is derived in the section Continuous Infusion later in this lesson.)

There are a number of conditions that may increase or decrease drug clearance. Agents that change renal blood flow directly affect the clearance of drugs excreted by the kidneys. Renal clearance may decrease when agents that compete for active renal secretion are administered concomitantly (such as penicillin with probenecid). For drugs that are eliminated hepatically, clearance may be altered by drugs or conditions that increase or decrease liver blood flow. Some conditions (such as hepatitis or cirrhosis) also may decrease the

capability of liver enzymes to metabolize drugs. Drug clearance may increase when organ function improves after healing, with concomitant drug administration, or under conditions that increase organ blood flow or the activity of metabolic enzymes.

Changes in drug clearance affect steady-state plasma drug concentrations. If the dose, dosing interval, and the volume of distribution are all unchanged but clearance increases, plasma drug concentrations will decrease because the drug is being removed at a faster rate. Conversely, if clearance decreases, plasma concentrations will increase because the drug is being removed at a slower rate (Figure 5-6).

This can also be demonstrated by the modification of the equation presented above:

$$C_{ss} = K_0/Cl_t$$

where K_0 = the rate of drug infusion and Cl_t = total body clearance. (Note: This equation is also derived in the section Continuous Infusion.)

As with volume of distribution, the effect of changes in clearance on plasma drug concentrations can be easily estimated for most drugs. When drug clearance increases by a factor of two, the average steady-state plasma drug concentration decreases by half. Conversely, if drug clearance decreases by half, the average steady-state plasma drug concentration would increase by a factor of two.

■ CLINICAL CORRELATE

One condition that may substantially alter the volume of distribution is severe traumatic or burn injury. Severely traumatized or burned patients often have a cytokine-induced, systemic inflammatory response syndrome (SIR), which results in decreased plasma proteins (i.e., albumin) and thus an accumulation of fluid in tissues. An average-weight person (70 kg) may gain as much as 20 kg in fluid over a few days. In comparison to the extra fluid, the body has decreased albumin for binding, and with the accumulation of fluid, due to this SIR, free drug shifts from the plasma into the extravascular fluid causing drugs that are primarily distributed into body water to have an increased volume of distribution.

Continuous Infusion

As stated previously, repeated doses of a drug (i.e., intermittent infusions) result in fluctuations in the plasma concentration over time. For some drugs, maintenance of a consistent plasma concentration is advantageous because of a desire to achieve a consistent effect. To maintain consistent plasma drug concentrations, continuous IV infusions are often used. Continuous IV infusion can be thought of as the administration of small amounts of drug at infinitely small dosing intervals. If administration is begun and maintained at a constant rate, the plasma drug concentration versus time curve in Figure 5-7 will result.

The plasma concentrations resulting from the continuous IV infusion of drug are determined by the rate of drug input (rate of drug infusion, K_0), volume of distribution (V), and drug clearance (Cl_t). The relationship among these parameters is:

$$C_t = \frac{K_0}{VK}(1 - e^{-Kt})$$

where t is the time since the beginning of the drug infusion. This equation shows that the plasma concentration is determined by the rate of drug infusion (K_0) and the clearance of drug from the body (remember, $VK = Cl_t$). The equation is used to find a concentration at a time before steady-state is reached.

TABLE 5-1.
Changes in Factor $(1 - e^{-Kt})$ Over Time

Time after Starting Infusion (hours)	Value of $(1 - e^{-Kt})$	Drug Half-Lives Elapsed
4	0.29	0.5
8	0.50	1.0
16	0.75	2.0
24	0.88	3.0
40	0.97	5.0
60	0.99	7.5

The term $(1 - e^{-Kt})$ gives the fraction of steady-state concentration achieved by time t after the infusion is begun. For example, when t is a very low number, just after an infusion is begun, $K_0(1 - e^{-Kt})$ is also very small. When t is very large, $(1 - e^{-Kt})$ approaches 1, so $K_0(1 - e^{-Kt})$ approaches K_0 and plasma concentration approaches steady state.

Suppose that a drug has a half-life of 8 hours (then $K = 0.087$ hr^{-1}). Table 5-1 shows how the factor $(1 - e^{-Kt})$ changes with time. When $(1 - e^{-Kt})$ approaches 1 (at approximately five half-lives), steady-state concentrations are approximately achieved.

In Figure 5-7, steady state is attained where the horizontal portion of the curve begins. With a drug such as theophylline, given by continuous IV infusion, the average half-life in adults is approximately 7 hours. Therefore, it will take 35 hours (5 × 7 hours) to reach approximate steady-state plasma concentrations.

When steady state is achieved, the factor $(1 - e^{-Kt})$ approximately equals 1, and then:

$$C_{ss} = \frac{K_0}{Cl_t}(1-e^{-\infty}) = \frac{K_0}{Cl_t}(1-0) = \frac{K_0}{Cl_t}$$

At steady state, the plasma concentration of drug is directly proportional to the rate of administration (assuming clearance is unchanged). If the infusion is increased, the steady-state plasma concentration (C_{ss}) will increase proportionally. Clearance is the pharmacokinetic parameter that relates the rate of drug input (dosing or infusion rate) to plasma concentration. The actual plasma concentration attained with a continuous IV infusion of drug depends on the following two factors:

- rate of drug infusion (K_0), and
- clearance of the drug (Cl_t).

If we know from previous data that a patient receiving IV theophylline (or aminophylline) has a half-life of

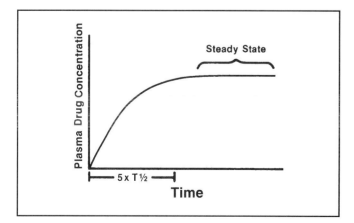

FIGURE 5-7.
Plasma drug concentrations over time with a continuous intravenous infusion.

6 hours ($K = 0.116$ hr^{-1}) and a volume of distribution of 30 L (clearance then equals 3.48 L/hour), we can predict the steady-state plasma concentration for a continuous IV theophylline infusion of 50 mg/hour:

$$C_{ss} = \frac{K_0}{VK} = \frac{50 \text{ mg/hr}}{30 \text{ L} \times 0.116 \text{ hr}^{-1}} = 14.4 \text{ mg/L}$$

If we wish to increase the steady-state theophylline plasma concentration to 18 mg/L, we would use the same equation to determine K_0:

$$18 \text{ mg/L} = \frac{K_0}{30 \text{ L} \times 0.116 \text{ hr}^{-1}}$$

$$K_0 = (18 \text{ mg/L})(30 \text{ L} \times 0.116 \text{ hr}^{-1}) = 62.6 \text{ mg/hr}$$

Or, as concentration and infusion rate are directly proportional, the following equation may be used to find a new infusion rate to obtain a desired steady-state concentration:

$$K_{0(new)} = \frac{C_{ss(desired)}}{C_{ss(measured)}} \times K_{0(original)}$$

$$= \frac{18 \text{ mg/L}}{14.4 \text{ mg/L}} \times 50 \text{ mg/hr}$$

$$= 62.5 \text{ mg/hr}$$

The continuous IV infusion of drugs is an important method of drug administration. With this method, it is sometimes necessary to predict drug plasma concentrations at times other than at steady state. In the following section, we examine some of these situations (Figure 5-8).

The equation predicting plasma concentrations with continuous IV infusion can be used to estimate plasma drug concentrations at times before steady state, as stated previously in the lesson:

$$C_t = \frac{K_0}{VK}(1 - e^{-Kt})$$

(Remember, $VK = Cl_t$)

For example, if Cl_t for a drug is known to be 4.5 L/hour (with $K = 0.15$ hr^{-1}) and this drug is given at a rate of 50 mg/hour, then the plasma concentration 8 hours after starting the infusion would be:

$$C_{8 hr} = \frac{50 \text{ mg/hr}}{4.5 \text{ L/hr}}(1 - e^{-(0.15 \text{ hr}^{-1})(8 \text{ hr})})$$

$$= \frac{50 \text{ mg/hr}}{4.5 \text{ L/hr}}(0.70)$$

$$= 7.8 \text{ mg/L}$$

If this infusion is continued, the steady-state concentration would be:

$$C_{ss} = \frac{K_0}{Cl_t} = \frac{50 \text{ mg/hr}}{4.5 \text{ L/hr}} = 11.1 \text{ mg/L}$$

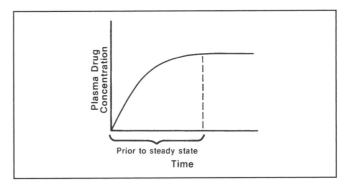

FIGURE 5-8.
Plasma drug concentrations over time with a continuous intravenous infusion.

Remember that with a continuous infusion, the steady-state plasma concentration is determined by the rate of drug going into the body (K_0) and drug clearance from the body (Cl_t). At steady state, the amount of drug going into the body per hour equals the amount of drug being removed per hour.

You have learned that it takes approximately five drug half-lives to reach steady state. Each time the infusion rate is changed, five half-lives will be required to attain a new steady-state concentration. For example, for a patient receiving IV theophylline at 20 mg/hour, the steady-state plasma concentration is 7.5 mg/L, and 25 hours is required to reach steady state ($T^{1/2} = 5$ hours, $K = 0.139$ hr^{-1}). If the infusion rate is increased to 40 mg/hour, an additional 25 hours will be required to attain the new steady-state concentration of 15 mg/L (Figure 5-9). If a dosing rate is changed, it takes one half-life to reach 50% of the difference between the old concentration and the new, two half-lives to reach 75% of the difference, three half-lives to reach 87.5%, etc.

If we wish to calculate the plasma concentration before the new steady state is achieved, we can use the factor given before: $(1 - e^{-Kt})$, where t is the time after beginning the new infusion rate and the resulting frac-

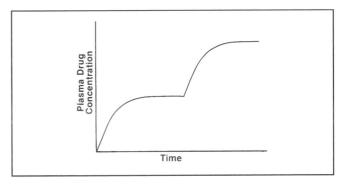

FIGURE 5-9.
Changing plasma drug concentrations with increased drug infusion rate.

tion is the relative "distance" between the old and new steady-state concentrations. For the example above (where K = 0.139 hr^{-1}), 8 hours after the infusion rate is increased:

$$(1 - e^{-Kt}) = 1 - e^{(-0.139 \text{ hr}^{-1})(8 \text{ hr})}$$
$$= 0.67$$

So at 8 hours, the concentration would be approximately two-thirds (67%) of the way between 7.5 and 15.0 mg/L (about 12.5 mg/L).

If an infusion is stopped before steady state is reached, the concentration could be determined:

$$C_t = (K_0/Cl_t)(1 - e^{-Kt})$$

where t = the duration of the infusion.

Another important situation occurs when continuous infusion is stopped after steady state is achieved. To predict plasma drug concentrations at some time after the infusion is stopped (Figure 5-10), the concentration at steady state (C_{ss}) is treated as if it were a peak concentration after an IV injection (C_0). In this situation, plasma concentrations after C_0 are predicted by:

$$C_t = C_0 e^{-Kt} \quad \text{(See \textbf{Equation 3-2}.)}$$

where t in this case is time after C_0, which is the time after the infusion is stopped.

In the case of continuous infusions:

$$C_t = C_{ss} e^{-Kt}$$

where t is time after the infusion is stopped. If, as in the previous example, K = 0.139 hr^{-1} and C_{ss} = 15 mg/L, the plasma concentration 12 hours after discontinuing the infusion would be:

$$C_{12 \text{ hr}} = (15 \text{ mg/L})e^{(-0.139 \text{ hr}^{-1})(12 \text{ hr})}$$
$$= 15 \text{ mg/L} (0.19)$$
$$= 2.9 \text{ mg/L}$$

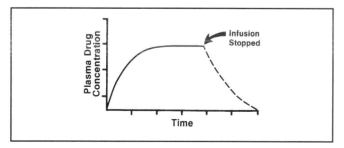

FIGURE 5-10.
Plasma drug concentrations after discontinuation of an intravenous infusion.

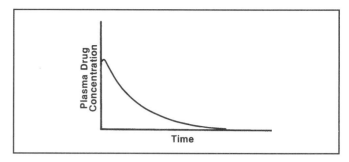

FIGURE 5-11.
Plasma drug concentrations resulting from an intravenous loading dose.

Loading Dose

As stated previously, after a continuous IV infusion of drug is begun, five drug half-lives are needed to achieve steady state. If an immediate effect is desired, that may be too long to reach the therapeutic range. Sometimes a "loading dose" is administered at the initiation of the infusion so that the therapeutic range is maintained from the outset. This loading bolus IV dose is usually relatively large and may produce immediate therapeutic plasma concentrations (Figure 5-11). Note that a loading dose should not be used if substantial side effects occur with large doses of the drug. Also, sometimes clinicians desire for drugs to accumulate slowly rather than to achieve therapeutic concentrations immediately so that the patient may have adequate time to develop tolerance to the initial side effects (e.g., tricyclic antidepressants).

The desired loading dose for many drugs can be derived from the definition of the volume of distribution. As shown previously, $V = X_0/C_0$ (see **Equation 1-1**) for a drug described by a one-compartment model. Rearranging this equation, we see that the loading dose equals the desired concentration multiplied by the volume of distribution:

$$X_0 = C_{0(desired)}V \quad \text{(See \textbf{Equation 1-1}.)}$$

Note that C_0 in this case is equivalent to the desired steady-state concentration.

We know that an IV loading dose produces plasma concentrations as shown in Figure 5-11, and the continuous infusion produces plasma concentrations as shown in Figure 5-12. If both the loading bolus injection and the continuous IV infusion are given, the net effect should be a fairly steady plasma concentration, as depicted by the bold line in Figure 5-13. Before the constant IV infusion has reached steady state, the bolus loading dose has produced a nearly steady-state drug concentration, and when the drug from the loading dose is almost eliminated, the constant IV infusion should be approximately at steady state. With lidocaine, heparin,

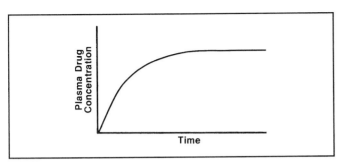

FIGURE 5-12.
Plasma drug concentrations over time resulting from a continuous intravenous infusion.

and theophylline, loading doses usually precede their continuous IV infusions, providing immediate as well as sustained effects that combine to produce a steady therapeutic plasma concentration.

Previously used equations can be combined to describe the plasma concentration resulting from a bolus injection with continuous infusion. With an IV injection, the equation describing the plasma concentration after a dose is:

$$C_t = \frac{X_0}{V} e^{-Kt}$$

where:
 t = time after dose,
 X_0 = initial loading dose,
 V = volume of distribution, and
 K = elimination rate constant.

With a continuous infusion, the plasma concentrations are described by:

$$C_t = \frac{K_0}{VK}(1 - e^{-Kt'})$$

where:
 t' = time after beginning infusion,
 K_0 = rate of drug infusion,

V = volume of distribution, and
K = elimination rate constant.

When both the injection and infusion are administered together, the plasma concentration after beginning the regimen is calculated by adding the two equations:

$$C_t = \frac{X_0}{V} e^{-Kt} + \frac{K_0}{VK}(1 - e^{-Kt'})$$

For example, an adult patient is estimated to have a theophylline half-life of 8 hours ($K = 0.087$ hr^{-1}) and a V of 30 L. These estimates are obtained from known information about this patient or from published reports of similar patients. If the patient is given a loading dose of 400 mg of theophylline, and a continuous infusion of 60 mg/hour is begun at the same time, what will the plasma concentration be 24 hours later?

$$C_t = \frac{X_0}{V} e^{-Kt} + \frac{K_0}{VK}(1 - e^{-Kt'})$$
$$= \frac{400 \text{ mg}}{30 \text{ L}} e^{-0.087 \text{ hr}^{-1}(24 \text{ hr})} + \frac{60 \text{ mg/hr}}{30 \text{ L} \times 0.087 \text{ hr}^{-1}}(1 - e^{-0.087 \text{ hr}^{-1}(24 \text{ hr})})$$
$$= \frac{400 \text{ mg}}{30 \text{ L}}(0.124) + \frac{60 \text{ mg/hr}}{30 \text{ L} \times 0.087 \text{ hr}^{-1}}(0.876)$$
$$= 1.6 \text{ mg/L} + 20.1 \text{ mg/L} = 21.7 \text{ mg/L}$$

In clinical practice, drugs such as theophylline usually are not given by IV bolus injection; not even loading doses. Loading doses usually are given as short infusions (often 30 minutes). Taking this procedure into account, we can further modify the above equations to predict plasma concentrations.

For the loading dose:

$$Cpeak_{ss} = \frac{X_0/t}{VK}(1 - e^{-Kt})$$

where:
 X_0 = dose;
 t = infusion period (e.g., 0.5 hour);
 K = elimination rate constant; and
 V = volume of distribution.

Multiple Intravenous Infusions (Intermittent Infusions)

In Lesson 4, we discussed multiple-dose IV bolus drug administration. With multiple-dose IV administration, we assumed that the drug was administered by rapid IV injection. However, rapid IV injections are not usually used for most drugs because of increased risks of adverse effects.

Most IV drugs are given over 30–60 minutes or longer. This method of giving multiple doses by infusion at specified intervals (τ), called *intermittent IV infusion*, changes the plasma concentration profile from what

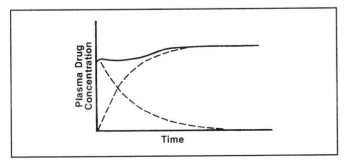

FIGURE 5-13.
Plasma drug concentrations resulting from an intravenous loading dose given with a continuous infusion.

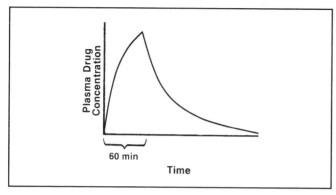

FIGURE 5-14.
Plasma drug concentrations resulting from a short intravenous infusion.

would be seen with multiple rapid IV injections. Therefore, a new model must be created to predict plasma drug concentrations after multiple-dose intermittent IV infusions. This model combines the approaches just presented for multiple-dose injections and continuous infusions.

Let's assume that a drug is given intravenously over 1 hour every 8 hours. For the first in a series of IV infusions lasting 60 minutes each, the plasma concentrations will be similar to those observed during the first 60 minutes of a continuous infusion. Then, when the infusion is stopped, plasma concentrations will decline in a first-order process, just as after IV injections (Figure 5-14).

The peak (or maximum) plasma concentration after the first infusion (C_{max1}) is estimated by:

$$C_{max1} = \frac{K_0}{VK}(1 - e^{-Kt})$$

where:
   C = concentration in plasma,
   K_0 = rate of drug infusion (dose/time of infusion),
   V = volume of distribution,
   K = elimination rate constant, and
   t = time (duration) of infusion.

This equation was used above to describe plasma drug concentrations with continuous infusion before steady state.

The trough concentration after the first dose (C_{min1}) occurs at the end of the dosing interval (τ) directly before the next dose.

C_{min1} is calculated by multiplying C_{max1} by $e^{-K\tau}$.

$$C_{min1} = (K_0/VK)(1 - e^{-Kt})(e^{-K\tau})$$

By the principle of superposition (see Lesson 4), C_{max2} can be estimated:

$$C_{max2} = C_{max1} + C_{min1}$$
$$= \frac{K_0}{VK}\left(1 - e^{-Kt}\right) + \frac{K_0}{VK}\left(1 - e^{-Kt}\right)\left(e^{-K\tau}\right)$$
$$= \frac{K_0}{VK}\left(1 - e^{-Kt}\right)\left(1 + e^{-K\tau}\right)$$

C_{min2} can be calculated:

$$C_{min2} = C_{max2} \times e^{-K\tau}$$
$$= \frac{K_0}{VK}\left(1 - e^{-Kt}\right)\left(1 + e^{-K\tau}\right)\left(e^{-K\tau}\right)$$
$$= \frac{K_0}{VK}\left(1 - e^{-Kt}\right)\left(e^{-K\tau} + e^{-2K\tau}\right)$$

This expansion of the equation can continue as in Lesson 4 until n number of infusions have been given:

$$C_{max\ n} = \frac{K_0}{VK}\left[\frac{(1 - e^{-Kt})(1 - e^{-nK\tau})}{(1 - e^{-K\tau})}\right]$$

As n becomes very large, $(1 - e^{-nK\tau})$ approaches 1, and the equation becomes:

⚠ 5-1
$$C_{maxss} = \frac{K_0}{VK}\left[\frac{(1 - e^{-Kt})}{(1 - e^{-K\tau})}\right]$$

Then, to determine the concentration at any time (t') after the peak, the following multiple IV infusion at steady-state equation can be used:

$$C = \frac{K_0}{VK}\left[\frac{(1 - e^{-Kt})}{(1 - e^{-K\tau})}\right]e^{-Kt'}$$

where t' = total hours drug was allowed to be eliminated. A practical example for this equation is shown below to determine the C_{pmin} or trough concentration of a drug given by intermittent infusion.

$$C_{min(steady\ state)} = \frac{K_0}{VK}\left[\frac{(1 - e^{-Kt})}{(1 - e^{-K\tau})}\right]e^{-Kt'}$$

where $t' = \tau - t$.

The equation for $C_{min(steady\ state)}$ is very important in clinical practice. It can be used to predict plasma concentrations for multiple intermittent IV infusions of any drug that follows first-order elimination (assuming a one-compartment model). It also can be used to predict plasma concentrations at any time between C_{max} and C_{min}, where t' equals the time between the end of the infusion and the determination of the plasma concentration. For application of this method, refer to cases that include IV intermittent infusions such as Lesson 12 (Aminoglycosides) and Lesson 13 (Vancomycin).

CLINICAL CORRELATE

Here is one way the relationship can be used. Suppose a patient with severe renal dysfunction receives a 1-g dose of vancomycin, and a peak concentration, drawn 2 hours after the end of the infusion, is 40 mg/L. (For vancomycin, "peak" concentrations are determined at least 2 hours after administration to allow time for distribution into tissues.) A concentration determined 24 hours later is 34 mg/L, but we want to wait until the concentration reaches 10 mg/L before administering a second dose. When will the concentration reach 10 mg/L?

First, K can be calculated using:

$$C_t = C_{peak}e^{-Kt}$$

$$34 \text{ mg/L} = (40 \text{ mg/L})e^{-K(24 \text{ hr})}$$

$$\frac{34 \text{ mg/L}}{40 \text{ mg/L}} = e^{-K(24 \text{ hr})}$$

$$0.85 = e^{-K(24 \text{ hr})}$$

$$\ln 0.85 = -K(24 \text{ hr})$$

$$-0.163 = -K(24 \text{ hr})$$

$$\frac{0.163}{24 \text{ hr}} = K$$

$$K = 0.0068 \text{ hr}^{-1}$$

Knowing K, we can calculate the time (t) required for the concentration to decrease to 10 mg/L:

$$C_t = C_{peak}e^{-Kt}$$

$$10 \text{ mg/L} = (40 \text{ mg/L})\, e^{(-0.0068 \text{ hr}^{-1})t}$$

$$\frac{10 \text{ mg/L}}{40 \text{ mg/L}} = e^{(-0.0068 \text{ hr}^{-1})t}$$

$$0.25 = e^{(-0.0068 \text{ hr}^{-1})t}$$

$$\ln 0.25 = (-0.0068 \text{ hr}^{-1})t$$

$$-1.39 = (-0.0068 \text{ hr}^{-1})t$$

$$\frac{-1.39}{-0.0068 \text{ hr}^{-1}} = t$$

$$t = 204 \text{ hr}^{-1}$$

Therefore, it will take approximately 8.5 days after the peak concentration for the concentration to reduce to 10 mg/L

■ Review Questions

5-1.   For a drug regimen, if the elimination rate (K) of a drug is reduced while V, X_0, and τ remain constant, the peak and trough concentrations will:

A. increase.

B. decrease.

5-2.   An increase in drug dose will result in higher plasma concentrations at steady state but will not change the time to reach steady state.

A. True

B. False

5-3.   Giving which of the following dosing techniques results in greater fluctuation between peak and trough plasma levels?

A. small doses very frequently

B. large doses relatively less frequently

5-4.   When the volume of distribution increases (and clearance remains the same), steady-state plasma concentrations will have more peak-to-trough variation.

A. True

B. False

5-5.   When drug clearance decreases (while volume of distribution remains unchanged), steady-state plasma concentrations will:

A. increase.

B. decrease.

5-6.   Steady-state plasma concentration is approximately reached when the continuous infusion has been given for at least how many half-lives of the drug?

A. two

B. three

C. five

D. ten

5-7.   If you double the infusion rate of a drug, you should expect to see a twofold increase in the drug's steady-state concentration. Assume that clearance remains constant.

A. True

B. False

5-8.   Theophylline is administered to a patient at 30 mg/hour via a constant IV infusion. If the patient has a total body clearance for theophylline of 50 mL/minute, what should this patient's steady-state plasma concentration be?

A. 0.625 mg/L

B. 10.0 mg/L

C. 0.1 mg/L

5-9.   With a continuous IV infusion of drug, the steady-state plasma concentration is directly proportional to:

A. clearance.

B. volume of distribution.

C. drug infusion rate.

D. K.

5-10.   If a drug is given by continuous IV infusion at a rate of 25 mg/hour and produces a steady-state plasma concentration of 10 mg/L, what infusion rate will result in a new C_{ss} of 20 mg/L?

A. 30 mg/hour

B. 35 mg/hour

C. 50 mg/hour

D. 75 mg/hour

5-11.   For a continuous infusion, given the equation $C = K_0(1 - e^{-Kt})/Cl_t$, at steady state the value for t approaches infinity and e^{-Kt} approaches infinity

A. True

B. False

This case applies to questions 5-12 and 5-13. A patient is to be started on a continuous infusion of a drug. To achieve an immediate effect, a loading dose is to be administered over 30 minutes and then the continuous infusion is to be begun. From a previous regimen of the same drug, you estimate that the patient's $K = 0.07$ hr^{-1} and $V = 40$ L. Assume that none of this drug has been administered in the last month, so the plasma concentration before therapy is 0 mg/L.

5-12.   If the $C_{ss(desired)}$ is 15 mg/L, what should the loading dose be?

A. 15 mg

B. 42 mg

C. 600 mg

D. 1200 mg

5-13. What rate of infusion (K_0) should result in a C_{ss} of 15 mg/L?

A. 0.2 mg/hour

B. 42 mg/hour

C. 600 mg/hour

Refer to this equation when working questions 5-14 through 5-16:

$$C = \frac{K_0}{VK}\left[\frac{\left(1 - e^{-nKt}\right)}{\left(1 - e^{-K\tau}\right)}\right]e^{-Kt'}$$

5-14. A patient is to be given 100 mg of gentamicin intravenously over 1 hour every 8 hours. If the patient is assumed to have a K of 0.20 hr^{-1} and a V of 15 L, how long will it take to reach steady state?

A. 3.5 hours

B. 5 hours

C. 17 hours

D. 34 hours

5-15. For the patient in the question above, what will the peak plasma concentration be after 20 doses?

A. 7.6 mg/L

B. 15.2 mg/L

C. 29.8 mg/L

D. 42 mg/L

5-16. For the patient in the previous question, calculate the trough plasma concentration after 20 doses.

A. 0.54 mg/L

B. 1.12 mg/L

C. 1.87 mg/L

D. 2.25 mg/L

▌ Answers

5-1. A. CORRECT ANSWER. This can be determined by examination of the equation from Lesson 4:

$$C_{peak(steady\ state)} = \frac{X_0}{V}\left[\frac{1}{(1 - e^{-K\tau})}\right]$$

B. Incorrect answer

5-2. A. CORRECT ANSWER. The time to reach steady state is determined by K.

B. Incorrect answer

5-3. A. Incorrect answer. Because the time interval would be relatively short, there would not be as much time for plasma concentrations to decline.

B. CORRECT ANSWER

5-4. A. Incorrect answer

B. CORRECT ANSWER. A larger volume of distribution will result in the same amount of drug distributing in a greater volume, which would result in a lower peak-to-trough variation.

5-5. A. CORRECT ANSWER. When clearance decreases, plasma concentrations will increase because drug is administered at the same rate (dose and dosing interval) but is being removed at a lower rate.

B. Incorrect answer

5-6. A. Incorrect answer. Only 75% of the steady-state concentration would be reached by two half-lives.

B. Incorrect answer. Only 87.5% of the steady-state concentration would be reached by three half-lives.

C. CORRECT ANSWER. At five half-lives, approximately 97% of the steady-state concentration has been reached.

D. Incorrect answer. This is much longer than necessary.

5-7. A. CORRECT ANSWER. The changes in the infusion rate will directly affect plasma concentrations, if other factors remain constant.

B. Incorrect answer

5-8. A, C. Incorrect answers

B. CORRECT ANSWER. The equation $C_{ss} = K_0/Cl_t$ should be used. The value for K_0 is 30 mg/hour. The value for Cl_t must be converted from 50 mL/minute to 3 L/hour.

5-9. A. Incorrect answer. As clearance increases the steady-state plasma concentration decreases.

B. Incorrect answer. If volume of distribution increased, the steady-state plasma concentration would decrease.

C. CORRECT ANSWER. The steady-state concentration is directly proportional to the drug infusion rate.

D. Incorrect answer. If K (the elimination rate constant) increased, the steady-state plasma concentration would decrease.

5-10. A, B, D. Incorrect answers

C. CORRECT ANSWER

5-11. A. Incorrect answer. As t becomes larger, the term e^{-Kt} becomes smaller, and the term $1 - e^{-Kt}$ approaches 1.

B. CORRECT ANSWER. To double the steady-state plasma concentration from 10 to 20 mg/L, the infusion rate should be doubled to 50 mg/hour.

5-12. A, B, D. Incorrect answers

C. CORRECT ANSWER. The loading dose is determined by multiplying the desired concentration (15 mg/L) by the volume of distribution: $C_{ss(desired)} \times V = 15$ mg/L $\times 40$ L $= 600$ mg. Note that the units cancel out to yield milligrams.

5-13. A, C. Incorrect answers

B. CORRECT ANSWER. The infusion rate is related to Cl_t and C_{ss} as follows: $C_{ss} = K_0/Cl_t$. Cl_t can be determined by multiplying $V \times K = 2.8$ L/hour. So, rearranging, $K_0 = C_{ss} \times Cl_t = 15$ mg/L $\times 2.8$ L/hour $= 42$ mg/hour.

5-14. A, B, D. Incorrect answers

C. CORRECT ANSWER. One half-life is calculated as follows: $T^{1/2} = 0.693/K$. Steady state is reached by five half-lives, or 17 hours.

5-15. A. CORRECT ANSWER. By 20 doses, steady state would have been reached, and the equation below would be used:

$$C_{max(steady\ state)} = \frac{K_0\left(1 - e^{-Kt}\right)}{VK\left(1 - e^{-K\tau}\right)}$$

$$= \frac{(100\ mg/hr)(0.181)}{(3.0\ L/hr)(0.798)}$$

$$= 7.6\ mg/L$$

B, C, D. Incorrect answers

5-16. A, B, D. Incorrect answers

C. CORRECT ANSWER. The trough concentration is calculated from the peak value as follows:

$$C_{trough} = C_{peak} \times e^{-K(t - \tau)}$$

$$= 7.6\ mg/L \times e^{-0.2\ hr^{-1}(8hr - 1hr)}$$

$$= 7.6\ mg/L \times 0.247 = 1.87\ mg/L.$$

Discussion Points

D-1.   Explain how changing the dosing interval (τ) influences the time to reach steady state when multiple doses are administered.

D-2.   If clearance is reduced to 25% of the initial rate and all other factors (such as dose, dosing interval, and volume of distribution) remain constant, how will steady-state plasma concentrations change?

D-3.   Theophylline is to be administered at a constant rate of 25 mg/hour. The following pharmacokinetic parameters are estimated for this patient: Cl_t = 15 mL/minute, V = 31.5 L, and K = 0.029 hr^{-1}. Calculate this patient's plasma concentrations at 6 and 12 hours after the infusion is begun. If the infusion is continued to steady state, what would C_{ss} be? If the infusion is stopped after steady state is reached, what would the concentration be 24 hours later?

D-4.   A loading dose of 1000 mg is infused over 30 minutes and a continuous infusion is begun when the loading infusion is stopped. The clearance is 2.5 L/hour, the volume of distribution is 50 L, and the infusion rate is 50 mg/hour. What will the plasma concentration be 12 hours after beginning the constant infusion?

D-5.   What is the following portion of the multiple-dose equation called, and why is it called that?

$$1/(1 - e^{-K\tau})$$

D-6.   Explain why, for most drugs, the increase in drug plasma concentrations resulting from a single dose will be the same magnitude whether it is the first or the tenth dose.

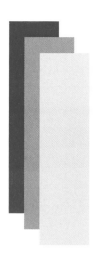

LESSON
6

Two-Compartment Models

 OBJECTIVES

After completing Lesson 6, you should be able to:

1. Describe when to use back-extrapolation versus method of residuals.

2. Calculate a residual line.

3. Calculate alpha (α), beta (β), and intercepts A and B for a drug conforming to a two-compartment model.

4. Describe when to use a monoexponential versus a biexponential equation.

5. Calculate V_c, V_{area} (also known as V_β), and V_{ss} (using both methods) for a two-compartment model.

Prior lessons focused on one-compartment models, but many drugs are characterized better by multicompartment models. In this lesson, we briefly discuss multicompartment models and present a few applications. Multicompartment models are not used as frequently as the one-compartment model in therapeutic drug monitoring, partly because they are more difficult to construct and apply.

Generally, multicompartment models are applied when the natural log of plasma drug concentration versus time curve is not a straight line after an intravenous dose or when the plasma concentration versus time profile cannot be characterized by a single exponential function (i.e., $C_t = C_0 e^{-Kt}$). When the natural log of plasma drug concentration versus time curve is not a straight line, a multicompartment model must be constructed to describe the change in concentration over time (Figure 6-1).

Of the multicompartment models, the two-compartment model is most frequently used. This model usually consists of a central compartment of the well-perfused tissues and a peripheral compartment of less well-perfused tissues (such as muscle and fat). Figure 6-2 shows a diagram of the two-compartment model after an intravenous bolus dose, where:

X_0 = dose of drug administered
X_c = amount of drug in central compartment
X_p = amount of drug in peripheral compartment
K_{12} = rate constant for transfer of drug from the central compartment to the peripheral compartment. (The subscript 12 indicates transfer from the first [central] to the second [peripheral] compartment.)
K_{21} = rate constant for transfer of drug from the peripheral compartment to the central compartment. (The subscript 21 indicates transfer from the second [peripheral] to the first [central] compartment. *Note*: Both K_{12} and K_{21} are called *microconstants*.)
K_{10} = first-order elimination rate constant (similar to the K used previously), indicating elimination of drug out of the central compartment into urine, feces, etc.

A natural log of plasma drug concentration versus time curve for a two-compartment model shows a curvilinear profile—a curved portion followed by a straight line. This biexponential curve can be described by two exponential terms (Figure 6-3). The phases of the curve may represent rapid distribution to organs with high blood flow (central compartment) and

FIGURE 6-1.
Concentration (Conc.) versus time plot for one- versus two-compartment (CMPT) model.

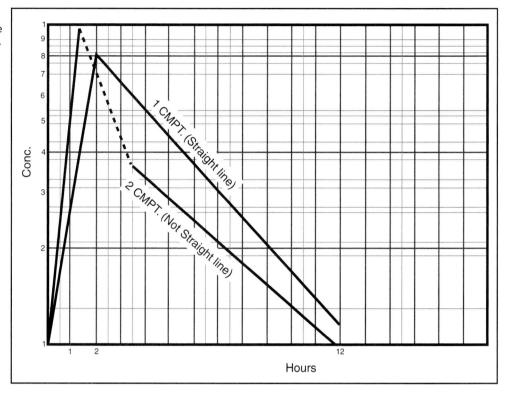

slower distribution to organs with less blood flow (peripheral compartment).

After the intravenous injection of a drug that follows a two-compartment model, the drug concentrations in all fluids and tissues associated with the central compartment decline more rapidly in the distribution phase than during the post-distribution phase. After some time, a pseudoequilibrium is attained between the central compartment and the tissues and fluids of the peripheral compartment; the plasma drug concentration versus time profile is then characterized as a linear process when plotted on semilog paper (i.e., terminal or linear elimination phase). For many drugs, such as aminoglycosides, the distribution phase is very short (e.g., 15–20 minutes). If plasma concentrations are measured after this phase is completed, the central compartment can be ignored and a one-compartment model adequately repre-

sents the plasma concentrations observed. However, for drugs such as vancomycin, the distribution phase lasts 1–4 hours. If plasma concentrations of vancomycin are determined within the first few hours after a dose is given, the nonlinear (multiexponential) decline of vancomycin concentrations must be considered when calculating half-life and other parameters.

▌ CLINICAL CORRELATE

Digoxin is a drug that, when administered as a short intravenous infusion, is best described by a two-compartment model. After the drug is infused, the distribution phase is apparent for 4–6 hours (Figure 6-4). Digoxin distributes extensively into muscle tissue (the peripheral compartment) and out of plasma (the central compartment). After the initial distribution phase, a pseudoequilibrium in distribution is achieved between the central and peripheral compartments. Because the site of digoxin effect is in muscle (specifically, the myocardium), the plasma concentrations observed after completion of the distribution phase more accurately reflect concentrations in the tissue and pharmacodynamic response. For patients receiving digoxin, blood should be drawn for plasma concentration determination after completion of the distribution phase; thus, trough digoxin concentrations

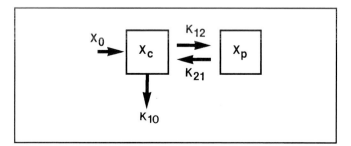

FIGURE 6-2.
Graphic representation of a two-compartment model.

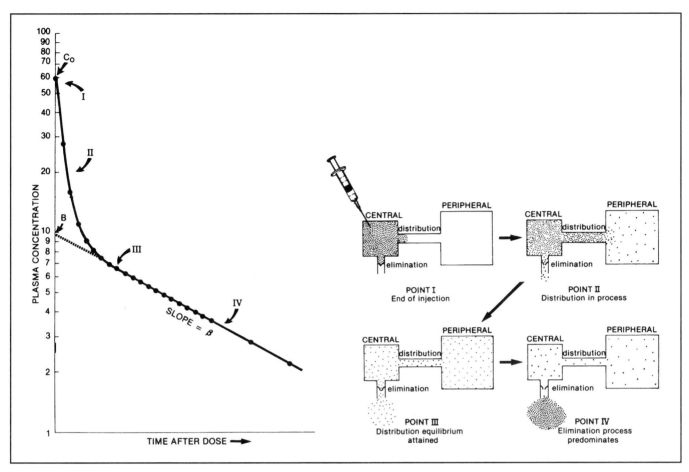

FIGURE 6-3.
Four stages of drug distribution and elimination after rapid intravenous injection. Points I, II, III, and IV (*right*) correspond to the points on the plasma concentration curve (*left*). **Point I:** The injection has just been completed, and drug density in the central compartment is highest. Drug distribution and elimination have just begun. **Point II:** Midway through the distribution process, the drug density in the central compartment is falling rapidly, mainly because of rapid drug distribution out of the central compartment into the peripheral compartment. The density of drug in the peripheral compartment has not yet reached that of the central compartment. **Point III:** Distribution equilibrium has been attained, and drug densities in the central and peripheral compartments are approximately equal. Drug distribution in both directions continues to take place, but the ratio of drug quantities in the central and peripheral compartments remains constant. At this point, the major determinant of drug disappearance from the central compartment becomes the elimination process; previously, drug disappearance was determined mainly by distribution. **Point IV:** During this elimination phase, the drug is being "drained" from both compartments out of the body (via the central compartment) at approximately the same rate. **Source:** Reprinted with permission from Greenblatt DJ and Shrader RI. *Pharmacokinetics in Clinical Practice*. Philadelphia, PA: Saunders; 1985.

are usually used clinically when monitoring digoxin therapy.

Vancomycin is another drug that follows a two-compartment model with an initial 2- to 4-hour α-distribution phase followed by a linear terminal elimination phase. As described later in the vancomycin cases (see Lesson 13) peak vancomycin concentrations must be drawn approximately 2 hours after the **end** of a vancomycin infusion to avoid obtaining a peak concentration during the initial distribution phase (see Figure 13-3).

CALCULATING TWO-COMPARTMENT PARAMETERS

In this section, we apply mathematical principles to the two-compartment model to calculate useful pharmacokinetic parameters.

From discussion of the one-compartment model, we know that the elimination rate constant (K) is estimated from the slope of the natural log of plasma drug concentration versus time curve. However, in a two-compartment model, in which that plot is curvilinear, the slope varies, depending on which portion of the curve is examined (Figure 6-5). The slope of the initial portion is

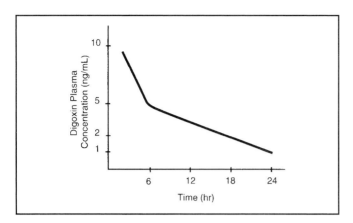

FIGURE 6-4.
Digoxin plasma concentration versus time.

determined primarily by the distribution rate while the slope of the terminal portion is determined primarily by the elimination rate.

The linear (or post-distributive) terminal portion of this curve may be back-extrapolated to time zero (t_0). The negative slope of this line is referred to as *beta* (β), and like K in the one-compartment model, β is an elimination rate constant. β is the terminal elimination rate constant, which means it applies after distribution has reached pseudoequilibrium. The y-intercept of this line (B) is used in various equations for two-compartment parameters.

As in the one-compartment model, a half-life (the beta half-life) can be calculated from β:

$$T\tfrac{1}{2} = \frac{0.693}{\beta} \qquad T\tfrac{1}{2} = \frac{0.693}{K}$$

Throughout the time that drug is present in the body, distribution takes place between the central and peripheral compartments. We can calculate a rate of distribution using the method of residuals, which separates the effects of distribution and elimination. This method

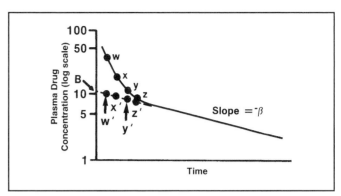

FIGURE 6-6.
Method of residuals.

estimates the effect of distribution on the overall plasma concentration curve and uses the difference between the effect of elimination and the actual plasma concentrations to determine the distribution rate.

To apply the method of residuals, we use the back-extrapolated line used to determine β and B (Figure 6-6). If w, x, y, and z are actual, determined concentration time points, let w', x', y', and z' represent points on the new (extrapolated) line at the same times that the actual concentrations were observed. These newly generated points represent the effect of elimination alone, as if distribution had been instantaneous. Subtraction of the extrapolated points from the corresponding actual points ($w–w'$, $x–x'$, etc.) yields a new set of plasma concentration points for each time point. If we plot these new points, we generate a new line, the residual line (Figure 6-7). The negative slope of the residual line is referred to as *alpha* (α), and α is the distribution rate constant for the two-compartment system. The y-intercept of the residual line is A.

Let's proceed through an example, applying the method of residuals. Draw the plot for the following example on semilog graph paper. A dose of drug is administered by rapid intravenous injection, and the concentrations shown in Table 6-1 result.

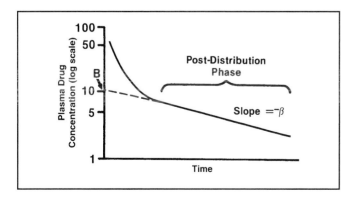

FIGURE 6-5.
Plasma drug concentrations with a two-compartment model after an intravenous bolus dose.

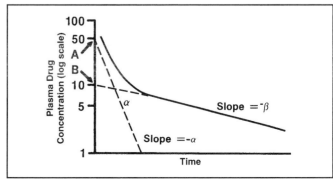

FIGURE 6-7.
Determination of the residual line.

TABLE 6-1.
Plasma Drug Concentrations after Rapid Intravenous Injection

Time after Dose (hours)	Plasma Concentration (mg/L)
0.25	43.0
0.5	32.0
1.0	20.0
1.5	14.0
2.0	11.0
4.0	6.5
8.0	2.8
12.0	1.2
16.0	0.52

TABLE 6-2.
Residual Concentration Points

Time after Dose (hours)	Plasma Concentration (mg/L)		
	Actual	Extrapolated	Residual
0.25	43	14.5	28.5
0.5	32	13.5	18.5
1.0	20	12.3	7.7
1.5	14	11.0	3.0
2.0	11	10.0	1.0

The last four points form a straight line, (similar to Figure 6-5) so back-extrapolate a line that connects them to the *y*-axis. Then, for the first five points, extrapolated values can be estimated at each time (0.25, 0.5, 1.0, 1.5, and 2.0 hours) where the time intersects the new line (similar to Figure 6-6). Subtracting the extrapolated values from the actual plasma concentrations yields a new set of residual concentration points, similar to those values shown in Table 6-2.

Plot the residual concentrations (on the same semilog paper) versus time and draw a straight line connecting all of your new points (similar to Figure 6-7). Determine that the slope of that plot equals –1.8 hours^{-1}.

$$\text{Slope } (\alpha) = \frac{\ln C_1 - \ln C_0}{t_1 - t_0} = \frac{(\ln 3 - \ln 18.5)}{(1.5 \text{ hr} - 0.5 \text{ hr})} = -1.8 \text{ hr}^{-1}$$

(distribution rate)

(See **Equation 3-1.**)

When the negative is dropped, this slope equals α; we observe from the plot that the intercept (*A*) of the residual line is 45 mg/L. We also can estimate β (0.21 hour^{-1}) from the slope of the terminal straight-line portion.

$$\text{Slope } (\beta) = \frac{\ln C_1 - \ln C_0}{t_1 - t_0} = \frac{(\ln 2.8 - \ln 6.5)}{(8 \text{ hr} - 4 \text{ hr})} = -0.21 \text{ hr}^{-1}$$

(elimination rate)

Inspection of the extrapolated portion yields a value for *B* (15 mg/L).

Note that α must be greater than β, indicating that drug removal from plasma by distribution into tissues proceeds at a greater rate than does drug removal from plasma by eliminating organs (e.g., kidneys and liver). The initial portion of the plot is steeper than the terminal portion.

BIEXPONENTIAL EQUATION AND VOLUMES OF DISTRIBUTION

The estimations of *A*, *B*, α, and β performed above are useful for predicting plasma concentrations of drugs characterized by a two-compartment model. For a one-compartment model (Figure 6-8), we know that the plasma concentration (*C*) at any time (*t*) can be described by:

$$C_t = C_0 e^{-Kt} \quad \text{(See **Equation 3-2.**)}$$

where C_0 is the initial concentration and *K* is the elimination rate. The equation is called a *monoexponential equation* because the line is described by one exponent.

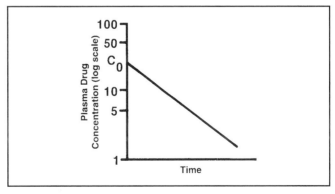

FIGURE 6-8.
Plasma drug concentrations with a one-compartment model after an intravenous bolus dose (first-order elimination).

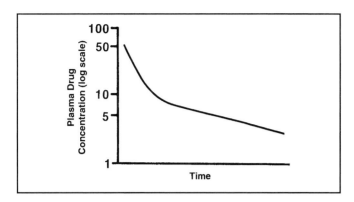

FIGURE 6-9.
Plasma drug concentrations with a two-compartment model after an intravenous bolus dose (first-order elimination).

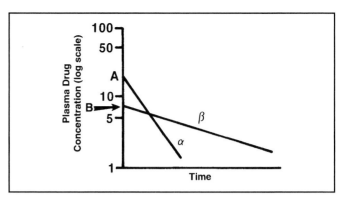

FIGURE 6-10.
Linear components of a two-exponential (two-compartment) model.

The two-compartment model (Figure 6-9) is the sum of two linear components, representing distribution and elimination (Figure 6-10), so we can determine drug concentration (C) at any time (t) by adding those two components. In each case, A or B is used for C_0, and α or β is used for K. Therefore:

$$C_t = Ae^{-\alpha t} + Be^{-\beta t}$$

This equation is called a *biexponential equation* because two exponents are incorporated.

For the two-compartment model, different volume of distribution parameters exist: the central compartment volume (V_c), the volume by area (V_{area}, also known as V_β), and the steady-state volume of distribution (V_{ss}). Each of these volumes relates to different underlying assumptions.

As in the one-compartment model, a volume can be calculated by:

$$V_c = \frac{dose}{A + B} = \frac{dose}{C_0}$$

For the two-compartment model, this volume would be equivalent to the volume of the central compartment (V_c). The V_c relates the amount of drug in the central compartment to the concentration in the central compartment. In the two-compartment model, C_0 is equal to the sum of intercepts A and B.

If another volume (V_{area} or V_β) is determined from the area under the plasma concentration versus time curve and the terminal elimination rate constant (β), this volume is related as follows:

$$V_{area} = V_\beta = \frac{dose}{\beta \times AUC} = \frac{Cl}{\beta}$$

This calculation is affected by changes in clearance (Cl). The V_{area} relates the amount of drug in the body to the

concentration of drug in plasma in the post-absorption and post-distribution phase.

A final volume term is the volume of distribution at steady state (V_{ss}). Although it is not affected by changes in drug elimination or clearance, it is more difficult to calculate. One way to estimate V_{ss} is to use the two-compartment microconstants:

$$V_{ss} = V_c + \frac{K_{12}}{K_{21}} V_c$$

or it may be estimated by:

$$V_{ss} = \frac{dose\left(\dfrac{A}{\alpha^2} + \dfrac{B}{\beta^2}\right)}{\left(\dfrac{A}{\alpha} + \dfrac{B}{\beta}\right)^2}$$

using A, B, α, and β.

Because different methods can be used to calculate the various volumes of distribution of a two-compartment model, you should always specify the method used. When reading a pharmacokinetic study, pay particular attention to the method for calculating the volume of distribution.

◼ CLINICAL CORRELATE

Here is an example of one potential problem when dealing with drugs exhibiting biexponential elimination. If plasma concentrations are determined soon after an intravenous dose is administered (during the distribution phase) and a one-compartment model is assumed, then the patient's drug half-life would be underestimated and β would be overestimated (Figure 6-11). Recall that

$$\text{Slope } (\beta \text{ or } K) = \frac{\ln C_1 - \ln C_0}{t_1 - t_0}$$

A steeper slope equals a faster rate of elimination resulting in a shorter half-life.

If a terminal half-life is being calculated for drugs such as vancomycin, you must be sure that the distribution phase is completed (approximately 3–4 hours after the dose) before drawing plasma levels.

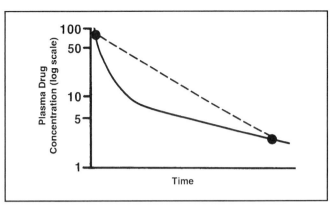

FIGURE 6-11.

Biexponential elimination.

■ Review Questions

6-1. In the two-compartment model, X_p represents the:

    A. amount of drug in the body.

    B. amount of drug in the peripheral compartment.

    C. fraction of the dose distributing to the peripheral compartment.

    D. parenteral drug dose.

6-2. The plasma drug concentration versus time curve for a two-compartment model is represented by what type of curve?

    A. biexponential

    B. monoexponential

6-3. With a two-compartment model, the term "K_{12}" represents the:

    A. first portion of the natural log of plasma drug concentration versus time curve, where the log concentration rapidly declines.

    B. elimination rate constant.

    C. rate constant for drug transfer from compartment 1 (central) to compartment 2 (peripheral).

    D. rate constant for drug transfer from compartment 2 (peripheral) to compartment 1 (central).

6-4. Which of the following is the best definition of beta (β)?

    A. initial rate constant of elimination

    B. terminal half-life

    C. average elimination rate constant

    D. terminal elimination rate constant

6-5. For a two-compartment model, which of the following is the term for the residual y-intercept for the terminal portion of the natural-log plasma-concentration versus time line?

    A. A

    B. B

    C. α (alpha)

    D. β (beta)

6-6. The method of back-extrapolation is used to calculate:

    A. the rate constant of drug elimination from the body.

    B. the area under the plasma-concentration versus time curve.

    C. the amount of drug present in specific organs.

6-7. Which equation below correctly represents the two-compartment model?

    A. $C_t = A + B(e^{-Kt})$

    B. $C_t = Ae^{-\beta t} + Be^{-\alpha t}$

    C. $C_t = Ae^{-\alpha t} + Be^{-\beta t}$

6-8. The equation describing elimination after an intravenous bolus dose of a drug characterized by a two-compartment model requires two exponential terms.

    A. True

    B. False

6-9. A patient is given a 500-mg dose of drug by intravenous injection and the following plasma concentrations result.

Plasma Concentration (mg/L)	Time after Dose (hours)
72.0	0.25
46.0	0.5
33.0	0.75
26.3	1.0
20.0	1.5
16.6	2.0
12.2	3.0
9.9	4.0
5.0	6.0
2.7	8.0
0.82	12.0

Which answer below is the best estimate for α and β (alpha, beta)?

    A. 0.30 hr^{-1}, 3.17 hr^{-1}

    B. 3.17 hr^{-1}, 0.3 hr^{-1}

    C. 2.1 hr^{-1}, 0.6 hr^{-1}

    D. 0.6 hr^{-1}, 2.1 hr^{-1}

Answers

6-1. A, C, D. Incorrect answers

B. CORRECT ANSWER. X represents amount of drug and p represents the peripheral compartment.

6-2. A. CORRECT ANSWER. A two-compartment model is best represented by a biexponential curve.

B. Incorrect answer

6-3. A, B, D. Incorrect answers

C. CORRECT ANSWER. K_{12} represents the rate constant for drug transfer from compartment 1 (central) to compartment 2 (peripheral).

6-4. A, B, C. Incorrect answers

D. CORRECT ANSWER. β (beta) is the terminal elimination rate constant.

6-5. A. CORRECT ANSWER. The y-intercept associated with the residual portion of the curve (which has a slope of $-\alpha$) is A.

B, C, D. Incorrect answers

6-6. A. CORRECT ANSWER. It can be used to calculate rate of drug elimination.

B, C. Incorrect answers

6-7. A, B. Incorrect answers

C. CORRECT ANSWER. The correct equation is: $C_t = Ae^{-\alpha t} + Be^{-\beta t}$

6-8. A. CORRECT ANSWER. One for distribution phase and the other for elimination or post-distribution phase.

B. Incorrect answer

6-9. A. Incorrect answer

B. CORRECT ANSWER. See table below for result (your numbers may vary slightly).

Time (hours)	Actual (mg/L)	−	Extrapolated (mg/L)	=	Residual (mg/L)
0.25	72.0		27.8		44.2
0.5	46.0		25.5		20.5
0.75	33.0		24.8		8.2
1.0	26.3		22.2		4.1
1.5	20.0		18.9		1.1

The slope of the residual line is determined to calculate α. Two residual points are selected, such as 0.25 and 1.0 hour:

$$\text{slope} = \frac{\Delta x}{\Delta y} = \frac{\ln C_2 - \ln C_1}{t_2 - t_1}$$

$$= \frac{\ln 4.1 - \ln 44.2}{1.0\ \text{hr} - 0.25\ \text{hr}}$$

$$= \frac{1.41 - 3.79}{0.75\ \text{hr}}$$

$$= -3.17\ \text{hr}^{-1}$$

$$\alpha = -\text{slope} = 3.17\ \text{hr}^{-1}$$

β can be determined from the slope of the terminal straight-line portion of the plot. For example, the points at 3 and 12 hours may be selected:

$$\text{slope} = \frac{\Delta x}{\Delta y} = \frac{\ln C_2 - \ln C_1}{t_2 - t_1}$$

$$= \frac{\ln 0.82 - \ln 12.2}{12\ \text{hr} - 3\ \text{hr}}$$

$$= \frac{-0.198 - 2.5}{9\ \text{hr}} = \frac{-2.698}{9\ \text{hr}}$$

$$= -0.30\ \text{hr}^{-1}$$

$$\beta = -\text{slope} = 0.30\ \text{hr}^{-1}$$

C, D. Incorrect answers

Discussion Points

D-1.   Describe situations for which it would be better to use a two-compartment model rather than a one-compartment model.

D-2.   What is the minimum number of plasma-concentration data points needed to calculate parameters for a two-compartment model?

Practice Set 2

The following problems are for your review. Definitions of symbols and key equations are provided here:

K = elimination rate constant
C_0 = plasma drug concentration just after a single intravenous injection
e = base for the natural log function = 2.718
τ = dosing interval
K_0 = rate of dose administration (may be expressed as milligrams per hour in the sense of a continuous infusion or as drug dose divided by infusion time for intermittent infusions)
V = volume of distribution
C_{peak} = peak plasma drug concentration at steady state
C_{trough} = trough plasma drug concentration at steady state
t = duration of intravenous infusion

For multiple-dose, intermittent, intravenous bolus injection at steady state:

$$C_{peak} = \frac{X_0}{V}\left(\frac{1}{1-e^{-K\tau}}\right)$$
$$C_{trough} = C_{peak}\,e^{-K\tau}$$

For multiple-dose, intermittent, intravenous infusion:

$$C_{peak} = \frac{K_0}{VK}\left(\frac{1-e^{-Kt}}{1-e^{-K\tau}}\right)$$
$$C_{trough} = C_{peak}\,e^{-K(\tau-t)}$$

For continuous infusion before steady state is reached:

$$C = \frac{K_0}{VK}(1-e^{-Kt})$$

For continuous infusion at steady state:

$$C_{ss} = \frac{K_0}{VK} = \frac{K_0}{Cl_t}$$

The following applies to questions PS2-1 to PS2-6 below: A 60-kg patient is begun on a continuous intravenous infusion of theophylline at 40 mg/hour. Forty-eight hours after beginning the infusion, the plasma concentration is 12 mg/L.

QUESTIONS

PS2-1. If we assume that this concentration is at steady state, what is the theophylline clearance?

   A. 3.3 L/hour

   B. 0.3 L/hour

   C. 33 L/hour

   D. 198 L/hour

PS2-2. If the volume of distribution is estimated to be 30 L, what is the half-life?

   A. 1.7 hours

   B. 6.3 hours

   C. 13.3 hours

   D. 22.1 hours

PS2-3. As we know V and K, what would the plasma concentration be 10 hours after beginning the infusion?

   A. 3.2 mg/L

   B. 4.8 mg/L

   C. 8.1 mg/L

   D. 11.0 mg/L

PS2-4. If the infusion is continued for 3 days and then discontinued, what would the plasma concentration be 12 hours after stopping the infusion?

   A. 1.2 mg/L

   B. 3.2 mg/L

   C. 7.6 mg/L

   D. 8.1 mg/L

PS2-5. If the infusion is continued for 3 days at 40 mg/hour and the steady-state plasma concentration is 12 mg/L, what rate of drug infusion would likely result in a concentration of 18 mg/L?

A. 46 mg/hour

B. 56 mg/hour

C. 60 mg/hour

D. 80 mg/hour

PS2-6. After the increased infusion rate above is begun, how long would it take to reach a plasma concentration of 18 mg/L?

A. 6.3 hours

B. 12.6 hours

C. 18.9 hours

D. 31.5 hours

The following pertains to questions PS2-7 to PS2-10: A 60-kg patient is started on 80 mg of gentamicin every 6 hours given as 1-hour infusions.

PS2-7. If this patient is assumed to have an "average" V of 15 L and a normal half-life of 3 hours, what will be the peak plasma concentration at steady state?

A. 6.3 mg/L

B. 8.9 mg/L

C. 12.2 mg/L

D. 15.4 mg/L

PS2-8. After the fifth dose, a peak plasma concentration (drawn at the end of the infusion) is 5 mg/L and the trough concentration (drawn right before the sixth dose) is 0.9 mg/L. What is the patient's actual gentamicin half-life?

A. 1 hour

B. 2 hours

C. 4 hours

D. 8 hours

PS2-9. What would be the volume of distribution?

A. 7.6 L

B. 10.2 L

C. 15.5 L

D. 22.0 L

PS2-10. For this patient, what dose should be administered to reach a new steady-state peak gentamicin concentration of 8 mg/L?

A. 64 mg

B. 82 mg

C. 95 mg

D. 128 mg

ANSWERS

PS2-1. A. CORRECT ANSWER. $Cl_t = K_0 / C_{ss}$ = 40 mg/hour / 12 mg/L = 3.3 L/hour

B. Incorrect answer. You may have inverted the formula.

C, D. Incorrect answers

PS2-2. A, C, D. Incorrect answers

B. CORRECT ANSWER. First, K can be calculated from the equation $Cl_t = KV$. Rearranged, $K = Cl_t/V$ = 3.3 L/hour / 30 L = 0.11 hr^{-1}. Then $T\frac{1}{2} = 0.693 /K$ = 6.3 hours.

PS2-3. A, B, D. Incorrect answers

C. CORRECT ANSWER. To calculate the plasma concentration with a continuous infusion before steady state is reached, the following equation can be used:

$$C = \frac{K_0}{VK}(1 - e^{-Kt})$$

where t = 10 hr. Then:

$$C = \frac{40 \text{ mg/hr}}{30 \text{ L} \times 0.11 \text{ hr}^{-1}}(1 - e^{-0.11 \text{ hr}^{-1}(10 \text{ hr})})$$

$$= \frac{40 \text{ mg/hr}}{30 \text{ L} \times 0.11 \text{ hr}^{-1}}(0.667)$$

$$= 8.1 \text{ mg/L}$$

PS2-4. A, C, D. Incorrect answers

B. CORRECT ANSWER. If the continuous intravenous infusion is continued for 3 days, steady state would have been reached, so the plasma concentration would be 12 mg/L. When the infusion is stopped, the declining drug concentration can be described just as after an intravenous injection:

$$C_t = C_{ss}e^{-Kt}$$

where:

C_t = plasma concentration after infusion has been stopped for t hour,

C_{ss} = steady-state plasma concentrations from continuous infusion, and K = elimination rate constant.

So, when t = 12 hours:

$$C_{12 \text{ hr}} = (12 \text{ mg/L})(e^{-0.11 \text{ hr}^{-1}(12 \text{ hr})})$$

$$= (12 \text{ mg/L})(0.267)$$

$$= 3.2 \text{ mg/L}$$

PS2-5. A, B, D. Incorrect answers

C. CORRECT ANSWER. The patient's theophylline clearance equals 3.3 L/hour. Then remember that at steady state:

$$C_{ss} = K_0 / Cl_t$$

or, rearranged: $C_{ss} \times Cl_t = K_0$

If the desired C_{ss} equals 18 mg/L, then:

$$k_0 = 18 \text{ mg/L} \times 3.3 \text{ L/hour}$$

$$= 59.4 \text{ mg/hour (round to 60)}$$

or

$$K_{0(new)} = \frac{C_{ss(desired)}}{C_{ss(measured)}} \times K_{0(original)}$$

$$= 18/12 \times 40 = 60 \text{ mg/hour}$$

Note that the above answer could be obtained by a direct proportion from the initial K_0, C, and the new K_0:

$$\frac{K_{0(new)}}{K_{0(initial)}} = \frac{C_{ss(new)}}{C_{ss(initial)}}$$

$$\frac{K_{0(new)}}{40 \text{ mg/hr}} = \frac{18 \text{ mg/L}}{12 \text{ mg/L}}$$

Rearranging gives:

$$K_{0(new)} = \frac{40 \text{ mg/hr} \times 18 \text{ mg/L}}{12 \text{ mg/L}}$$

$$= 60 \text{ mg/hr}$$

PS2-6. A, B, C. Incorrect answers

D. CORRECT ANSWER. Whenever the infusion rate is changed to a new rate (increased or decreased), it will take approximately five half-lives to achieve a new steady state. So it will take 5 × 6.3 hours = 31.5 hours.

PS2-7. A. CORRECT ANSWER. First, recall that the multiple-dose infusion equation should be used:

$$C_{peak} = \frac{K_0(1 - e^{-Kt})}{VK(1 - e^{-K\tau})}$$

where: K_0 = 80 mg/1 hour (because the dose is given over 1 hour). As given, V = 15 L, τ = 6 hours, and $T^{1/2}$ = 3 hours. So:

$$K = \frac{0.693}{3 \text{ hr}} = 0.231 \text{ hr}^{-1}$$

Then:

$$C_{peak} = \frac{(80 \text{ mg/hr})(1 - e^{-0.231 \text{ hr}^{-1}(1 \text{ hr})})}{(15 \text{ L} \times 0.231 \text{ hr}^{-1})(1 - e^{-0.231 \text{ hr}^{-1}(6 \text{ hr})})}$$

$$= \frac{(80 \text{ mg/hr})(0.206)}{(15 \text{ L} \times 0.231 \text{ hr}^{-1})(0.75)}$$

$$= 6.34 \text{ mg/L}$$

B, C, D. Incorrect answers

PS2-8. A, C, D. Incorrect answers

B. CORRECT ANSWER. The half-life can be calculated from the concentrations given. Recall that there are two concentrations on a straight line, where K is the slope of the line. The slope equals the change in the y-axis divided by the change in the x-axis. The time between the end of one infusion and the start of the next is 5 hours. Therefore:

$$K = -\text{slope} = -\frac{\Delta y}{\Delta x}$$

$$= -\frac{(\ln 5 \text{ mg/L} - \ln 0.9 \text{ mg/L})}{0 - 5 \text{ hr}}$$

$$= \frac{-[1.61 - (-0.11)]}{-5 \text{ hr}} = \frac{1.72}{5 \text{ hr}}$$

$$= 0.344 \text{ hr}^{-1}$$

Then:

$$T\tfrac{1}{2} = \frac{0.693}{K} = \frac{0.693}{0.344 \text{ hr}^{-1}} = 2.01 \text{ hr}$$

PS2-9. A, B, D. Incorrect answers

C. CORRECT ANSWER. To calculate V, the multiple-dose infusion equation can be used, where:

$$C_{peak} = \frac{K_0(1 - e^{-Kt})}{VK(1 - e^{-K\tau})}$$

and:

C_{peak} = 5 mg/L

K_0 = 80 mg/hour

K = 0.344 hr^{-1}

t = 1 hour

τ = 6 hours

By substituting, we get:

$$5\,\text{mg/L} = \frac{(80\,\text{mg/hr})(1 - e^{-0.344\,\text{hr}^{-1}(1\,\text{hr})})}{(V \times 0.344\,\text{hr}^{-1})(1 - e^{-0.344\,\text{hr}^{-1}(6\,\text{hr})})}$$

Rearranging gives:

$$V = \frac{(80\,\text{mg/hr})(1 - e^{-0.344\,\text{hr}^{-1}(1\,\text{hr})})}{(5\,\text{mg/L} \times 0.344\,\text{hr}^{-1})(1 - e^{-0.344\,\text{hr}^{-1}(6\,\text{hr})})}$$

$$= \frac{(80\,\text{mg/hr})(0.291)}{(5\,\text{mg/L} \times 0.344\,\text{hr}^{-1})(0.873)}$$

$$= 15.5\,\text{L}$$

PS2-10. A, B, C. Incorrect answers

D. CORRECT ANSWER. To calculate a new dose, we would use the same equation as above but would now include the known V and desired C_{peak} and then solve for K_0:

$$K_0 = \frac{C_{\text{peak}} V K (1 - e^{-K\tau})}{(1 - e^{-Kt})}$$

$$= \frac{(8\,\text{mg/L})(15.5\,\text{L})(0.344\,\text{hr}^{-1})(0.873)}{(0.291)}$$

$$= 128\,\text{mg over 1 hr}$$

So, in practical terms, a 125-mg dose would be infused over 1 hour to attain a peak of approximately 8 mg/L.

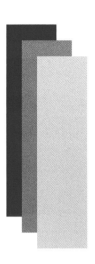

LESSON
7

Biopharmaceutics: Absorption

 OBJECTIVES

After completing Lesson 7, you should be able to:

1. Define and understand the factors that comprise the term *biopharmaceutics.*

2. Describe the effects of the extent and rate of absorption of a drug on plasma concentrations and area under the curve (AUC).

3. Name factors that can affect a drug's oral bioavailability and explain the relationship of bioavailability to drug absorption and AUC.

4. Calculate an *F* factor for a drug given its intravenous (IV) and oral absorption time versus concentration AUCs.

5. Use the oral absorption model to calculate pharmacokinetic parameters.

6. Describe the pharmacokinetic differences and clinical utility of controlled-release products and the several techniques used in formulating controlled-release drugs.

7. Calculate dose and clearance of controlled-release products given plasma concentration, volume of distribution, and elimination rate constant.

INTRODUCTION TO BIOPHARMACEUTICS

The effect of a drug depends not only on the drug's characteristics but also on the nature of the body's systems. The drug enters the body by some route of administration and is subjected to processes such as absorption, distribution, metabolism, and excretion (Figure 7-1).

The concepts used in pharmacokinetics enable us to understand what happens to a drug when it enters the body. Unless a drug is given intravenously or is absorbed cutaneously, it must be absorbed into the systemic circulation to exert its effect. After entering the systemic circulation, the drug is distributed to various tissues and fluids. Plasma and tissue protein binding affect the volume of distribution, transport to and from sites of action or metabolism, and elimination. While the drug is distributing into tissues and producing an effect, the body is working to eliminate the drug and terminate its effect.

A term often used in conjunction with pharmacokinetics is *biopharmaceutics,* which is the study of the relationship between the nature and intensity of a drug's effects and various drug formulations or administration factors. These factors include the drug's chemical nature, inert formulation substances, pharmaceutical processes used to manufacture the dosage form, and routes of administration.

For an orally administered drug, the absorption process depends on the drug dissociating from its dosage form, dissolving in body fluids, and then diffusing across the biologic membrane barriers of the gut wall into the systemic circulation (Figure 7-2). Different drugs or different formulations of the same drug can vary considerably in both the rate and extent of absorption. The extent of absorption depends on the nature of the drug itself (e.g., its solubility and pKa) as well as the physiologic environment (pH, gastrointestinal [GI] motility, and muscle vascularity). Most drugs given orally are not fully absorbed into the systemic circulation. The differ-

FIGURE 7-1.
Disposition of drug in the body.

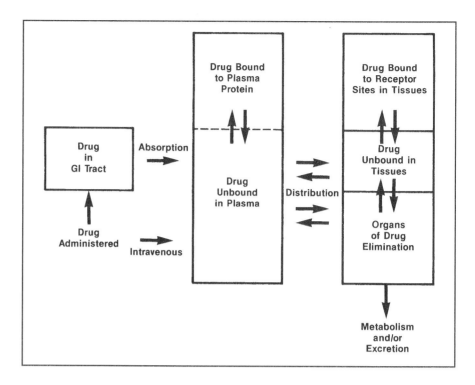

ence in absorption rates of drugs has important therapeutic implications. Assuming that concentration correlates with effect, if one drug is absorbed at a faster rate than another similar drug, the first drug may produce a higher peak concentration, which may lead to a clinical effect sooner than the second drug (Figure 7-3).

When drug absorption is delayed (usually through manipulation of the rate of drug release from the formulation), a prolonged or sustained effect can be produced. For certain drugs (e.g., most oral analgesics and hypnotics), rapid absorption is preferable. For other agents (e.g., antiarrhythmics and bronchodilators), a slower rate of absorption with a stable effect over a longer time may be desirable.

The amount of the drug dose that reaches the systemic circulation determines its bioavailability. Factors that can affect a drug's oral bioavailability include the drug's absorption characteristics, drug metabolism within the intestinal wall, and hepatic first-pass metabolism of a drug. Therefore, overall oral bioavailability can be described by the following equation, which shows the combination of all these factors:

$$F_{oral} = F_{abs} \times F_{gut} \times F_{hepatic}$$

where F is a fraction.

A product with poor bioavailability is not completely absorbed into the systemic circulation or is eliminated by the liver before it reaches the systemic circulation. Differences in bioavailability may be evident between two products (A and B) containing the same drug but

FIGURE 7-2.
Processes involved in drug absorption after oral administration.

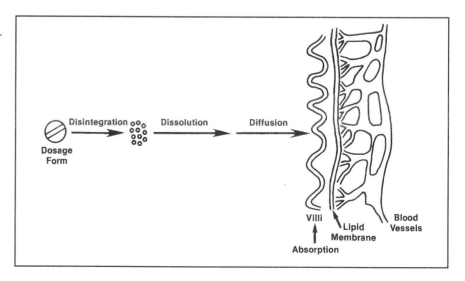

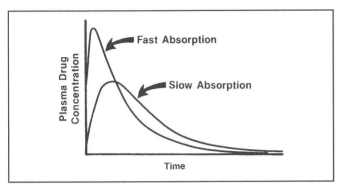

FIGURE 7-3.
Typical effect of absorption rate on plasma drug concentrations.

producing different plasma concentrations (Figure 7-4). Although these products may contain the same amount of drug, their formulations are different (e.g., tablet and capsule). Different formulations may have different absorption characteristics and result in different plasma concentrations. Because product B is not absorbed to the same extent as product A, lower plasma concentrations result for product B.

The AUC of a plasma drug concentration versus time plot reflects the total amount of drug reaching the systemic circulation. Because bioavailability describes the extent of drug eventually reaching the systemic circulation, comparison of the AUCs of various dosage forms of a drug would compare their bioavailabilities.

In Figure 7-4, a drug is given in a similar dose (e.g., 100 mg) in two different oral dosage products (A and B). The AUC for product A is greater than that for product B, indicating that the bioavailability of product A is greater than that of product B. When comparing AUCs to assess bioavailability, we assume that the clearance of drug with each dosage form is the same, so differences in the AUC are directly related to the amount of drug that enters the systemic circulation. For a specific drug, the AUC is determined by the amount of drug that

enters the systemic circulation and its clearance from circulation.

In discussing drug absorption and bioavailability, we should recognize that absorption from the GI tract is not always desirable. For some agents, the intended effects are limited to the lumen of the GI tract, so absorption may be undesirable. Examples would be anthelmintics and antibiotics, such as neomycin, given to decrease gut bacterial counts.

A term used to express bioavailability is F. It is a number less than or equal to 1 that indicates the fraction of drug reaching the systemic circulation. F is often erroneously referred to as the fraction of a drug absorbed—it actually represents the *fraction of a drug that reaches the systemic circulation* and can be affected by not only absorption, but that fraction of drug that escapes both pre-systemic (i.e., intestinal wall) and systemic first-pass metabolism. For instance, for oral formulations of a drug:

$$F = \frac{\text{amount of drug reaching systemic circulation}}{\text{total amount of drug}}$$

Usually, F is determined by comparing the AUC for the oral dosage form with the AUC for IV administration of the same dose. The AUC for IV administration is used because when a drug is given intravenously, it bypasses absorption. The total amount of drug goes into the systemic circulation. A typical value for F is 0.70 for digoxin tablets, and it may be higher for digoxin elixir. This indicates that more of the drug reaches systemic circulation when administered as the elixir. The F term gives no indication how fast a drug is absorbed. Proper studies of drug product bioavailability examine both the rate and extent of absorption.

■ CLINICAL CORRELATE

Absorption of a drug whose bioavailability is low due to a low F factor is erratic and is more likely to be affected by disease-related changes in absorption (e.g., rapid GI transit times, short bowel syndromes).

BIOAVAILABILITY

We next examine a one-compartment model in which the drug is given orally and absorbed from the GI tract. This example would also apply to intramuscular administration as the drug must undergo absorption from the muscle to produce a therapeutic effect. Let us assume that:

- The drug is 100% absorbed ($F = 1$).
- The absorption rate is much greater than the elimination rate.

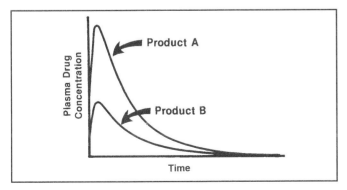

FIGURE 7-4.
Typical effect of different extents of absorption on plasma drug concentrations.

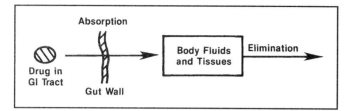

FIGURE 7-5.
First-order elimination.

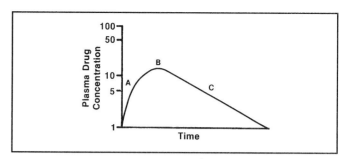

FIGURE 7-7.
Effects of both absorption and elimination on concentration versus time curve.

- Distribution to all tissues and fluids is instantaneous (a one-compartment model).
- The drug follows first-order elimination (Figure 7-5).

Continuous measurement of plasma drug concentrations would probably produce a plot similar to that shown in Figure 7-6 when plotted using semilog graph paper. By knowing F to be 1 in this example and the drug concentrations over time, we can calculate the pharmacokinetic parameters of elimination rate (K), volume of distribution (V), half-life ($T\frac{1}{2}$), and total clearance (Cl_t). In many cases, the actual F is not known, so these parameters can only be calculated in terms of their relationship to F (e.g., Cl_t/F, V/F). But first, let's examine the plot more closely. The initial uphill portion of the graph indicates drug absorption. Of course, elimination of drug also begins as soon as some drug is in the body. But in the initial portion of the curve (A), the rate of drug absorption is greater than the rate of elimination, so there is an increase in the plasma drug concentration (Figure 7-7). As the amount of drug in the GI tract (or in the muscle with intramuscular administration) decreases, the rate of absorption begins to taper off; at point B, the rate of absorption equals the rate of elimination. On the downhill portion of the curve (C), elimination predominates and absorption is nearly complete.

If the drug follows first-order elimination, the terminal portion of the plasma drug concentration versus time curve should theoretically be a straight line on semilog graph paper (Figure 7-8). The slope of the straight-line portion of the curve is related to the elimination rate constant (K). To calculate K or $T\frac{1}{2}$, we use the techniques described previously, but the calculations are made from the terminal portion (straight-line portion) of the curve.

$$\text{slope} = \frac{\ln C_2 - \ln C_1}{t_2 - t_1} = -K$$

(See **Equation 3-1**.)

$$T\frac{1}{2} = \frac{0.693}{K}$$

(See **Equation 3-3**.)

For most drugs, absorption after oral administration is usually nearly complete by 1–2 hours. After that time, plasma concentrations should reflect the effect of elimination. For sustained-release products, however, significant drug absorption can continue for considerably longer than 2 hours.

Let's calculate the volume of distribution after oral or intramuscular administration. This calculation can be performed as follows:

$$V = \frac{\text{amount of drug administered}}{K \times \text{AUC}}$$

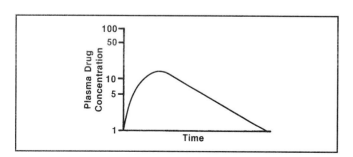

FIGURE 7-6.
Typical plasma drug concentration versus time curve resulting from an oral formulation.

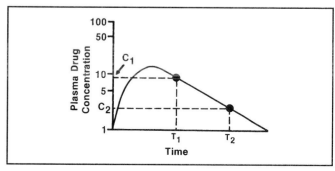

FIGURE 7-8.
Determination of slope (and K) from terminal portion of plasma drug concentration curve.

(assuming $F = 1$), using the trapezoidal rule to calculate the AUC.

Terms in the equation:

$$\frac{mg}{hr^{-1} \times (mg/L) \times hr}$$

can be canceled, leaving us with a unit for volume of distribution—liters. It is referred to as the V_{area}. Once we have the values of volume of distribution (V) and elimination rate constant (K), the total body clearance (Cl_t) can be calculated as follows:

$$Cl_t = V \times K \quad \text{(See Equation 3-4.)}$$

When drug is absorbed from outside the systemic circulation, as with oral and intramuscular doses, the peak plasma drug concentration occurs sometime after time zero rather than at time zero, as with an IV drug injection. The peak plasma concentration occurs at the point where the amount eliminated and the amount absorbed are equal (Figure 7-9).

CLINICAL CORRELATE

When a drug is absorbed more slowly, such as after an intramuscular injection, it will have a smaller peak concentration and a slightly longer duration of action than the IV administration of the same drug. Because of the slower absorption of intramuscularly administered drugs, it will take longer to reach peak concentrations than with IV administration. Consequently, a therapeutic peak concentration may not be attained. To obtain a correct peak concentration time for intramuscularly administered drugs, the measurement must be made in the appropriate time frame. For example, a drug that reaches its peak concentration after 1 hour should not be sampled after 20 minutes; otherwise, a false value will be obtained because absorption is not complete. In addition, because intramuscular absorption occurs more slowly, allowing

significant drug elimination to occur before absorption is complete, peak concentrations after an intramuscular injection can yield a lower value than that seen with IV administration. The time to peak is the time corresponding with that peak concentration. The time required to reach the peak plasma concentration depends on the relative rates of absorption and elimination. A rapidly absorbed drug has a short time to peak concentration.

ORAL ABSORPTION MODEL

The elimination rate constant has been denoted by the symbol K. The absorption rate constant will be represented by K_a. This value indicates the fraction of drug present at the absorption site (usually the GI tract) that is absorbed per unit of time. The usual measurement of K_a is the percentage of drug absorbed per unit of time. If K_a is greater than one in a time unit, almost all the drug would be absorbed over that time interval.

A high K_a (over 1.0 hr^{-1}) indicates rapid absorption. For this explanation, we will assume that first-order absorption or elimination rates do not change with time. Although the rates do not change, the amount of drug absorbed or eliminated changes.

CLINICAL CORRELATE

Some drug absorption rates (K_a) change when large doses of the drug are administered as a single oral dose—the percentage of the total dose absorbed is smaller with a large dose than with a smaller dose of the same drug. Gabapentin (Neurontin), which is actively absorbed via L-amino acid transport system in the gut, is a common example of this absorption phenomenon. Consequently, the daily dose must sometimes be given in divided doses, depending on the total daily dose desired.

With an orally administered drug, K is measured by the slope of the terminal portion of the plasma drug concentration versus time curve, the time when absorption no longer has an appreciable effect (Figure 7-10). In the first part of the curve (the uphill portion), absorption is occurring, but K_a cannot be measured directly because the curve demonstrates the effects of both absorption and elimination.

Elimination processes begin immediately after the drug is given. A steeper uphill portion indicates a K_a much greater than K, but visual inspection does not provide an accurate assessment of K_a.

One way to calculate K_a is to use the method of residuals. This method estimates what the plasma drug con-

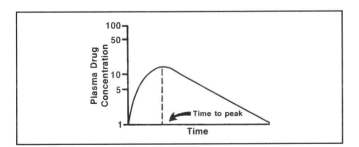

FIGURE 7-9.
Time to peak for oral or intramuscular concentration versus time curve.

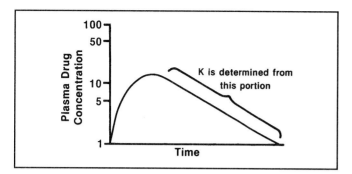

FIGURE 7-10.
Plasma drug concentration versus time for a typical oral formulation.

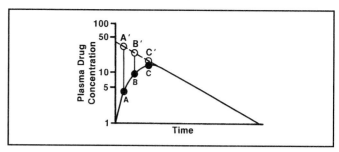

FIGURE 7-12.
Back-extrapolated concentrations.

centration plot would look like if absorption were instantaneous and then uses the difference between the actual and estimated concentrations to determine K_a. We first estimate (by back-extrapolation) the straight-line portion of the curve (Figure 7-11). The extrapolated portion represents the effect of elimination alone—as if absorption had been instantaneous.

Let us suppose that A, B, and C are actual measured concentrations and that A', B', and C' are extrapolated concentrations for the same times (Figure 7-12). Points on the extrapolated line can be determined visually from the graph or with the following equation:

$$C = (y\text{-intercept}) \times e^{-Kt}$$

Subtraction of the actual points on the uphill portion from the corresponding points on the extrapolated line (e.g., $A' - A$, $B' - B$, and $C' - C$) will yield a new set of plasma drug concentrations for each time point. These values can be plotted with the appropriate times, and a line is then drawn that best fits the new points. This new line is called the *residual* (Figure 7-13).

The slope of the line for these new points gives an estimate of the absorption rate. Just as the negative slope of the terminal portion of the plasma concentration curve equals K, the negative slope of the residual line equals K_a.

The technique of residuals attempts to separate the two processes of absorption and elimination. These concepts become important when different dosage forms of a drug are evaluated. They can also be used to evaluate the absorption of different brands of the same drug in the same dosage form. A higher K_a indicates a faster absorption rate. This factor is only one component of such evaluations, but it is often important to know how rapidly a drug is made available to the systemic circulation. An overriding assumption of this technique for calculating K_a is that $K_a >>> K$.

Determination of K and K_a can also be used to predict the resulting plasma drug concentrations after an oral drug dose. If K, K_a, and the intercepts of the back-extrapolated line from the drug elimination phase (B) and the residual line (A) are known, the plasma drug concentration (C), which represents the y-intercept, at any time after a single dose (t) can be calculated:

$$C = Be^{-Kt} - Ae^{-K_a t}$$

Although this equation is similar to the one for a single IV injection in a one-compartment model described previously, it accounts for drug yet to be absorbed ($-Ae^{-K_a t}$).

Plasma drug concentration can also be calculated for any given single dose (X_0) when K and K_a are known and

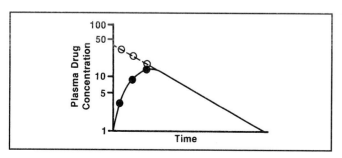

FIGURE 7-11.
Back-extrapolation.

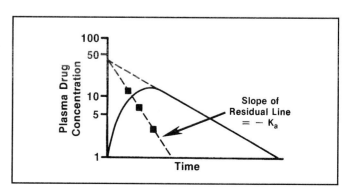

FIGURE 7-13.
Residual line.

estimates of the bioavailability (*F*) and volume of distribution (*V*) are available:

$$C_t = \frac{F\,X_0\,K_a}{V(K_a - K)}(e^{-Kt} - e^{-K_a t})$$

X_0 = amount of drug given orally,
C_t = concentration at time t,
F = bioavailability,
K_a = absorption rate constant,
V = volume of distribution,
t = time after dose has been given,
K = elimination rate constant

Just as with multiple IV doses, multiple oral doses result in increasing drug concentrations until steady state is reached (Figure 7-14). If *K*, K_a, *V*, and *F* are known, the steady-state plasma drug concentration at any time (*t*) after a dose (X_0) is given can also be calculated:

$$C_t = \frac{F\,X_0\,K_a}{V(K_a - K)}\left[\left(\frac{1}{1-e^{-K\tau}}e^{-Kt} - \frac{1}{1-e^{-K_a\tau}}\right)e^{-K_a t}\right]$$

These equations are presented to demonstrate that plasma drug concentrations after oral doses can be predicted, but they are infrequently applied in clinical practice.

CONTROLLED-RELEASE PRODUCTS

In our discussions of drug absorption so far, it was assumed that the drug formulations used were relatively rapidly absorbed from the GI tract into the systemic circulation. In fact, most drugs are absorbed relatively rapidly from the GI tract. With rapid drug absorption, a peak plasma concentration of drug is evident soon after drug administration (often within 1 hour) and plasma concentrations may decline relatively soon after dose administration, particularly with

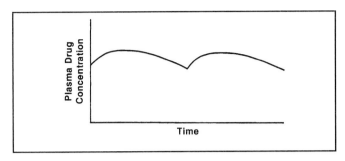

FIGURE 7-15.
Typical plasma drug concentration versus time curve at steady state for a controlled-release oral formulation.

drugs having short elimination half-lives. When drugs are eliminated rapidly from the plasma, a short dosing interval (e.g., every 6 hours) may be required to maintain plasma concentrations within the therapeutic range.

To overcome the problem of frequent dosage administration with drugs having short elimination half-lives, products have been devised that release drug into the GI tract at a controlled rate. These controlled-release products (or sustained-release products) usually allow for less frequent dosage administration. As opposed to the first-order absorption that occurs with most rapidly absorbed oral drug products, some controlled-release drug products approximate zero-order drug absorption. With zero-order absorption, the amount of drug absorbed in a given time remains constant for much of the dosing interval. The result of zero-order absorption is a more consistent plasma concentration (Figure 7-15).

Many types of controlled-release drug products have been produced. Products from different manufacturers (e.g., theophylline products) that contain the same drug entity may have quite different absorption properties, resulting in different plasma concentration versus time curves.

Controlled-release products include enteric-coated products that delay absorption until the drug reaches the small intestine. Enteric-coated products, however, do not necessarily have prolonged action. Other controlled-release products include:

- repeat-action formulations, which release an initial dose of drug and then, at some later time, release a second dose into the GI tract;
- sustained-release formulations, which release an initial drug dose followed by a slower, constant release of drug;
- prolonged-action formulations, which provide a slow but continuous release of drug over an extended time; and
- drugs designed to be released in specific parts of the small or large intestine.

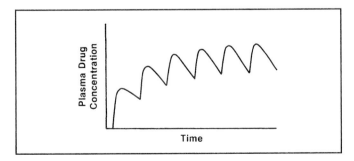

FIGURE 7-14.
Plasma drug concentration versus time for a typical oral formulation given in multiple doses.

TABLE 7-1.
Examples of Controlled-Release Formulations

Drug	Formulation
Potassium chloride	Wax matrix tablet
Theophylline	Coated pellets in tablet
Decongestants	Coated pellets in capsule
Aspirin	Microencapsulation
Nifedipine	Osmotic pump

Controlled-release formulations incorporate various techniques to slow drug absorption. These techniques include the application of coatings that delay absorption, the use of slowly dissolving salts or esters of the parent drug, the use of ion-exchange resins that release drug in either acidic or alkaline environments, and the use of gel, wax, or polymeric matrices. Examples of available drugs in controlled-release formulations are shown in Table 7-1.

A few features of controlled-release products must be considered in therapeutic drug monitoring:

1. When multiple doses of a controlled-release drug product are administered, before reaching steady state, the difference between peak and trough plasma concentrations is not as great as would be evident after multiple doses of rapidly absorbed drug products (Figure 7-16).
2. Because drug may be absorbed for most of a dosing interval, an elimination phase may not be as apparent—that is, the log of plasma drug concentration versus time curve may not be linear for any part of the dosing interval.

Because, with controlled-release formulations, drug may be absorbed continuously from the GI tract over the dosing interval, it is often not possible to calculate a drug's half-life.

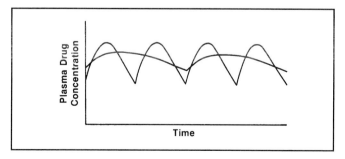

FIGURE 7-16.
Plasma drug concentrations over time with controlled-release and rapid-release products.

Some predictions can be made about plasma drug concentrations with controlled-release preparations. For preparations that result in continued release of small drug doses, the plasma drug concentration can be estimated as follows:

$$\text{average steady-state plasma concentration} = \frac{\text{dose} \times \text{fraction reaching systemic circulation}}{\text{dosing interval} \times \text{clearance}}$$

or:

$$\bar{C} = \frac{X_0 \times F}{\tau \times Cl_t}$$

(See **Equation 4-3**.)
Given this equation, the dose, the amount entering the systemic circulation, dosing interval, and clearance can be used to predict the average steady-state plasma drug concentration. Also, if the average plasma drug concentration is estimated (determined approximately halfway through a dosing interval), drug clearance can be determined using the same formula. Finally, the effect of changing the dose or dosing interval on plasma drug concentration can be estimated.

For example, if it is known from previous regimens that a patient has a theophylline half-life of 7 hours ($K = 0.1$ hr^{-1}) and a volume of distribution of 30 L, what dose of a sustained-release preparation given every 12 hours will be required to achieve an average plasma concentration of 12 mg/L? Assume that the product is 90% absorbed.

First, theophylline clearance must be estimated as follows:

$$Cl_t = K \times V$$
$$= 0.1 \text{ } hr^{-1} \times 30 \text{ L}$$
$$= 3.0 \text{ L/hr}$$

Then the known variables can be applied:

$$\bar{C} = \frac{X_0 \times F}{\tau \times Cl_t}$$

$$12 \text{ mg/L} = \frac{X_0 \times 0.9}{12 \text{ hr} \times 3 \text{ L/hr}}$$

Rearranging gives:

$$X_0 = \frac{3\ \text{L/hr} \times 12\ \text{hr} \times 12\ \text{mg/L}}{0.9}$$

$$= 480\ \text{mg given every 12 hr}$$

$$\text{(may be rounded to 500 mg)}$$

This same equation could be used to estimate drug clearance if a steady-state plasma drug concentration at the midpoint of a dosing interval is known.

Another feature of sustained-release dosage products is that the drug dose is directly related to the area under the plasma drug concentration versus time curve (AUC), just as for rapidly absorbed products. If rapid- and sustained-release products of the same drug are absorbed to the same extent, then the resulting AUC at steady state for a similar time will be equivalent for each product if the same daily dosages are given. For example, if 500 mg of a sustained-release drug product is given every 12 hours and 250 mg of a rapidly absorbed formulation of the same drug is given every 6 hours, the AUC over 12 hours (two dosing intervals for the rapidly absorbed product) should be the same. Again, the assumption is that the bioavailability (F) is the same for each product.

The AUC after administration of a controlled-release dosage formulation is related to drug dosage; the relating factor is drug clearance, as discussed previously:

$$\text{AUC} = \frac{\text{dose} \times F}{\text{clearance}}$$

(See **Equation 3-5**.)

or:

$$\text{clearance} = \frac{\text{dose} \times F}{\text{AUC}}$$

So if the AUC, dose administered, and fraction reaching the systemic circulation are known, drug clearance can be estimated.

The considerations for controlled-release dosage forms will become increasingly important as more drugs are being formulated into preparations that can be administered at convenient intervals (daily or even less frequently).

■ CLINICAL CORRELATE

The importance of the absorption rate depends to some extent on the type of illness being treated. For example, when treating pain it is usually desirable to use an analgesic that is rapidly absorbed (i.e., has a high absorption rate constant) so that drug effect may begin as soon as possible. For chronic diseases, such as hypertension, it is more desirable to have a product that results in a lower absorption rate and more consistent drug absorption over time, so that blood pressure does not change over the dosing interval.

▮ Review Questions

7-1. Absorption of a drug from a tablet form involves dissolution of the solid dosage form into GI fluids and diffusion through body fluids and membranes.

A. True

B. False

7-2. The extent to which a drug is absorbed partially determines its:

A. elimination rate.

B. bioavailability.

C. half-life.

D. volume of distribution.

7-3. Which of the following statements best describes F?

A. rate of absorption of the administered drug into the systemic circulation

B. amount of administered drug that reaches the systemic circulation

C. speed at which the administered drug reaches the systemic circulation

D. fraction of the administered drug that reaches the systemic circulation

7-4. If 500 mg of a drug is given orally and 250 mg is absorbed into the systemic circulation, what is F?

A. 0.6

B. 0.5

C. 3

D. 1.66

7-5. A drug given intravenously results in an AUC of 400 (mg/L) × hour. If the same dose of drug is given orally and the resulting AUC is 300 (mg/L) × hour, what percentage of the oral dose reaches the systemic circulation, and what is the F value?

A 75%, $F = 0.75$

B. 33%, $F = 0.33$

C. 50%, $F = 0.5$

D. 0.5%, $F = 0.005$

7-6. Two generic brands of equal strength of a drug (as a tablet) are given orally. Tablet A results in an AUC of 600 (mg/L) × hour, while Tablet B results in an AUC of 400 (mg/L) × hour. Which product has the better bioavailability?

A. tablet A

B. tablet B

7-7. For Figure 7-7 (p. 90), match the sequence of parts of the plasma concentration curve (i.e., A, B, or C) with the following description sequences: (1) The rate of drug absorption is less than the rate of excretion. (2) The rate of drug excretion is less than the rate of absorption. (3) The rate of drug excretion equals the rate of absorption.

A. A, C, B

B. C, A, B

C. C, B, A

D. A, C, B

Use the following information for questions 7-8 through 7-10: A 500-mg oral dose of drug X is given, and the following plasma concentrations result:

Plasma Concentration (mg/L)	Time after Dose (hours)
0	0
4.0	0.5
7.3	1.0
9.0	1.5
8.4	2.0
4.6	4.0
2.5	6.0

7-8. Calculate the elimination rate constant (K) and the half-life ($T\frac{1}{2}$).

A. $K = 0.30$ hr^{-1}; $T\frac{1}{2} = 2.31$ hours

B. $K = 0.030$ hr^{-1}; $T\frac{1}{2} = 23.1$ hours

C. $K = 0.50$ hr^{-1}; $T\frac{1}{2} = 1.41$ hour

D. $K = 0.20$ hr^{-1}; $T\frac{1}{2} = 3.4$ hours

7-9. Calculate the AUC (from $t = 0 \rightarrow \infty$).

A. 8.33 (mg/L) × hour

B. 32.33 (mg/L) × hour

C. 40.71 (mg/L) × hour

D. 7.1 (mg/L) × hour

7-10. Calculate the V_{area} given the above AUC, K, and dose.

A. 24.5 L

B. 51.5 L

C. 409 L

D. 40.9 L

7-11. If two formulations of the same drug are tested and product A has a faster absorption rate than product B, product A will take a shorter amount of time to reach peak concentration.

A. True

B. False

7-12. Refer to Figure 7-17. The plasma concentrations and times observed for several points are as follows:

Observed Plasma Concentration (mg/L)	Time after Dose (hours)
3.8	0.25
7.3	0.5
9.1	0.75
9.7	1.0

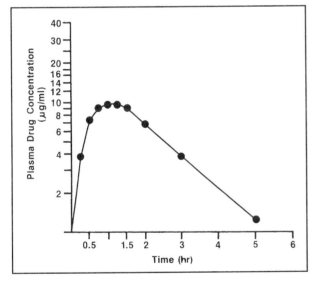

FIGURE 7-17.
Oral absorption plot.

On semilog graph paper, draw the back-extrapolated line from the terminal portion of the curve. Next, using a ruler, draw a line directly upward from the times of 0.25, 0.5, 0.75, and 1.0 hour; then estimate, on the concentration scale (*y*-axis), the concentrations from the extrapolated line at the following times after drug administration: 0.25, 0.5, 0.75, and 1.0 hour. Which choice below represents these extrapolated values from each time point?

A. 16.0, 14.0, 12.0, and 10.0 mg/L

B. 20.4, 18.0, 16.0, and 14.1 mg/L

C. 18.4, 17.0, 15.0, and 13.1 mg/L

D. 18.4, 16.0, 14.0, and 12.1 mg/L

For each of the four times used in the previous question, calculate the corresponding concentrations for the residual line in questions 7-13 through 7-16.

7-13. Time = 0.25 hour

A. 14.6 mg/L

B. 8.7 mg/L

C. 4.9 mg/L

D. 2.4 mg/L

7-14. Time = 0.5 hour

A. 14.6 mg/L

B. 8.7 mg/L

C. 4.9 mg/L

D. 2.4 mg/L

7-15. Time = 0.75 hour

A. 14.6 mg/L

B. 8.7 mg/L

C. 4.9 mg/L

D. 2.4 mg/L

7-16. Time = 1.0 hour

A. 14.6 mg/L

B. 8.7 mg/L

C. 4.9 mg/L

D. 2.4 mg/L

The following applies to questions 7-17 through 7-20 below. You wish to begin a patient on a sustained-release preparation of drug Y and to maintain an average plasma drug concentration of 20 mg/L. From published data, you estimate V and K for this drug to be 10 L and 0.3 hr^{-1} in this patient, respectively.

7-17. If the fraction of drug absorbed is assumed to be 1.0 and the drug is to be given every 12 hours, what dose should be administered?

A. 500 mg

B. 720 mg

C. 2400 mg

D. 360 mg

7-18. After 5 days (assume steady state has been reached), the mid-dose (average) plasma drug concentration is 13 mg/L. What is the patient's actual drug clearance?

A. 780 L

B. 20 L

C. 6.42 L

D. 4.62 L

7-19. What should the new daily dose be to result in an average plasma drug concentration of 25 mg/L?

A. 720 mg

B. 552 mg

C. 1109 mg

D. 2772 mg

7-20. Finally, plot the residual concentration points on graph paper and use the first and last sets of time/concentration pairs to calculate the slope of this line, which also represents K_a.

A. 2.41 hr^{-1}

B. 4.21 hr^{-1}

C. 3.21 hr^{-1}

D. 6.21 hr^{-1}

▪ Answers

7-1. A. CORRECT ANSWER. Drug must disintegrate before dissolution.

B. Incorrect answer

7-2. A. Incorrect answer. Elimination only occurs after drug is absorbed.

B. CORRECT ANSWER

C. Incorrect answer. Half-life is related to elimination rate and occurs only after drug is absorbed.

D. Incorrect answer. Distribution occurs only after drug is absorbed.

7-3. A, B, C. Incorrect answers

D. CORRECT ANSWER

7-4. A, C, D. Incorrect answers

B. CORRECT ANSWER. F = mg absorbed/ total dose, F = 250 mg/500 mg = 0.5.

7-5. A. CORRECT ANSWER. Percentage of dose reaching blood stream = $AUC_{po\ dose}/AUC_{IV\ dose}$, % = (300 mg/L × hour)/400 mg/L × hour) = 75%

B, C, D. Incorrect answers

7-6. A. CORRECT ANSWER

B. Incorrect answer

7-7. A, C, D. Incorrect answers

B. CORRECT ANSWER

7-8. A. CORRECT ANSWER.

$$K = \frac{\ln 8.4\ mg/L\ -\ \ln 2.5\ mg/L}{6\ hr\ -\ 2\ hr}$$

$$= \frac{1.21}{4\ hr} = 0.30\ hr^{-1}$$

$$T\ \tfrac{1}{2} = \frac{0.693}{0.30\ hr^{-1}} = 2.31\ hr$$

B, C, D. Incorrect answers

7-9. A, B, D. Incorrect answers

C. CORRECT ANSWER. Remember that the AUC equals the area under the curve from time zero to 6 hours plus the area under the curve from 6 hours to infinity. The AUC (6 hours to infinity) is obtained by dividing the 6-hour concentration by the elimination rate constant (K) from above.

AUC from 0 to 6 hours is:

$$\frac{0 + 4}{2} \times 0.5 = 1$$

$$\frac{4 + 7.3}{2} \times 0.5 = 2.83$$

$$\frac{7.3 + 9}{2} \times 0.5 = 4.10$$

$$\frac{9 + 8.4}{2} \times 0.5 = 4.35$$

$$\frac{8.4 + 4.6}{2} \times 2 = 13.0$$

$$\frac{4.6 + 2.5}{2} \times 2 = 7.1$$

$$AUC_{0\rightarrow6\ hr} = 1 + 2.83 + 4.10 + 4.35 + 13.0 + 7.1 =$$
$$32.38\ (mg/L) \times\ hr$$

To this value is added $AUC_{6\ hr\rightarrow\infty}$, which is calculated:

$$\frac{C_{6\ hr}}{K} = \frac{2.5\ mg/L}{0.30\ hr^{-1}} = 8.33\ (mg/L) \times\ hr$$

$$AUC_{0\rightarrow\infty} = AUC_{0\rightarrow6\ hr} + AUC_{6\ hr\rightarrow\infty}$$
$$= 32.38 + 8.33\ (mg/L) \times\ hr$$
$$= 40.71\ (mg/L) \times\ hr$$

7-10. A, C. Incorrect answers. Did you use $K = 0.3$ hr^{-1}?

B. Incorrect answer. Did you use AUC = 40.71 (mg/L) × hour?

D. CORRECT ANSWER.

$$V_{area} = \frac{dose}{AUC \times K}$$

$$= \frac{500 \text{ mg}}{40.71 \text{ (mg/L} \times \text{hr)} \times 0.30 \text{ hr}^{-1}} = 40.93 \text{ L}$$

You can see that this value differs considerably from V_{extrap}; V_{area} is usually a better estimate.

7-11. A. CORRECT ANSWER. Drugs that are absorbed more quickly also reach a higher peak concentration.

B. Incorrect answer

7-12. A, B, C. Incorrect answers

D. CORRECT ANSWER. Residual concentration = back-extrapolated concentration minus actual concentration.

7-13. A. CORRECT ANSWER. Residual concentration = back-extrapolated concentration minus actual concentration.

B, C, D. Incorrect answers

7-14. A, C, D. Incorrect answers

B. CORRECT ANSWER. Residual concentration = back-extrapolated concentration minus actual concentration.

7-15. A, B, D. Incorrect answers

C. CORRECT ANSWER. Residual concentration = back-extrapolated concentration minus actual concentration.

7-16. A, B, C. Incorrect answers

D. CORRECT ANSWER. Residual concentration = back-extrapolated concentration minus actual concentration.

7-17. A, C, D. Incorrect answers

B. CORRECT ANSWER.

clearance = VK

$= 0.3 \text{ hr}^{-1} \times 10 \text{ L} = 3.0 \text{ L/hr}$

Then, the equations below can be used to estimate the dose:

$$\bar{C} = \frac{X_0 \times F}{Cl_t \times \tau}$$

$$20 \text{ mg/L} = \frac{X_0 \times 1.0}{3.0 \text{ L/hr} \times 12 \text{ hr}}$$

Rearranging gives:

$$X_0 = \frac{20 \text{ mg/L} \times 3.0 \text{ L/hr} \times 12 \text{ hr}}{1.0} = 720 \text{ mg}$$

(given every 12 hr)

7-18. A, B, C. Incorrect answers

D. CORRECT ANSWER.

We know the following:

τ = 12 hours
X_0 = 720 mg
F = 1.0
$\bar{C}$ = 13 mg/L

And since:

$$\bar{C} = \frac{X_0 \times F}{Cl_t \times \tau}$$

$$13 \text{ mg/L} = \frac{720 \text{ mg} \times 1.0}{Cl_t \times 12 \text{ hr}}$$

Rearranging gives:

$$Cl_t = \frac{720 \text{ mg} \times 1.0}{13 \text{ mg/L} \times 12 \text{ hr}} = 4.62 \text{ L/hr}$$

7-19. A, B, C. Incorrect answers

D. CORRECT ANSWER.

$$\bar{C} = \frac{X_0 \times F}{Cl_t \times \tau}$$

$$25 \text{ mg/L} = \frac{X_0 \times 1.0}{4.62 \text{ L/hr} \times 12 \text{ hr}}$$

Rearranging gives:

$$X_0 = \frac{4.62 \text{ L/hr} \times 12 \text{ hr} \times 25 \text{ mg/L}}{1.0} = 1386 \text{ mg}$$

(given every 12 hr)

7-20. A. CORRECT ANSWER. K_a = –slope = (ln 14.6 – ln 2.4)/(1 hour – 0.25 hour) = 2.41 hr^{-1}.

B, C, D. Incorrect answers

Discussion Points

D-1. Plot (not to scale) the concentration versus time curves for 100 mg of the following four oral formulations of a drug and then rank (from highest to lowest) their relative peak concentrations and AUCs. Describe the effects of variation in these two factors (K_a and F) on the concentration versus time curves.

A. $F = 1$, $K_a = 1$ hr^{-1}

B. $F = 0.7$, $K_a = 1$ hr^{-1}

C. $F = 1$, $K_a = 0.4$ hr^{-1}

D. $F = 0.7$, $K_a = 0.4$ hr^{-1}

D-2. Look up the bioavailability for the three dosage forms of Lanoxin (tablet, elixir, and liquid filled capsule) and then plot representation concentration versus time curves for all three products at the same dose. Discuss all pharmacokinetic differences observed from these plots.

D-3. For the example above (D-2), discuss potential advantages and disadvantages of all three dosage forms. Also, list specific situations in which one dosage form might be preferred or not preferred in a clinical dosing situation.

D-4. Find bioavailability data for at least two different brands of the same drug (brand vs. generic, if possible) and describe the bioavailability comparisons made for each product.

D-5. For the drug products researched in question D-4 above, research the U.S. Food and Drug Administration's bioequivalence statement. Can these drugs be generically substituted and, if so, what data are used to support this claim?

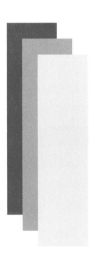

LESSON 8

Drug Distribution and Protein Binding

☑ OBJECTIVES

After completing Lesson 8, you should be able to:

1. Describe the major factors that affect drug distribution.
2. Explain the relative perfusion (i.e., high or low) characteristics of various body compartments (e.g., kidneys, fat tissue, lungs).
3. Describe the three main proteins that bind various drugs.
4. List the major factors that affect drug protein binding.
5. Describe the dynamic processes involved in drug protein binding.
6. Compare perfusion-limited distribution and permeability-limited distribution.
7. Calculate the volume of distribution based on drug protein binding data.

Once a drug begins to be absorbed, it undergoes various transport processes, which deliver it to body areas away from the absorption site. These transport processes are collectively referred to as *drug distribution* and are evidenced by the changing concentrations of drug in various body tissues and fluids.

Information concerning the concentration of a drug in body tissues and fluids is limited to only a few instances in time (i.e., we know the precise plasma drug concentration only at the few times that blood samples are drawn). Usually, we only measure plasma concentrations of drug, recognizing that the drug can be present in many body tissues.

For most drugs, distribution throughout the body occurs mainly by blood flow through organs and tissues. However, many factors can affect distribution, including:

- differing characteristics of body tissues,
- disease states that alter physiology,
- lipid solubility of the drug,

- regional differences in physiologic pH (e.g., stomach and urine), and
- extent of protein binding of the drug.

BODY TISSUE CHARACTERISTICS

To understand the distribution of a drug, the characteristics of different tissues must be considered. Certain organs, such as the heart, lungs, and kidneys, are highly perfused with blood; fat tissue and bone (not the marrow) are much less perfused. Skeletal muscle is intermediate in blood perfusion. The importance of these differences in perfusion is that for most drugs the rate of delivery from the circulation to a particular tissue depends greatly on the blood flow to that tissue. This is called *perfusion-limited distribution*. Perfusion rate limitations occur when the membranes present no barrier to distribution. The rate-limiting step is how quickly the drug gets to the tissue. If the blood flow rate increases, the distribution of the drug to the tissue increases. Therefore, drugs apparently distribute more rapidly to areas with higher blood flow.

Highly perfused organs rapidly attain drug concentrations approaching those in the plasma; less well-perfused tissues take more time to attain such concentrations. Furthermore, certain anatomic barriers inhibit distribution, a concept referred to as *permeability-limited distribution*. This situation occurs for polar drugs diffusing across tightly knit lipoidal membranes. It is also influenced by the oil/water partition coefficient and degree of ionization of a drug. For example, the blood–brain barrier limits the amount of drug entering the central nervous system from the bloodstream. This limitation is especially great for highly ionized drugs and for those with large molecular weights.

After a drug begins to distribute to tissue, the concentration in tissue increases until it reaches an equilibrium at which the amounts of drug entering and leaving the tissue are the same. The drug concentration in a tissue at equilibrium depends on the plasma drug concentration and the **rate** at which drug distributes into that tissue. In highly perfused organs, such as the liver, the distribution rate is relatively high; for most agents, the drug in that tissue rapidly equilibrates with the drug in plasma. For tissues in which the distribution rate is lower (e.g., fat), reaching equilibrium may take much longer (Figure 8-1).

DISEASE STATES AFFECTING DISTRIBUTION

Another major factor affecting drug distribution is the effect of various disease states on body physiology. In several disease states, such as liver, heart , and renal failure, the cardiac output and/or perfusion of blood to various tissues are altered. A decrease in perfusion to the tissues results in a lower rate of distribution and, therefore, a lower drug concentration in the affected tissues relative to the plasma drug concentration. When the tissue that receives poor perfusion is the primary eliminating organ, a lower rate of drug elimination results, which then may cause drug accumulation in the body.

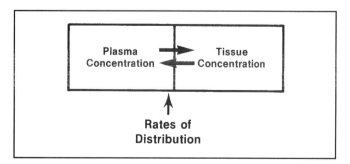

FIGURE 8-1.
Distribution rates.

LIPID SOLUBILITY OF THE DRUG

The extent of drug distribution in tissues also depends on the physiochemical properties of the drug as well as the physiologic functions of the body. A drug that is highly lipid soluble easily penetrates most membrane barriers, which are mainly lipid based, and distributes extensively to fat tissues. Drugs that are very polar and therefore hydrophilic (e.g., aminoglycosides) do not distribute well into fat tissues. This difference becomes important when determining loading dosage requirements of drugs in overweight patients. If total body weight is used to estimate dosage requirements and the drug does not distribute to adipose tissue, the dose can be overestimated.

> ### ■ CLINICAL CORRELATE
>
> In general, volume of distribution is based on ideal body weight for drugs that do not distribute well into adipose tissue and on total body weight for drugs that do. If a drug distributes partially into fat, an adjusted body weight between the patient's actual and ideal body weights is often used. Vancomycin is one notable exception to this rule; the patient's total body weight is usually used to calculate volume of distribution for vancomycin.

REGIONAL DIFFERENCES IN PHYSIOLOGIC pH

Another factor affecting drug distribution is the different physiologic pHs of various areas of the body. The difference in pH can lead to localization of drug in tissues and fluids. A drug that is predominantly in its ionized state at physiologic pH (7.4) does not readily cross membrane barriers and probably has a limited distribution. An example of this phenomenon is excretion of drugs in breast milk. Only un-ionized drug can pass through lipid membrane barriers into breast milk. Alkaline drugs, which would be mostly un-ionized at pH 7.4, pass into breast tissue. Once in breast tissue, the alkaline drugs ionize because breast tissue has an acidic pH; therefore, the drugs become trapped in this tissue. This same phenomenon can occur in the urine.

Due to the nature of biologic membranes, drugs that are un-ionized (uncharged) and have lipophilic (fat-soluble) properties are more likely to cross most membrane barriers. Several drugs (e.g., amphotericin) are formulated in a lipid emulsion to deliver the active drug to its intended site while decreasing toxicity to other tissues.

PHYSIOLOGIC MODEL

It is difficult to conceptualize the effect that the factors discussed above have on the volume of distribution of a drug. Many of these factors can be incorporated into a relatively simple physiologic model. This model describes the critical components that influence a drug's volume of distribution. The equation below represents this physiologic model and provides a conceptual perspective of the volume of distribution:

$$V = V_p + V_t(F_p/F_t)$$

where:
V = volume of distribution,
V_p = plasma volume,
V_t = tissue volume,
F_p = fraction of unbound drug in the plasma, and
F_t = fraction of unbound drug in the tissue.

From this model, it is evident that the volume of distribution is dependent on the volume of the plasma (3–5 L), the volume of the tissue, the fraction of unbound drug in the plasma, and the fraction of unbound drug in the tissue. A drug must have a distribution at least as large as the volume of plasma. The volume of the tissue is much more difficult to estimate. In contrast to plasma protein binding, tissue protein binding cannot be measured directly. Changes in any of these parameters can influence a drug's volume of distribution. We use this equation to help us understand why the volume of distribution of a drug may have changed as a consequence of drug interactions or disease states. Usually, changes in the volume of distribution of a drug can be attributed to alterations in the plasma or tissue protein binding of the drug. This topic is discussed in the next section, Protein Binding.

The clinical consequence of changes in the volume of distribution of a drug in an individual patient is obvious. Because the initial plasma concentration of the drug (C_0) is primarily dependent on the size of the loading dose and the volume of distribution (C_0 = loading dose/V), changes in any of these parameters could significantly alter the C_0 achieved after the administration of a loading dose. Therefore, one must carefully consider the loading dose of a drug for a patient whose volume of distribution is believed to be unusual. Phenytoin can be used to describe changes in the factors determining volume of distribution. For a typical 70-kg person, the volume of distribution for phenytoin is approximately 45 L. Generally, the unbound fraction of drug in plasma is approximately 0.1 (90% bound to albumin). If we assume that the plasma volume is 5 L, the tissue volume is 80 L, and the fraction unbound in tissue is 0.2, we can estimate how changes in plasma unbound fraction affect volume of distribution:

$$V = V_p + V_t(F_p/F_t)$$

$$= 5\ L + 80\ L\ (0.1/0.2)$$

$$= 45\ L$$

If the plasma fraction unbound increases to 0.2, which is possible for patients with hypoalbuminemia, the volume of distribution would change as shown:

$$V = V_p + V_t(F_p/F_t)$$

$$= 5\ L + 80\ L\ (0.2/0.2)$$

$$= 85\ L$$

So, by changing protein binding in the plasma, the volume of distribution has almost doubled.

PROTEIN BINDING

Another factor that influences the distribution of drugs is binding to tissues (nucleic acids, ligands, calcified tissues, and adenosine triphosphatase) or proteins (albumins, globulins, alpha-1-acid glycoprotein, and lipoproteins). It is the unbound or free portion of a drug that diffuses out of plasma. Protein binding in plasma can range from 0 to >99% of the total drug in the plasma and varies with different drugs. The extent of protein binding may depend on the presence of other protein-bound drugs and the concentrations of drug and proteins in the plasma.

The usual percentages of binding to plasma proteins for some commonly used agents are shown in Table 8-1.

Theoretically, drugs bound to plasma proteins are usually not pharmacologically active. To exert an effect, the drug must dissociate from protein (Figure 8-2).

TABLE 8-1.
Protein Binding

Drug	Binding (%)
Ampicillin	18
Chloramphenicol	53
Digoxin	25
Gentamicin	<10
Lidocaine	70
Phenytoin	89
Vancomycin	30

Source: Shargel L, Yu ABC. *Applied Biopharmaceutics and Pharmacokinetics.* 3rd ed. Norwalk, CT: Appleton & Lange; 1993. pp. 594–5.

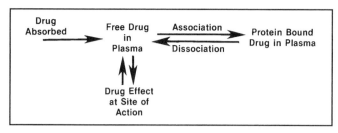

FIGURE 8-2.
Free drug is available to interact with receptor sites and exert effects.

Although only unbound drug distributes freely, drug binding is rapidly reversible (with few exceptions), so some portion is always available as free drug for distribution. The association and dissociation process between the bound and unbound states is very rapid and, we assume, continuous (Figure 8-3).

A drug's protein-binding characteristics depend on its physical and chemical properties. Hydrophobic drugs usually associate with plasma proteins. The binding of a drug to plasma proteins will primarily be a function of the affinity of the protein for the drug. The percentage of protein binding of a drug in plasma can be determined experimentally as follows:

$$\% \text{ protein binding} = \frac{[\text{total}] - [\text{unbound}] \times 100}{[\text{total}]}$$

where [total] is the total plasma drug concentration (unbound drug + bound drug) and [unbound] refers to the unbound or free plasma drug concentration.

Another way of thinking about the relationship between free and total drug concentration in the plasma is to consider the fraction of unbound drug in the plasma (F_p). F_p is determined by the following relationship:

$$F_p = \frac{[\text{unbound}]}{[\text{total}]}$$

Although the protein binding of a drug will be determined by the affinity of the protein for the drug, it will

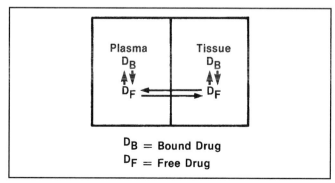

FIGURE 8-3.
Association and dissociation process.

TABLE 8-2.
Plasma Protein Plasma Concentrations

Protein	Normal Concentration	Type of Drugs Bound	Example
Albumin	3.5–4.5 g/L	Anionic, cationic	Phenytoin
Alpha-1-acid glycoprotein	0.4–1.0 g/L	Cationic	Lidocaine
Lipoproteins	Variable	Lipophilic	Cyclosporine

Source: Shargel L, Yu ABC. *Applied Biopharmaceutics and Pharmacokinetics.* 3rd ed. Norwalk, CT: Appleton & Lange; 1993. p. 93.

also be affected by the concentration of the binding protein. Two frequently used methods for determining the percentage of protein binding of a drug are equilibrium dialysis and ultrafiltration.

Three plasma proteins are primarily responsible for the protein binding of most drugs. They are shown in Table 8-2 with their normal plasma concentration ranges.

Although only the unbound portion of drug exerts its pharmacologic effect, most drug assays measure total drug concentration—both bound and unbound drug. Therefore, changes in the binding characteristics of a drug could affect pharmacologic response to the drug. For example, the anticonvulsant and toxic effects of phenytoin are more closely related to the concentration of free drug in plasma than to the concentration of total drug in plasma. In most patients, the free phenytoin concentration is approximately 10% of the total concentration. However, in patients with low serum albumin concentrations, a lower fraction of phenytoin is bound to protein, and the free portion is up to 20% of the total concentration (Table 8-3). With hypoalbuminemia, therefore, a patient with a total phenytoin concentration of 15 mg/L may experience side effects

TABLE 8-3.
Phenytoin Concentration with Regards to Serum Albumin Concentration

Phenytoin	Concentration (mg/L)
Total	15.0
Free (normal)	1.5
Free (hypoalbuminemia)	3.0

TABLE 8-4.
Plasma Concentration Changes

Condition	Albumin	Alpha-1-Acid Glycoprotein
Renal failure	↓	↑
Hepatic cirrhosis	↓	–
Arthritis	–	↑
Surgery	–	↑
Burns	↓	–
Myocardial infarction	–	↑
Stress/trauma	↓	↑
Pregnancy	↓	–

– = no data available; ↓ = decreased; ↑ = increased.
Sources: Shargel L, Yu ABC. *Applied Biopharmaceutics and Pharmacokinetics*. 3rd ed. Norwalk, CT: Appleton & Lange; 1993. p. 93; and Rowland M, Tozer TN. *Clinical Pharmacokinetics: Concepts and Applications*. 2nd ed. Philadelphia, PA: Lea & Febiger; 1989. p. 445.

(nystagmus and ataxia) usually seen at a total concentration of 30 mg/L. In these patients, a lower total phenytoin concentration may control seizures.

The plasma concentration of the two major plasma-binding proteins, albumin and alpha-1-acid glycoprotein, are known to be influenced by various disease states as illustrated in Table 8-4. Albumin is a high-capacity, low-affinity protein. Alpha-1-acid glycoprotein is a low-capacity, high-affinity protein. Obviously, such changes could have a significant impact on the plasma protein binding of many drugs.

■ CLINICAL CORRELATE

For certain drugs that are highly protein bound and have a narrow therapeutic index, it may be useful to obtain an unbound plasma drug concentration rather than a total plasma drug concentration. This will more accurately reflect the true concentration of active drug. An example of this is phenytoin.

The implications of protein binding are not fully understood. Warfarin, salicylates, and phenytoin are highly bound agents. The extent of protein binding does not consistently predict tissue distribution or half-life. In other words, because an agent has a high fraction bound to protein does not mean it achieves poor tissue penetration.

The distribution characteristics of a drug have implications for therapeutic drug monitoring. For drugs whose plasma concentrations are monitored, sites of action are usually recognized. It is important to understand the distribution of an agent from plasma to its site of action.

Protein binding is certainly an important consideration in the interpretation of plasma drug concentration data. However, a considerable amount of intra- and interpatient variability exists in the plasma concentration of binding proteins (albumin and alpha-1-acid glycoprotein) as well as their affinity for a specific drug. A major contributor to this variability is the presence of a disease or altered physiologic state, which can affect the plasma concentration or affinity of the binding protein. For example, albumin concentrations are decreased with hepatic or renal dysfunction, and alpha-1-acid glycoprotein concentrations are increased with myocardial infarction. Renal dysfunction may also decrease the affinity of albumin for phenytoin. In addition, concomitant administration of a displacer drug (i.e., an agent that competes with the drug of interest for common protein binding sites) can alter the protein binding of a drug. Examples of displacer drugs include salicylic acid and valproic acid.

These considerations are important because most plasma drug concentration data available to the clinician are measured as **total** plasma concentration (bound plus unbound). In addition, most of the therapeutic and toxic plasma concentration ranges available in reference texts are expressed in terms of **total** drug concentration. Consequently, proper interpretation of such information can only occur with a thorough knowledge of the drug's plasma protein binding. Free or unbound drug concentration analysis can also be done but often requires equipment and techniques to separate the protein from the plasma sample that is not available in smaller hospitals. Consequently, these requests may be sent to a reference laboratory, which may delay the final report. Free plasma drug concentrations are also much more expensive than the standard total drug concentrations.

Changes in plasma protein binding of drugs can have considerable influence on therapeutic or toxic effects that result from a drug regimen. Provided below are practical considerations regarding plasma protein binding, with examples of specific agents for which these considerations are important to therapeutics.

The following questions should be considered when assessing the clinical importance of protein binding for a given drug:

- Does the drug possess a narrow therapeutic index?
- Is a high fraction of the drug bound to plasma protein?
- Which plasma protein is primarily responsible for binding, and does it account for the majority of the drug's binding variability?

Answers to these questions will help you establish a basis on which to evaluate the clinical significance of changes in plasma protein binding due to drug–drug or drug–disease state interactions.

In addition to having an impact on the interpretation of a drug's steady-state plasma concentration data, changes in plasma and tissue protein binding can have a major influence on clearance and volume of distribution. The remainder of this lesson discusses the effect that changes in a drug's protein binding will have on the apparent volume of distribution of a drug. The ramifications of altered protein binding on drug clearance are discussed in Lesson 9.

The consequence of protein binding changes on volume of drug distribution was implied in this equation shown earlier in this lesson:

$$V = V_p + V_t(F_p/F_t)$$

where:

V = volume of distribution,
V_p = plasma volume,
V_t = tissue volume,
F_p = fraction of unbound drug in the plasma, and
F_t = fraction of unbound drug in the tissue.

How can a drug's volume of distribution be altered by the administration of other drugs, disease, or altered physiologic state? The unbound fraction in the plasma and tissue is dependent on both the quantity (concentration) and quality (affinity) of the binding proteins; therefore, changes in these parameters can alter the volume of distribution. Four examples are briefly discussed to demonstrate the potential consequences of altered protein binding on a drug's volume of distribution.

Example 1.

Plasma Protein Binding Drug Interaction: Effect of Valproic Acid Administration on Volume of Distribution of Phenytoin

Assuming that V_p and V_t are unchanged as a consequence of valproic acid administration, let's consider the effect of valproic acid on the protein binding of phenytoin. Both phenytoin and valproic acid are highly protein bound (approximately 90%) to the same site on the plasma albumin molecule. When these drugs are administered concomitantly, the protein binding of phenytoin is reduced (e.g., from 90% to 80%). This is an example of displacement, or reduction in the protein binding of a drug due to competition from another drug (i.e., the displacer). In this case, valproic acid has a higher affinity for the plasma protein binding site on the albumin molecule and competitively displaces

phenytoin, resulting in a high fraction of unbound phenytoin.

What is the consequence of phenytoin having a higher unbound fraction due to plasma protein binding displacement by valproic acid? The equation above would predict that an increase in the unbound fraction in the plasma would result in an increase in phenytoin's volume of distribution and result in a lower plasma drug concentration:

$$V_p(\leftrightarrow) + V_t(\leftrightarrow)\frac{F_p(\uparrow)}{F_t(\leftrightarrow)} = V(\uparrow)$$

Example 2.

Tissue Binding Drug Interaction: Effect of Quinidine Administration on Volume of Distribution of Digoxin

Assuming that V_p and V_t are unchanged as a result of quinidine administration, let's consider the consequences quinidine may have on the protein binding of digoxin. Digoxin is negligibly bound to plasma proteins (approximately 25%), whereas 70–90% of quinidine is bound to plasma albumin and alpha-1-acid glycoprotein. Digoxin normally has a very large apparent volume of distribution (4–7 L/kg),[1] which suggests extensive tissue distribution. Digoxin is significantly associated with cardiac muscle tissue, as demonstrated by a 70:1 cardiac muscle to plasma digoxin concentration ratio, which explains why its volume of distribution exceeds any normal physiologic space.[2]

When these drugs are administered concomitantly, the tissue binding of digoxin is reduced. This is also an example of displacement but, in this case, quinidine has a higher affinity for the tissue protein binding site and displaces digoxin, resulting in a high unbound fraction in the tissue. What are the consequences of digoxin having a higher unbound fraction in the tissue due to quinidine displacement? The equation listed previously predicts that an increase in the unbound fraction in the tissue would result in a decrease in the volume of distribution of digoxin, thus increasing digoxin's plasma drug concentration:

$$V_p(\leftrightarrow) + V_t(\leftrightarrow)\frac{F_p(\leftrightarrow)}{F_t(\uparrow)} = V(\downarrow)$$

Drug–drug interactions are not the only way a drug's apparent volume of distribution can be altered. We next consider the effect of a disease state (chronic renal failure) on the volume of distribution of phenytoin and digoxin.

Example 3.

Effect of Disease State on Volume of Distribution: Renal Failure and Volume of Distribution of Phenytoin

Assuming that V_p and V_t are unchanged as a consequence of renal failure, let's consider the consequences of this disease state on the protein binding of phenytoin. Phenytoin's plasma protein binding is dependent on both the quantity and quality of albumin. Because chronic renal failure reduces albumin concentrations as well as albumin's affinity for phenytoin, it is not surprising that the plasma protein binding of phenytoin could be reduced from approximately 90% to 80%. What is the consequence of phenytoin's higher unbound fraction (0.2 [renal failure] vs. 0.1 [normal]) due to renal failure? The equation below predicts that an increase in the unbound fraction in the plasma would result in an increase in the volume of distribution of phenytoin, which would increase the concentration of the active unbound phenytoin able to cross the blood–brain barrier. This increase could result in "supratherapeutic" unbound concentrations, even when the total concentration is within normal limits:

$$V_p(\leftrightarrow) + V_t(\leftrightarrow)\frac{F_p(\uparrow)}{F_t(\leftrightarrow)} = V(\uparrow)$$

Example 4.

Effect of Disease State on Volume of Distribution: Renal Failure and Volume of Distribution of Digoxin

Assuming that V_p and V_t are unchanged as a consequence of renal failure, let's consider the consequences of renal failure on the protein binding of digoxin. Because digoxin is negligibly bound to plasma proteins, changes in its concentration should not be of clinical significance. However, renal failure does reduce the cardiac muscle-to-plasma digoxin concentration ratio to 30:1. The mechanism by which renal failure alters the tissue protein binding of digoxin is presently not fully understood. What is the consequence of digoxin's higher unbound fraction in the tissue due to renal failure? The equation below predicts that an increase in the unbound fraction in the tissue would result in a decrease in the volume of distribution of digoxin and may cause an increased plasma digoxin drug concentration:

$$V_p(\leftrightarrow) + V_t(\leftrightarrow)\frac{F_p(\leftrightarrow)}{F_t(\uparrow)} = V(\downarrow)$$

In all these examples, the volume of distribution of the drug in question was altered as a consequence of a drug–drug or drug–disease state interaction. Consequently, the calculation of their loading dose ($X_0 = C_0V$) is influenced by changes in a drug's plasma or tissue protein binding. This must be considered in the development of a patient's drug dosing regimen.

REFERENCES

1. Kelly RA, Smith TW. Pharmacologic treatment of heart failure. In: Hardman JG, Limbird LE, editors. *Goodman & Gilman's: The Pharmacologic Basis of Therapeutics.* 9th ed. New York: McGraw-Hill; 1996. p. 814.
2. Hartel G, Kyllonen K, Merikallio E, et al. Human serum myocardial digoxin. *Clin Pharmacol Ther* 1976;19:153–7.

▌ Review Questions _____

8-1.   Drugs that are very lipid soluble tend to distribute well into body tissues.

   A. True

   B. False

8-2.   Drugs that are predominantly un-ionized at physiologic pH (7.4) have a limited distribution when compared to drugs that are primarily ionized.

   A. True

   B. False

8-3.   Drugs are generally less well distributed to highly perfused tissues (compared with poorly perfused tissues).

   A. True

   B. False

8-4.   Estimate the volume of distribution for a drug when the volume of plasma and tissue are 5 and 20 L, respectively, and the fraction of drug unbound in plasma and tissue are both 0.7.

   A. 18.5 L

   B. 100 L

   C. 30 L

   D. 25 L

8-5.   The portion of drug that is *not* bound to plasma protein is pharmacologically active.

   A. True

   B. False

8-6.   Penetration of drug into tissues is directly related to the extent bound to plasma proteins.

   A. True

   B. False

8-7.   Cationic drugs and weak bases are more likely to bind to:

   A. globulin

   B. alpha-1-acid glycoprotein

   C. lipoprotein

   D. A and C

8-8.   Anionic drugs and weak acids are more likely to bind to:

   A. albumin

   B. globulin

   C. alpha-1-acid glycoprotein

   D. lipoprotein

8-9.   Predict how the volume of distribution (V) would change if the phenytoin unbound fraction in plasma decreased from 90% to 85%. Assume that unbound fraction in tissues (F_t) and volumes of plasma (V_p) and tissues (V_t) are unchanged.

   A. increase

   B. no change

   C. decrease

   D. cannot be predicted with the information provided

8-10.   A new drug has a tissue volume (V_t) of 15 L, an unbound fraction in plasma (F_p) of 5%, and an unbound fraction in tissues (F_t) of 5%. What will be the resulting volume of distribution if the plasma volume (V_p) is reduced from 5 to 4 L?

   A. 13 L

   B. 19 L

   C. 18 L

   D. 5 L

8-11.   How is the volume of distribution (V) of digoxin likely to change if a patient has been taking both digoxin and quinidine and the quinidine is discontinued? Assume that plasma volume (V_p), tissue volume (V_t), and unbound fraction of drug in plasma (F_p) are unchanged.

   A. increase

   B. no change

   C. decrease

   D. cannot be predicted with the information provided.

Answers

8-1. A. CORRECT ANSWER

B. Incorrect answer

8-2. A. Incorrect answer

B. CORRECT ANSWER

8-3. A. Incorrect answer

B. CORRECT ANSWER

8-4. A, B, C. Incorrect answers

D. CORRECT ANSWER.

$$V = V_p + V_t \left(\frac{F_p}{F_t} \right)$$

$$= 5 \, L + 20 \, L \left(\frac{0.7}{0.7} \right) = 25 \, L$$

8-5. A. CORRECT ANSWER

B. Incorrect answer

8-6. A. Incorrect answer

B. CORRECT ANSWER

8-7. A, C, D. Incorrect answers

B. CORRECT ANSWER

8-8. A. CORRECT ANSWER

B, C, D. Incorrect answers

8-9. A, B, D. Incorrect answers

C. CORRECT ANSWER. If fraction bound decreases, then V will also decrease:

$$V = V_p + V_t \left(\frac{F_p}{F_t} \right)$$

If F_p is decreased,

$$V_p(\leftrightarrow) + V_t(\leftrightarrow) \frac{F_p(\downarrow)}{F_t(\leftrightarrow)} = V(\downarrow)$$

8-10. A, C, D. Incorrect answers

B. CORRECT ANSWER. Solve the equation using $V_p = 5$ L, then re-solve using 4 L and compare:

$$V = V_p + V_t \left(\frac{F_p}{F_t} \right)$$

$$= 5 \, L + 15 \, L \left(\frac{0.05}{0.05} \right) = 20 \, L$$

If V_p is decreased to 4 L,

$$V = 4 \, L + 15 \, L \left(\frac{0.05}{0.05} \right) = 19 \, L$$

8-11. A. CORRECT ANSWER. Remember, when quinidine is administered concomitantly with digoxin, quinidine competes with digoxin for tissue binding sites and increases the unbound fraction of digoxin in the tissues (F_t). Therefore, assuming V_p and V_t remain unchanged, the effect of quinidine is shown below:

$$V_p(\leftrightarrow) + V_t(\leftrightarrow) \frac{F_p(\leftrightarrow)}{F_t(\uparrow)} = V(\downarrow)$$

When quinidine is discontinued, the unbound fraction of digoxin in the tissues (F_t) decreases as the tissue binding sites formerly occupied by quinidine become available.

$$V_p(\leftrightarrow) + V_t(\leftrightarrow) \frac{F_p(\leftrightarrow)}{F_t(\downarrow)} = V(\uparrow)$$

Therefore, the volume of distribution will increase.

B, C, D. Incorrect answers

Discussion Points

D-1. Draw representative concentration versus time curves for: (*a*) a drug that diffuses into highly vascularized tissue before equilibrating in all body compartments, and (*b*) a drug that distributes equally well into all body compartments. Describe how these curves differ and discuss potential clinical implications.

D-2. Discuss major physiologic and physiochemical factors that affect a drug's distribution and comment on how these factors can affect the pharmacokinetic variable "apparent volume of distribution."

D-3. Describe how knowledge of a drug's distribution and lipid solubility affect the calculation of a drug's loading dose. Clinically, what type of loading dose adjustments can be made to account for these factors?

D-4. A patient has a total plasma phenytoin concentration of 19 mcg/mL with a serum albumin concentration of only 2.5 g/dL. Estimate this patient's bound and unbound phenytoin concentration.

D-5. In the same patient as described in discussion point D-4, calculate a new total phenytoin concentration that would yield a therapeutic unbound phenytoin concentration.

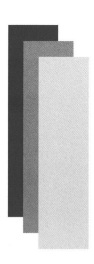

LESSON
9

Drug Elimination Processes

 OBJECTIVES

After completing Lesson 9, you should be able to:

1. Describe the impact of disease and altered physiologic states on the clearance and dosing of drugs.
2. Identify the various routes of drug metabolism and excretion.
3. Explain the two general types (phase I and II) of drug metabolism.
4. Define the methods of hepatic drug metabolism and the approaches used to quantitate and characterize this metabolism.
5. Describe the effects of a drug's hepatic extraction ratio on that drug's removal via the liver's first-pass metabolism.
6. Explain the various processes involved in renal elimination (i.e., filtration, secretion, and reabsorption).
7. Define both the physiologic and mathematical relationship of drug clearance to glomerular filtration.

DRUG ELIMINATION

The liver and kidneys are the two major organs responsible for eliminating drugs from the body. Although both organs share metabolic and excretory functions, the liver is principally responsible for metabolism and the kidneys for elimination. The importance of these organs cannot be overestimated in determining the magnitude and frequency of drug dosing. Additionally, an appreciation of the anatomy and physiology of these organs will provide insight into the impact of disease and altered physiologic states, as well as concomitant drug administration, on the clearance and dosing of drugs.

The physical and chemical properties of a drug are important in determining drug disposition. For example, lipophilic drugs (compared with hydrophilic drugs) tend to be:

• bound to a greater extent to plasma proteins,

• distributed to a greater extent throughout the body, and
• metabolized to a greater extent in the liver.

Hydrophilic drugs, particularly ionized species, tend to have more limited distribution and more rapid elimination (often by renal excretion).

Drug elimination from the body can be very complex. As mentioned previously, drugs undergo biotransformation and/or excretion. Metabolism (also known as *biotransformation*) involves conversion of the administered drug into another substance. Metabolism can result in the formation of either an active or inactive metabolite, which is then eliminated from the body faster than the parent drug.

Two examples of drugs with active metabolites are the antiarrhythmic drugs procainamide and encainide. For both drugs, the metabolites formed are active and may contribute significantly to the patient's pharmacologic response. Consequently, the plasma concentration of an active metabolite must be considered in addition to that of the parent compound when predicting overall pharmacologic response. In this case, the active metabolites formed have a longer half-life than that of the parent compound. In addition, many drugs are actually "pro-drugs," which require activation to their active forms. Examples of pro-drugs include many 3-hydroxy-3-methyl-glutaryl-coenzyme A reductase inhibitors and angiotensin-converting enzyme inhibitors.

Let's next explore two introductory concepts with regard to metabolite pharmacokinetics. Consider the following situation:

$$\text{drug X} \xrightarrow[K_m]{\text{liver}} \text{metabolite Y} \xrightarrow[K_r]{\text{kidney}} \text{excreted Y}$$

where drug X represents the intravenous bolus administration of the compound and K_m and K_r represent the elimination rate constants for hepatic metabolism of drug X and renal excretion of metabolite Y, respectively.

Figure 9-1 shows the decline in plasma concentration of parent drug X (assuming a one-compartment model after intravenous administration). Now consider the profile of metabolite Y after the same dose of drug X (Figure 9-2). If the excretion rate constant of metabolite Y (K_r) is much greater than the elimination rate constant of drug X (K_m), the terminal slope of the natural log of concentration of metabolite Y versus time plot will be K_m and not K_r. This result occurs because the plasma concentration of metabolite Y is determined by the rate of formation from drug X (the slower rate constant).

On the other hand, if K_r is much less than K_m, the terminal slope of the plasma metabolite Y concentration versus time plot will be K_r (Figure 9-3). In this case, the relatively slow renal elimination of metabolite Y determines the resulting plasma concentrations. Although the liver is the major organ of drug biotransformation, the intestines, kidneys, and lungs may also metabolize

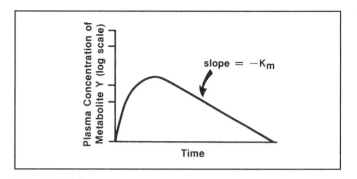

FIGURE 9-2.
Plasma concentrations of metabolite Y (from drug X) when the elimination rate constant (K_r) of metabolite Y is greater than the rate constant for metabolism (K_m) of drug X.

some drugs. Before we can develop the concepts of drug metabolism, we must first examine the anatomy, physiology, and fundamental functions of the liver. The adult liver weighs 1400–1600 g and is uniquely situated between the gastrointestinal (GI) tract and the systemic circulation (Figure 9-4).

The basic functional unit of the liver is the liver lobule (Figure 9-5). The human liver contains approximately 50,000–100,000 such lobules. The liver lobule is constructed around a central vein, which empties into the hepatic veins and the vena cava. Therefore, the hepatic cells (hepatocytes), which are principally responsible for metabolic functions (including drug metabolism), are exposed to portal blood.

The liver (ultimately the liver lobule) receives its blood supply from two separate sources: the portal vein and the hepatic artery. The liver receives approximately 1100 mL/minute of blood from the portal vein and 350 mL/minute of blood from the hepatic artery. Consequently, blood flow in a normal 70-kg adult is approximately 1450 mL/minute.

After entering the liver, blood flows in the veins and arteries of the portal triads, enters the sinusoidal spaces

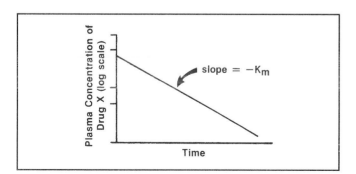

FIGURE 9-1.
Plasma concentration versus time curve for drug X, primarily metabolized by the liver.

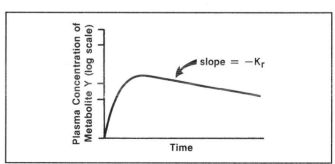

FIGURE 9-3.
Plasma concentrations of metabolite Y (from drug X) when the elimination rate constant (K_r) of metabolite Y is less than the rate constant for metabolism (K_m) of drug X.

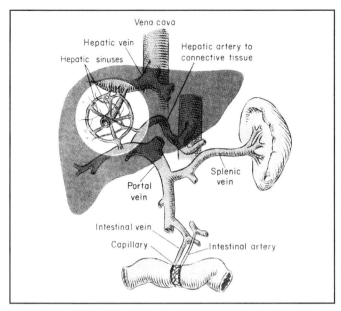

FIGURE 9-4.
Portal and hepatic circulations. **Source:** Reproduced with permission from Guyton AC. *Textbook of Medical Physiology.* 7th ed. Philadelphia, PA: WB Saunders; 1986.

of the liver, and exits via the central hepatic vein. In the sinusoids, the drug is transferred from the blood to the hepatocytes, where it is metabolized or excreted unchanged into the biliary system (Figure 9-6).

The liver is involved in numerous functions, including storage and filtration of blood, secretion and excretion processes, and metabolism. In clinical pharmacokinetics, we are primarily interested in the last role, drug metabo-

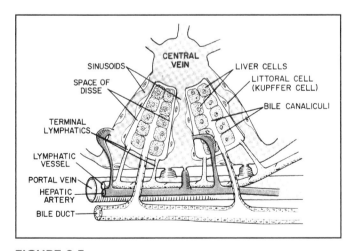

FIGURE 9-5.
Basic structure of a liver lobule showing the hepatic cellular plates, blood vessels, bile-collecting system, and lymph flow system comprised of the spaces of Disse and interlobular lymphatics. **Source:** Reproduced with permission from Guyton AC. *Textbook of Medical Physiology.* 7th ed. Philadelphia, PA: WB Saunders; 1986.

lism, and the factors that influence it. It is generally recognized that wide interpatient and intrapatient variability exists in the biotransformation of most drugs. It is also accepted that changes in liver function may greatly alter the extent of drug elimination from the body. To appreciate the importance of these functions and patient factors in the metabolism of a specific drug, it is necessary to understand the mechanisms involved in hepatic drug metabolism and the relative ability of the liver to extract the particular drug from the blood into the hepatocyte.

Within the liver, hundreds of enzyme systems metabolize drugs. Most of these metabolic processes are classified as either phase I or phase II reactions. Drugs may be subjected to either type of reaction, but commonly drugs undergo phase I reactions followed by phase II reactions. Phase I reactions, called *preparatory reactions*, include oxidations, reductions, and hydrolyses that allow a drug to be processed more readily in phase II reactions.

The major hepatic enzyme system responsible for phase I metabolism is called the *cytochrome P450 enzyme* or *mixed function oxidase system*, which contains many isoenzyme subclasses with varying activity and specificity in phase I drug metabolism processes. Cytochrome P450 isoenzymes are grouped into families according to their genetic similarities. Enzymes with greater than 40% of their genes in common are considered to be from the same family and are designated by an arabic number (i.e., 1, 2, 3), and those enzymes within each family that

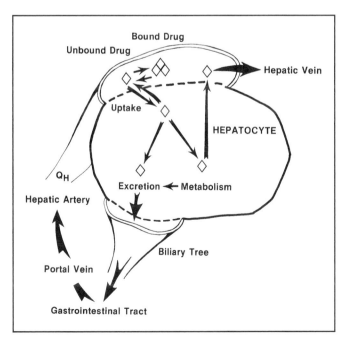

FIGURE 9-6.
Representation of drug metabolism and excretion by the hepatocyte. Q_H = hepatic blood flow.

TABLE 9-1.
Drug-Metabolizing Enzymes and Selected Inhibitors and Inducers

Isozyme	Drug	Inhibitors	Inducers
CYP1A2	Caffeine, tacrine, theophylline, lidocaine, R-warfarin	Cimetidine, ciprofloxacin, erythromycin, tacrine	Omeprazole, smoking
CYP2B6	Cocaine, ifosfamide, cyclophosphamide	Chloramphenicol	Phenobarbital
CYP2C9/10	S-warfarin, phenytoin, tolbutamide, diclofenac, piroxicam	Amiodarone, fluconazole, lovastatin	Rifampin, phenobarbital
CYP2C19	Diazepam, omeprazole, mephenytoin	Fluvoxamine, fluoxetine, omeprazole	Rifampin, phenobarbital
CYP2D6	Codeine, haloperidol, dextromethorphan, tricyclic antidepressants, phenothiazines, metoprolol, propranolol, risperidone, paroxetine, sertraline, venlafaxine	Quinidine, fluoxetine, sertraline, amiodarone, propoxyphene	None known
CYP2E1	Acetaminophen, alcohol	Disulfiram	Isoniazid, alcohol
CYP3A3/4	Nifedipine, verapamil, cyclosporine, carbamazepine, astemizole, tacrolimus, midazolam, alfentanil, diazepam, verapamil, loratadine, ifosfamide, cyclophosphamide	Erythromycin, cimetidine, clarithromycin, fluvoxamine, fluoxetine, ketoconazole, itraconazole, grapefruit juice, metronidazole, ritonavir, indinavir, mibefradil	Rifampin, phenytoin, carbamazepine

contain greater than 55% common genes are given a sub-family designation using a capital letter (i.e., A, B, C). Finally, those enzymes with greater than 97% common genes are further classified with another arabic number and often represent a very specific drug-metabolizing enzyme. The cytochrome P450 enzymes most important in human drug metabolism are CYP1, CYP2, and CYP3. In addition to the action on specific drug substrates, these isoenzymes can also be either induced or inhibited by other drugs, thus increasing or decreasing the plasma concentration of the drug it metabolizes. This can have clinical significance for drugs whose concentration-dependent effects are significantly affected by enzyme inhibition or induction. Table 9-1 lists common drug-metabolizing isoenzymes and the drugs most commonly affected as well as other drugs that can either inhibit or induce the drug's metabolism by this enzyme.

Phase II reactions, also called *synthetic* (or *conjugation*) *reactions*, result in very polar compounds that are easily excreted in the urine. Examples of drugs that undergo phase I or phase II reactions are shown in Table 9-2.

Understanding whether a drug undergoes phase I or phase II biotransformation may be helpful in predicting how it will be affected by a certain disease state. For example, liver disease and the aging process appear to reduce the elimination of drugs that undergo phase I

TABLE 9-2.
Drugs Undergoing Phase I or II Metabolizing Reactions

Phase I Reactions	Examples
Oxidation:	
Hydroxylation	Phenytoin, acetaminophen (also phase II)
Dealkylation	Diazepam, phenacetin
Deamination	Amphetamine
Sulfoxidation	Chlorpromazine
Reduction	Sulfasalazine, chloramphenicol
Hydrolysis	Aspirin, phenacetin

Phase II Reactions	Examples
Glucuronidation	Acetaminophen (also phase I), chloramphenicol
Methylation	Norepinephrine
Acetylation	Procainamide, isoniazid

metabolism more than those dependent on conjugation (phase II) reactions.

BIOTRANSFORMATION

Biotransformation processes are affected by many factors. The functioning of metabolic enzyme systems may be quite different at the extremes of age. Neonates are at risk of toxicity from chloramphenicol because they do not conjugate this drug efficiently. Also, the social habits of a patient may affect drug elimination. Alcohol use and smoking may increase hepatic clearance of some drugs by inducing metabolic enzymes. Obviously, disease states such as cirrhosis and hepatitis and conditions that decrease liver blood flow (e.g., heart failure) significantly affect drug metabolism. Finally, concomitant drug use may affect drug metabolism. Certain drugs, such as phenobarbital, induce hepatic enzymes; others, such as cimetidine, may inhibit them.

Even in healthy individuals, in the absence of hepatic enzyme inducers or inhibitors, the ability to metabolize drugs may vary considerably. For example, investigators have shown that two distinct subpopulations have varying capacities for drug acetylation (phase II reaction). These differences are the result of genetic variations. "Fast acetylators" have a greater rate of elimination for drugs such as isoniazid and hydralazine. For "slow acetylators," the usual doses of these agents may result in excessive plasma concentrations and, therefore, increased drug toxicities.

HEPATIC CLEARANCE

Now let's focus on hepatic drug metabolism and the approaches used to quantitate and characterize this process. Depending on physical and chemical properties, each drug is taken up or extracted by the liver to different degrees. Knowledge of the affinity of a drug for extraction by the liver is important in anticipating the influence of various factors on drug metabolism. Generally, drugs are characterized as possessing a low to high affinity for extraction by the liver. Briefly, drugs with a low hepatic extraction ($< 20\%$) tend to be more available to the systemic circulation and have a low systemic clearance. Drugs with a high hepatic extraction ($> 80\%$) tend to be less available to the systemic circulation and have a high systemic clearance. Drugs with extraction ratios between 20 and 80 are termed *intermediate-extraction drugs*. These points will become more apparent as we develop a mathematical model to relate a drug's hepatic clearance to hepatic physiology.

The efficiency of the liver in removing drug from the bloodstream is referred to as the *extraction ratio* (*E*), the fraction of drug removed during one pass through the liver. The value of *E* theoretically ranges from 0 to 1. With high-extraction drugs, *E* is closer to 1, and with low extraction drugs, *E* is closer to zero. The reader may wish to refer back to the discussion of *E* in Lesson 2.

In Lesson 1, we learned that the concentration of drug in the body was dependent on the dose of the drug administered and the volume into which the agent distributed. This was represented by the equation:

$$C = \frac{X}{V}$$

(See **Equation 1-1**.)

In Lesson 2, we further discovered that steady-state plasma drug concentrations are affected by several variables, including the rate at which a drug is administered and the drug's clearance. This relationship is demonstrated in the following equation:

$$C_{ss} = \frac{K_0}{Cl_t}$$

where Cl_t represents the total body clearance of the drug, K_0 is the drug infusion rate, and C_{ss} is the steady-state plasma drug concentration.

The factors that determine the extraction ratio and its relationship to overall hepatic clearance can be shown mathematically as:

$$E = \frac{Cl_i}{Q_h + Cl_i}$$

(See **Equation 2-2**.)

where Cl_i = intrinsic clearance and Q_h = hepatic blood flow.

Because $Cl_h = Q_h \times E$, then:

$$Cl_h = \frac{Q_h \times Cl_i}{Q_h + Cl_i}$$

The systemic clearance of a drug relates dosing rate to a steady-state plasma drug concentration. The systemic clearance of a drug equals the hepatic clearance when the liver is the sole organ responsible for elimination. Another way of looking at this relationship is to remember that clearance terms are additive. Therefore:

$$Cl_t = Cl_h + Cl_r + Cl_{other\ organs} \quad \text{(See Equation 2-1.)}$$

and Cl_t is equal to Cl_h when Cl_r and $Cl_{other\ organs}$ are minimal.

For a drug that is totally dependent on the liver for its elimination, a number of useful mathematical models show critical relationships between systemic drug clearance and various physiologic functions. These models consider three factors:

- the liver's innate ability to remove unbound drug from plasma irreversibly,
- the fraction of drug unbound in the blood, and
- hepatic blood flow.

One practical and useful model is called the *jar, venous equilibrium*, or *well-stirred model*:

$$Cl_h = \frac{Q_h F_p Cl_i}{Q_h + F_p Cl_i}$$

where:

 Cl_h = hepatic drug clearance,
 F_p = fraction of free drug in plasma,
 Cl_i = intrinsic clearance, and
 Q_h = hepatic blood flow.

Recall that Cl_h equals Cl_t for drugs eliminated only by the liver. Therefore, changes in any of the parameters defined in the previous equation will have a considerable impact on Cl_t and, consequently, the steady-state drug plasma concentration produced by a given dosing regimen. In a normal 70-kg individual, Q_h (portal vein plus hepatic artery blood flows) should approach 1500 mL/minute. Obviously, changes in Q_h would change the rate of drug delivery to the liver and impact Cl_h. However, the magnitude of that impact would depend on the liver's ability to extract the drug. F_p is incorporated into the relationship because only free or unbound drug is available to be metabolized by the hepatocytes. Finally, intrinsic clearance (Cl_i) represents the liver's innate ability to clear unbound drug from intracellular water via metabolism or biliary excretion. Changes in Cl_i should have a profound effect on hepatic clearance. However, as with Q_h, the extent and magnitude of such an effect would depend on the extraction characteristics of the drug.

Examination of the equation for the venous equilibrium model at the extremes of intrinsic clearance values provides insight into the influences of hepatic blood flow and intrinsic clearance on drug dosing. For high intrinsic clearance drugs, Cl_i is much greater than Q_h; Q_h becomes insignificant when compared to Cl_i. Hepatic clearance of drugs with high extraction ratios (>0.8) is dependent on hepatic blood flow only. It is not influenced by protein binding or enzymes.

Therefore, when Cl_i is large, Cl_h equals Q_h, or hepatic clearance equals hepatic blood flow. Hepatic clearance is essentially a reflection of the delivery rate (Q_h) of the drug to the liver; changes in blood flow will produce similar changes in clearance. Consequently, after intravenous administration, the hepatic clearance of highly extracted compounds (e.g., lidocaine and propranolol) is principally dependent on liver blood flow and independent of both free fraction and intrinsic clearance. This particular commonly used model is best applied to intravenously administered drugs, as orally absorbed drugs with high extraction ratios may act more like low-extraction drugs. Other models may work better in these cases.

For low intrinsic clearance drugs, Q_h is much greater than Cl_i. Therefore, the hepatic clearance of compounds with a low extraction ratio (e.g., phenytoin and theophylline) is virtually independent of hepatic blood flow. Hepatic clearance for these drugs becomes a reflection of the drug's intrinsic clearance and the free fraction of drug in the plasma.

Some examples of individual intrinsic clearances are given in Table 9-3. However, there is no clear-cut division between the classes described; additional factors may need to be considered when predicting drug disposition.

TABLE 9-3.
High-, Intermediate-, and Low-Extraction Drugs

High Intrinsic Clearance ($Cl_i \gg Q_h$)	Intermediate Intrinsic Clearance	Low Intrinsic Clearance ($Cl_i \ll Q_h$)
Propranolol	Aspirin	Warfarin
Lidocaine	Quinidine	Phenytoin
Propoxyphene	Desipramine	Isoniazid
Morphine		Tolbutamide
Meperidine		Diazepam
Nitroglycerin		Phenylbutazone
Isoproterenol		Antipyrine
Pentazocine		Chloramphenicol
Verapamil		Erythromycin
		Phenobarbital
		Procainamide
		Theophylline

Source: Rogge MC, Solomon WR, Sedman AJ, et al. The theophylline–enoxacin interaction: II. Changes in the disposition of theophylline and its metabolites during intermittent administration of enoxacin. *Clin Pharmacol Ther* 1989;46:420–8.

▉ CLINICAL CORRELATE

If the liver's ability to metabolize a drug is increased, possibly due to enzyme induction, then the extraction ratio (E) is also increased. However, the magnitude of change in E depends on the initial value of the intrinsic clearance of the drug.

If Cl_i is small (low intrinsic clearance drug), then E is initially small. Increasing Cl_i causes an almost proportional increase in extraction and hepatic clearance. However, if Cl_i and E are already high, a further increase in intrinsic clearance does not greatly affect the extraction ratio or hepatic drug clearance.

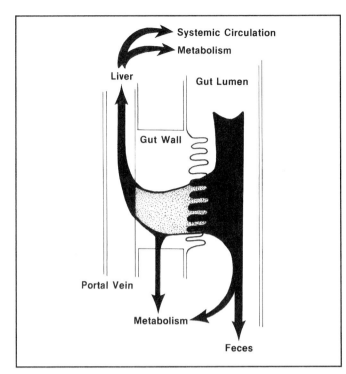

FIGURE 9-7.
Routes of drug disposition with GI drug administration.

FIRST-PASS EFFECT

An important characteristic of drugs having a high extraction ratio (e.g., propranolol) is that, with oral administration, a significant amount of drug is metabolized before reaching the systemic circulation (Figure 9-7). Drug removal by the liver after absorption is called the *first-pass effect*. The result can be that the amount of drug reaching the systemic circulation is considerably less than the dose given.

The first-pass effect becomes obvious when we examine comparable intravenous and oral doses of a drug with a high extraction ratio. For propranolol, plasma concentrations achieved after oral doses of 40–80 mg are equivalent to those achieved after intravenous doses of 1–2 mg. The difference in required dosage is not explained by low oral absorption but by liver first-pass metabolism. Anatomically, the liver receives the blood supply from the GI tract via the portal vein before its entrance into the general circulation via the hepatic vein. Therefore, the liver can metabolize or extract a certain portion of the drug before it reaches the systemic circulation. Also, enzymes in the gut wall can metabolize the drug before it reaches the liver.

Because the blood supply draining the GI tract passes through the liver first, the fraction of an oral dose (F) that reaches the general circulation (assuming the dose is 100% absorbed across the gut wall) is given by:

$$F = 1 - E$$

Remember, E is the extraction ratio that indicates the efficiency of the organ eliminating a drug. For example, if the drug is 100% absorbed across the gut wall and the liver extracts 70% before it reaches the systemic circulation, 30% of the dose finally reaches the bloodstream. Therefore:

$$E = 0.7$$
$$F = 1 - E$$
$$= 0.3$$

Again, F is the fraction of drug reaching the systemic circulation.

EFFECTS OF DISEASE STATES AND DRUG INTERACTIONS ON HEPATICALLY METABOLIZED DRUGS

It is important to appreciate the effect that a potential drug or disease state interaction may have on the pharmacologic response of a drug that is principally eliminated by the liver. Therefore, we will consider the potential impact that changes in Q_h, F_p, and Cl_i will have on the steady-state concentration of both total and free drug concentration. Remember, we will assume that Cl_t (total body clearance) equals Cl_h (hepatic clearance) and that steady-state free drug concentration is the major determinant of pharmacologic response.

When trying to assess clinical implications, always consider the following:

- route of administration (intravenous vs. oral),
- extraction ratio (high [>0.8] vs. low [<0.2]), and
- protein binding (high [>80%] vs. low [<50%]).

$$Cl_h = \frac{Q_h F_p Cl_i}{Q_h + F_p Cl_i}$$

and

$$C_{ss(total)} = \frac{K_0}{Cl_t} \text{ or } \frac{K_0}{Cl_h}$$

Then, substituting for $C_{ss(total)}$

$$C_{ss(free)} = F_p \times C_{ss(total)} = F_p \times \frac{K_0}{Cl_h}$$

where:
Cl_h = hepatic drug clearance,
F_p = fraction of drug unbound in plasma, and
K_0 = the drug infusion rate.

In the following three examples, we apply the previously described hepatic extraction equation to several cases involving a specific disease state effect or drug interaction.

Example 1.

Effect of Addition of Enzyme Inhibitor on Pharmacologic Response of Theophylline

Theophylline (which is metabolized primarily by CYP1A2 of the hepatic cytochrome P450 mixed function oxidase system) was administered to a patient via a constant intravenous infusion and produced a steady-state total plasma concentration of 15 mg/L (therapeutic range, 5–15 mg/L). Cimetidine, a known inhibitor of the hepatic cytochrome P450 enzyme system, was later added to this patient's drug dosing regimen. Assuming that cimetidine reduces the intrinsic clearance of theophylline by 50%, what impact should cimetidine administration have on this patient's pharmacologic response?

Considerations
- Theophylline (in this example) is administered via a constant intravenous infusion (K_0).
- Theophylline has a low extraction ratio.
- Theophylline possesses low protein binding.

Because theophylline has a low extraction ratio and is not extensively bound to proteins,

$$Cl_h = F_p \times Cl_i.$$

And

$$C_{ss(total)} = \frac{K_0}{Cl_h} \text{ or } \frac{K_0}{F_p Cl_i}$$

Then substituting for $C_{ss(total)}$

$$C_{ss(free)} = F_p \times C_{ss(total)} = F_p \times \frac{K_0}{F_p Cl_i} = \frac{K_0}{Cl_i}$$

Impact on $C_{ss(total)}$
Because K_0 and F_p are unchanged and Cl_i is reduced by 50%, $C_{ss(total)}$ should double.

Impact on $C_{ss(free)}$
Because K_0 is unchanged and Cl_i is reduced by 50%, $C_{ss(free)}$ should double.

Consequence
You should anticipate significant side effects as a consequence of a higher free steady-state concentration of theophylline (Figure 9-8). The dosing rate of theophylline should be reduced by 50% in this example.

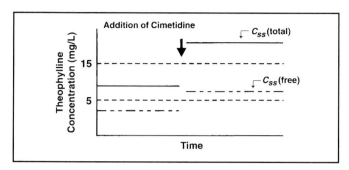

FIGURE 9-8.
Changes in free and total steady-state plasma theophylline concentrations with the addition of cimetidine.

Enoxacin is another enzyme inhibitor that reduces the clearance of theophylline. Figure 9-9 demonstrates changes in plasma theophylline concentrations when enoxacin is begun and then later discontinued.[1]

Example 2.

Effect of Decreased Protein Binding of Phenytoin Due to Renal Failure

Phenytoin (which is metabolized primarily by CYP2C9/10 of the hepatic cytochrome P450 mixed

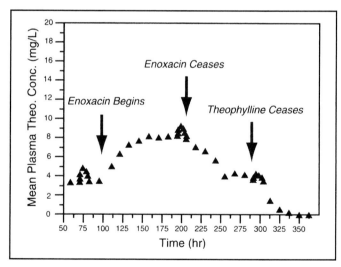

FIGURE 9-9.
Mean plasma theophylline concentration-time profile. The time period shown (60–360 hours) includes each of the three steady-state periods. Theophylline (Theo.) was administered as a Theo-Dur tablet, 150 mg, every 12 hours through 300 hours. Short-term rises in plasma theophylline concentrations (Conc.; 72–84, 192–204, and 288–300 hours) occurred during periods of frequent blood sampling after theophylline administration. **Source:** Reproduced with permission from Rogge MC, Solomon WR, Sedman AJ, et al. The theophylline–enoxacin interaction: II. Changes in the disposition of theophylline and its metabolites during intermittent administration of enoxacin. *Clin Pharmacol Ther* 1989;46:420–8.

function oxidase system) was administered to a patient by intermittent intravenous administration and produced a steady-state total plasma concentration of 15 mg/L (therapeutic range: 10–20 mg/L). The patient unexpectedly experienced acute renal failure. Renal failure is known to reduce the plasma protein binding of phenytoin from approximately 90% to about 80% but has minimal effect on phenytoin's intrinsic clearance. What impact should renal failure have on this patient's pharmacologic response?

Considerations
- Phenytoin is administered by intermittent intravenous administration.
- Phenytoin has a low extraction ratio.
- Phenytoin possesses high protein binding.
- Because phenytoin has a low extraction ratio and is extensively bound to proteins, $Cl_h = F_p \times Cl_i$

$$C_{ss(total)} = \frac{K_0}{Cl_h} \text{ or } \frac{K_0}{F_p Cl_i}$$

Substituting for $C_{ss(total)}$

$$C_{ss(free)} = F_p \times C_{ss(total)} = F_p \times \frac{K_0}{F_p Cl_i} = \frac{K_0}{Cl_i}$$

Impact on $C_{ss(total)}$
Because K_0 and Cl_i are unchanged and F_p is doubled, $C_{ss(total)}$ should decrease by half.

Impact on $C_{ss(free)}$
Because K_0 and Cl_i are unchanged, $C_{ss(free)}$ should remain unchanged.

Consequence
You should anticipate no significant change in this patient's pharmacologic response (despite a significant drop in phenytoin's steady-state total concentration) because steady-state free drug concentrations remain unchanged (Figure 9-10). However, the total concentration necessary to achieve this therapeutic unbound concentration will be less than the normal reference range for phenytoin.

Example 3.

Effects of Increased Protein Binding of Lidocaine Due to Myocardial Infarction
Lidocaine (which is metabolized primarily by CYP1A2 of the hepatic cytochrome P450 mixed

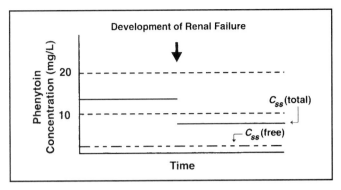

FIGURE 9-10.
Change in total steady-state plasma phenytoin concentration due to renal failure.

function oxidase system) was administered to a patient for a life-threatening ventricular arrhythmia via a constant intravenous infusion, producing a steady-state total plasma concentration of 4 mg/L (therapeutic range: 2–6 mg/L). The next day, the patient had a myocardial infarction. Myocardial infarctions are known to significantly increase the concentration of alpha-1-acid glycoprotein (a serum globulin) and the protein binding of drugs associated with it. The protein binding of lidocaine is known to be high and primarily dependent on alpha-1-acid glycoprotein. What impact should a myocardial infarction have on this patient's pharmacologic response (assuming that the myocardial infarction had no effect on hepatic blood flow)?

Considerations
- Lidocaine is administered via a constant intravenous infusion.
- Lidocaine has a high extraction ratio.
- Lidocaine possesses high protein binding to alpha-1-acid glycoprotein.

Because lidocaine has a high extraction ratio and binds extensively to alpha-1-acid glycoprotein, $Cl_h = Q_h$.

$$C_{ss(total)} = \frac{K_0}{Cl_h} \text{ or } \frac{K_0}{Q_h}$$

Substituting for $C_{ss(total)}$

$$C_{ss(free)} = F_p \times C_{ss(total)} = F_p \times \frac{K_0}{Q_h}$$

Impact on $C_{ss(total)}$
Because K_0 and Q_h are unchanged, $C_{ss(total)}$ should remain unchanged.

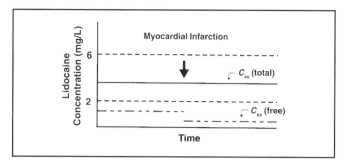

FIGURE 9-11.
Change in free steady-state plasma lidocaine concentrations due to myocardial infarction.

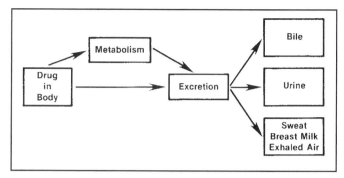

FIGURE 9-12.
Drug elimination.

Impact on $C_{ss(free)}$

Because K_0 and Q_h are unchanged and F_p is decreased, $C_{ss(free)}$ should decrease, which could result in a reduced pharmacologic response (Figure 9-11).

Consequence

Because only total (bound and unbound) lidocaine concentrations can be measured clinically, you should anticipate a reduced pharmacologic response despite similar steady-state total lidocaine concentrations. This reduced response may necessitate high total lidocaine concentrations and a higher dose to achieve the desired response.

■ CLINICAL CORRELATE

This reduced response is why lidocaine's dose is generally titrated to a clinical response based on electrocardiogram readings (i.e., decrease in arrhythmias) rather than dosed to a therapeutic concentration.

These three examples represent how the well-stirred model and knowledge of the pharmacokinetic characteristics of a drug can be used to predict the effect of changes in hepatic blood flow, protein binding, and intrinsic clearance. These same principles can be used to assess a wide variety of clinically relevant situations.

RENAL ELIMINATION

As stated previously, *drug elimination* refers to metabolism and excretion (Figure 9-12). Some drugs are primarily excreted unchanged; others are extensively metabolized before excretion. The fraction of drug metabolized is different for various agents. The overall elimination rate is the sum of all metabolism and excretion processes and is referred to as *total body elimination*:

total body elimination = drug excreted unchanged
+ drug metabolized

Excretion is the process that removes a drug from tissues and the circulation. A drug can be excreted through urine, bile, sweat, expired air, breast milk, or seminal fluid. The most important routes of excretion for many drugs and their metabolites are the urine and bile. For anesthetic gases, pulmonary excretion can play a significant role.

Excretion may occur for a biotransformed drug or for a drug that remains unchanged in the body. For example, penicillin G is primarily excreted unchanged in the urine. Elimination of this drug is thus dependent on renal function. Renal excretion is the net effect of three distinct mechanisms within the kidneys:

- glomerular filtration,
- tubular secretion, and
- tubular reabsorption.

With glomerular filtration, blood flows into the capsule of the glomerulus and there is a passive diffusion of fluids and solutes across the porous glomerular membrane (Figure 9-13). In a healthy adult, up to 130 mL of fluid may cross the glomeruli per minute (total of both kidneys). Three factors influence glomerular filtration:

- molecular size,
- protein binding, and
- glomerular integrity and total number of functioning nephrons.

Drugs dissolved in the plasma may be filtered across the glomerulus; drugs that are protein bound or have a molecular weight greater than 60,000 are not filtered. Pathophysiologic changes in the kidneys may also alter glomerular filtration.

Some drugs are actively secreted from the blood into the proximal tubule, which contains urine. These drugs (primarily weak organic acids and some bases) are

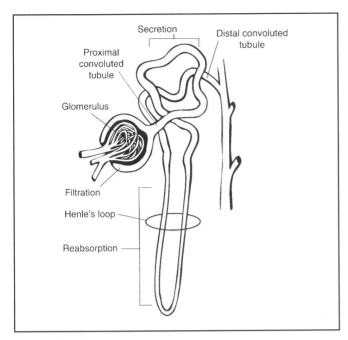

FIGURE 9-13.
Renal nephron.

excreted by carrier-mediated active processes that may be subject to competition from other substances in the body due to broad specificity of the carriers. For example, probenecid and penicillin are both actively secreted. If given together, probenecid competes with penicillin for secretion, so penicillin is secreted less rapidly (it has a longer half-life). This particular relationship can be used in therapeutic situations to extend the duration of penicillin action.

Most drugs also undergo tubular reabsorption back into the blood. This process occurs passively in the distal tubules for drugs that are lipid soluble or not highly ionized. For other agents, it can occur as an active process and (as with tubular secretion) is subject to competition from other agents. An example of reabsorption is glucose, which normally undergoes 100% reabsorption in the distal tubules of the kidneys. With renal dysfunction, glucose often is not reabsorbed and may appear in the urine. Other examples of agents that are actively reabsorbed include endogenous substances such as vitamins, electrolytes, and amino acids.

Tubular reabsorption is dependent on the physical and chemical properties of the drug and the pH of the urine. Drugs that are highly ionized in the urine have less tubular reabsorption; they tend to stay in the urine and are excreted. Drugs must be uncharged to pass easily through biologic membranes. Tubular reabsorption of some compounds may also be dependent on urine flow rate. Urea, for example, has a high tubular reabsorption at low urine flow rates and a low tubular reabsorption at high urine flow rates.

Because renal clearance is determined by filtration, active secretion, and reabsorption, it is fairly complicated. Total renal clearance, Cl_r, can be determined from the following equation:

$$Cl_r = \text{amount excreted in urine}_{(t_1 \rightarrow t_2)} / AUC_{(t \rightarrow t_2)}$$

where AUC is the area under the plasma concentration curve.

However, because it is not easy to differentiate these processes when measuring the amount of drug in the urine, renal clearance is calculated from the ratio of the urine excretion rate to the drug concentration in plasma:

$$Cl_r = \frac{\text{drug excretion rate}}{\text{drug plasma concentration}}$$

There are several different methods to calculate renal drug clearance. In one method, the excretion rate of the drug is estimated by determining the drug concentration in a volume of urine collected over short time periods after drug administration. This excretion rate is then divided by the plasma concentration of drug entering the kidneys at the midpoint of the urine collection period. To express this as an equation:

$$Cl_r = \frac{\text{amount of drug in urine from } t_1 \text{ to } t_2 / (t_2 - t_1)}{C_{midpoint}}$$

where t_1 and t_2 are the times of starting and stopping the collection, respectively, and C is the plasma concentration at the midpoint of t_1 and t_2. Therefore, overall renal clearance is calculated usually without differentiating among filtration, secretion, and reabsorption. This method is commonly used to calculate creatinine clearance when the "amount of drug" is the amount of creatinine that appears in the urine over 24 hours, $t_2 - t_1 = 24$ hours, and $C_{midpoint}$ is the serum creatinine determined at the midpoint of the urine collection period.

RELATIONSHIP BETWEEN RENAL CLEARANCE AND GLOMERULAR FILTRATION RATE

If a drug is exclusively eliminated renally and the only renal process involved is glomerular filtration, the relationship between total body clearance and glomerular filtration rate (GFR) is as shown in Figure 9-14. Creatinine clearance is commonly used as a measure of GFR. Remember that creatinine undergoes some tubular secretion and, therefore, GFR can sometimes be slightly overestimated. As GFR increases, clearance of drug increases. When GFR is zero, clearance is zero. Recall that the equation for the line is $Y = mX + b$. Then, the line in Figure 9-14 can be defined as:

$$\text{clearance} = (\text{slope})(GFR) + 0$$

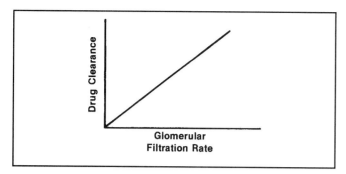

FIGURE 9-14.

Relationship between drug clearance and glomerular filtration rate for a drug that is exclusively eliminated by glomerular filtration.

or:

$$\text{clearance} = (\text{slope})\ (\text{GFR})$$

However, if a drug is excreted by glomerular filtration as well as some other route (e.g. biliary excretion), the relationship illustrated in Figure 9-15 could exist. As GFR increases, the clearance of drug increases; but when GFR is zero, clearance is still greater than zero. In this example, the equation for the line is:

$$\text{clearance} = \text{slope}\ (\text{GFR}) + y\text{-intercept}$$

$$Y = mX + b$$

and we see that when GFR is zero, clearance is the value of the y-intercept, which is nonrenal clearance.

This approach has been used to relate the aminoglycoside elimination rate constant (K) to creatinine clearance. When dosing these agents, we must consider the individual's GFR, as reflected by creatinine clearance. The relationship observed between K and creatinine clearance is shown in Figure 9-16.[2] Therefore, K can be predicted for aminoglycosides (such as gentamicin) based on an individual's creatinine clearance.

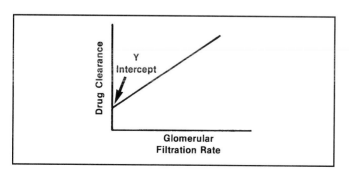

FIGURE 9-15.

Relationship between drug clearance and glomerular filtration rate for a drug that is eliminated by renal and nonrenal processes.

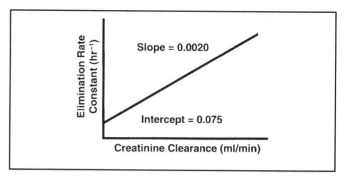

FIGURE 9-16.

Relationship between elimination rate constant and creatinine clearance for aminoglycosides.

With the equation for a line, $Y = mX + b$:

$$K = 0.00293\ \text{hr}^{-1} \times \text{creatinine clearance (in mL/minute)} + 0.014$$

■ CLINICAL CORRELATE

Note that drugs that are cleared almost solely by renal mechanisms will have a y-intercept of zero or very close to zero. Drugs that have extra-renal routes of elimination will have larger y-intercepts.

Determining patient-specific creatinine clearance can be accomplished by either direct measurement of the amount of creatinine contained in a 24-hour urine sample or by estimating this parameter using standard mathematical equations. Direct measurement is the most accurate of these. When using this method, creatinine clearance (CrCl) is determined as follows:

$$\text{CrCl} = \frac{UV}{P \times 1440}$$

where:
- U = urinary creatinine concentration,
- V = volume of urine collected,
- P = plasma creatinine concentration (taken at midpoint of urine collection), and
- 1440 = number of minutes in 24 hours.

Although there are several formulas for estimating creatinine clearance, the Cockcroft–Gault equation is commonly used[3]:

9-1 $$\text{CrCl}_{male} = \frac{(140 - \text{age})\text{IBW}}{72 \times \text{SCr}}$$

or

$$CrCl_{female} = \frac{(0.85)(140 - age)IBW}{72 \times SCr}$$

where:

CrCl = creatinine clearance (milliliters per minute per 1.73 m^2 body surface area),

age = patient's age (years),

IBW = ideal body weight (kilograms), and

SCr = serum creatinine concentration (milligrams per deciliter).

Adjusting this equation for a patient's body surface area is not necessary clinically.

This formula also requires the following patient data:

- ideal body weight (lean body weight) or adjusted body weight (AdjBW),
- age,
- sex, and
- steady-state serum creatinine concentration.

IBW may be estimated as follows:

⚠ IBW$_{males}$ = 50 kg + 2.3 kg for each inch
9-2   over 5 feet in height

IBW$_{females}$ = 45.5 kg + 2.3 kg for each inch over 5 feet in height

In obese patients, the use of total body weight (TBW) overestimates whereas the use of IBW underestimates creatinine clearance. In patients whose TBW is more than 20% over their IBW, adjusted body weight (AdjBW) should be used to estimate creatinine clearance:

⚠ AdjBW = IBW + 0.4 (TBW − IBW)
9-3

For a patient who weighs less than IBW, the actual body weight would be used.

It is important to note that the use of serum creatinine values less than 1 mg/dL will greatly elevate the calculated creatinine clearance value when using Equation 9-1. This is especially true in the elderly. In patients with serum creatinine values of less than 1 mg/dL, it has been recommended to either round the low serum creatinine value up to 1 mg/dL before calculating creatinine clearance, or round the final calculated creatinine clearance value down.

Creatinine clearance is more fully discussed in Lesson 12.

REFERENCES

1. Rogge MC, Solomon WR, Sedman AJ, et al. The theophylline–enoxacin interaction: II. Changes in the disposition of theophylline and its metabolites during intermittent administration of enoxacin. *Clin Pharmacol Ther* 1989; 46:420–8.

2. Matzke GR, Jameson JJ, Halstenson CE. Gentamicin distribution in young and elderly patients with various degrees of renal function. *J Clin Pharmacol* 1987;27:216–20.

3. Shargel L, Yu ABC. *Applied Biopharmaceutics and Pharmacokinetics.* 4th ed. Norwalk, CT: Appleton & Lange; 1999. p. 382.

■ Review Questions

9-1. The body converts a drug to a less active substance by a process called:

A. phosphorylation.

B. hydrogenation.

C. biotransformation.

D. distransformation.

9-2. Biotransformation is also known as:

A. hepatic clearance

B. elimination

C. renal excretion

D. metabolism

9-3. In total, hepatic elimination encompasses both the processes of:

A. biotransformation and excretion.

B. oxidation and glucuronidation.

C. hydroxylation and oxidation.

D. absorption and demethylation.

9-4. Glucuronidation is a phase II biotransformation process.

A. True

B. False

9-5. Biotransformation may be dependent on factors such as age,

A. height, and gender.

B. gender, and weight.

C. disease, and genetics.

D. disease, and gender.

9-6. Which of the following is not a phase I reaction?

A. oxidation

B. glucuronidation

C. reduction

D. hydrolysis

9-7. The basic functional unit of the liver is the:

A. renal lobule.

B. hepatocyte.

C. liver cell.

D. liver lobule.

9-8. The liver receives its blood from the:

A. portal artery and hepatic vein.

B. portal vein and hepatic artery.

C. vena cava and aorta.

D. portal artery and hepatic artery.

9-9. A drug administered orally must go through the liver before it is available to the systemic circulation.

A. True

B. False

9-10. Because the extraction ratio can maximally be 1, the maximum value that hepatic clearance can approach is that of:

A. creatinine clearance.

B. glomerular filtration.

C. renal blood filtration.

D. hepatic blood flow.

9-11. Intrinsic clearance is the maximal ability of the liver to eliminate drug in the absence of any blood flow limitations.

A. True

B. False

9-12. Smoking is known to increase the enzymes responsible for theophylline metabolism (a drug with a low hepatic extraction). Would a patient with a history of smoking likely require a higher, lower, or equivalent theophylline total daily dose compared to a nonsmoking patient?

A. lower

B. higher

C. equivalent

9-13. Heart failure reduces cardiac output and hepatic blood flow. Consequently, the total daily dose of lidocaine may need to be decreased in a patient with heart failure who has a myocardial infarction.

A. True

B. False

9-14. Which of the following types of metabolism do drugs with a high extraction ratio undergo to a significant extent?

A. first-pass

B. zero-order

C. intraluminal

D. nonlinear

9-15. Significant first-pass metabolism means that much of the drug's metabolism occurs before its arrival at the:

A. hepatocyte.

B. systemic circulation.

C. portal blood.

D. liver lobule.

9-16. The liver receives blood supply from the GI tract via the:

A. portal vein.

B. hepatic artery.

C. hepatic vein.

D. portal artery.

9-17. For a drug that is totally absorbed without any pre-systemic metabolism and then undergoes hepatic extraction, which of the following is the correct equation for F?

A. $F = 1 - K_a$

B. $F = 1 - F_p$

C. $F = 1 - E$

D. $F = 1 -$ the fraction of the drug absorbed

9-18. Route of administration, extraction ratio, and protein binding are all factors that should be considered when trying to assess the effect of disease states on plasma concentrations of drugs eliminated by the liver.

A. True

B. False

9-19. Will drugs that inhibit the hepatic cytochrome P450 system likely increase or decrease the plasma clearance of theophylline?

A. increase

B. decrease

9-20. Disease states may increase or decrease drug protein binding.

A. True

B. False

9-21. Drug elimination encompasses both:

A. metabolism and excretion.

B. metabolism and biotransformation.

C. absorption and metabolism.

D. metabolism and distribution.

9-22. Two important routes of drug excretion are:

A. hepatic and tubular secretion

B. biliary and metabolic

C. renal and biliary

D. renal and metabolic

9-23. Fluid is filtered across the glomerulus through active transport.

A. True

B. False

9-24. Tubular secretion most often occurs with weak organic acids.

A. True

B. False

9-25. Which of the following statements about tubular reabsorption is *false*?

A. Tubular reabsorption depends on the pH of the urine.

B. Highly ionized drugs tend to remain in the urine.

C. Tubular reabsorption can only be an active transport process.

D. A and C.

9-26. Renal clearance can be calculated from the ratio of which of the following drug's rates to the drug's concentration in plasma?

A. tubular reabsorption rate

B. tubular secretion rate

C. glomerular filtration rate

D. excretion rate

9-27. For aminoglycoside doses, which of the following must be calculated to estimate an individual patient's drug elimination rate? An individual patient's:

A. pulmonary clearance

B. biliary clearance

C. creatinine clearance

D. A and C

9-28. For aminoglycosides, the terminal elimination rate constant can be estimated from the creatinine clearance by which of the following equations?

A. $K = 0.00293$ hr^{-1} × (creatinine clearance in mL/minute) + 1.4

B. $K = 0.00293$ hr^{-1} × (creatinine clearance in mL/minute) + 0.014

C. $K = 2.93$ hr^{-1} × (creatinine clearance in mL/minute)

D. $K = 0.00293$ hr^{-1} + (creatinine clearance in mL/minute)

▌Answers

9-1. A, B, D. Incorrect answers
      C. CORRECT ANSWER

9-2. A, B, C. Incorrect answers
      D. CORRECT ANSWER

9-3. A. CORRECT ANSWER
      B, C, D. Incorrect answers

9-4. A. CORRECT ANSWER
      B. Incorrect answer. Oxidation, reduction, and hydrolysis are examples of phase I reactions.

9-5. A, B, D. Incorrect answers
      C. CORRECT ANSWER

9-6. A, C, D. Incorrect answers
      B. CORRECT ANSWER

9-7. A, B, C. Incorrect answers
      D. CORRECT ANSWER

9-8. A, C, D. Incorrect answers
      B. CORRECT ANSWER

9-9. A. CORRECT ANSWER
      B. Incorrect answer

9-10. A, B, C. Incorrect answers
      D. CORRECT ANSWER

9-11. A. CORRECT ANSWER
      B. Incorrect answer

9-12. A, C. Incorrect answers
      B. CORRECT ANSWER. Smoking raises the concentrations of enzymes that also metabolize theophylline, so more theophylline would be metabolized, requiring a higher theophylline dose.

9-13. A. CORRECT ANSWER
      B. Incorrect answer

9-14. A. CORRECT ANSWER
      B. Incorrect answer. Zero-order processes are not determined by amount of hepatic extraction.
      C. Incorrect answer. Intraluminal metabolism is independent of hepatic extraction.
      D. Incorrect answer. Nonlinear metabolism only involves saturation of hepatic enzymes.

9-15. A, C, D. Incorrect answers
      B. CORRECT ANSWER

9-16. A. CORRECT ANSWER
      B, C, D. Incorrect answers

9-17. A, B, D. Incorrect answers
      C. CORRECT ANSWER. F represents the fraction of drug that reaches the systemic circulation; E is the extraction ratio.

9-18. A. CORRECT ANSWER
      B. Incorrect answer

9-19. A. Incorrect answer
      B. CORRECT ANSWER. Theophylline is a low-extraction drug and its clearance is roughly equal to intrinsic hepatic clearance (Cl_i), so the effect of cytochrome P450 enzyme induction is likely to decrease intrinsic and overall clearance.

9-20. A. CORRECT ANSWER
      B. Incorrect answer

9-21. A. CORRECT ANSWER
      B. Incorrect answer. Biotransformation is a type of metabolism.
      C. Incorrect answer. Absorption is not an elimination process.

D. Incorrect answer. Distribution is not an elimination process.

9-22. A, B, D. Incorrect answers

C. CORRECT ANSWER

9-23. A. Incorrect answer

B. CORRECT ANSWER

9-24. A. CORRECT ANSWER

B. Incorrect answer

9-25. A. Incorrect answer. Urine pH does affect tubular reabsorption.

B. Incorrect answer. Highly ionized drugs do remain in the urine because ionized forms of drugs do not cross membranes well.

C. CORRECT ANSWER

D. Incorrect answer

9-26. A. Incorrect answer. Tubular reabsorption rate cannot be directly measured.

B. Incorrect answer. Tubular secretion rate cannot be directly measured.

C. Incorrect answer. Glomerular filtration rate does not account for tubular secretion or reabsorption.

D. CORRECT ANSWER

9-27. A, B, C. Incorrect answers. Aminoglycosides are not eliminated hepatically.

D. CORRECT ANSWER

9-28. A. Incorrect answer. The y-intercept is wrong. Aminoglycosides undergo little if any extra-renal elimination and therefore the y-intercept value should be close to zero.

B. CORRECT ANSWER

C. Incorrect answer. The answer should represent the approximate fraction of drug excreted per hour, and this value should be less than one.

D. Incorrect answer. The correct answer should be expressed as a product, not a sum (i.e., A × B, not A + B).

Discussion Points

D-1. Research the metabolism of primidone and discuss the clinical significance of its metabolites. Discuss the proper method to monitor a patient receiving primidone.

D-2. Select several drugs whose prescribing information indicates that the dose should be decreased with hepatic impairment. Describe the pharmacokinetics of these drugs and discuss why this drug's dose should be decreased. Finally, indicate specifically how you would go about decreasing this dose.

D-3. Research the pharmacokinetics of carbamazepine and discuss its metabolism when given alone and when given with other enzyme inhibitors or inducers. Specifically, how would you begin a patient on carbamazepine and how would you monitor and adjust its dose?

D-4. Research the various oral fluoroquinolones to determine which can affect the metabolism of theophylline and to what extent. Discuss why some of these drugs affect theophylline and others do not.

D-5. Describe several clinical situations in which a drug's ability to compete for renal secretion with another drug can be either useful or harmful.

D-6. Describe situations in which alteration of urine pH with urine acidifier or alkalinizing agents can be used to enhance the clinical response of other drugs.

D-7. Look up and compare the various equations that can be used to calculate the elimination rate constant for gentamicin, tobramycin, and amikacin. Are these equations the same or different? Try to explain why they are either the same or different.

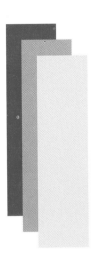

LESSON
10

Nonlinear Processes

 OBJECTIVES

After completing Lesson 10, you should be able to:

1. Describe the relationship of both drug concentration and area under the plasma drug concentration versus time curve (AUC) to the dose for a nonlinear, zero-order process.

2. Explain the various biopharmaceutic processes that can result in nonlinear pharmacokinetics.

3. Describe how hepatic enzyme saturation can result in nonlinear pharmacokinetics.

4. Use the Michaelis–Menten model for describing nonlinear pharmacokinetics.

5. Describe V_{max} and K_m.

6. Use the Michaelis–Menten model to predict plasma drug concentrations.

7. Use the $t_{90\%}$ equation to estimate the time required for 90% of the steady-state concentration to be reached.

Until now, we have used a major assumption in constructing models for drug pharmacokinetics: drug clearance remains constant with any size dose. This is the case only when drug elimination processes are first order (as described in previous lessons). With a first-order elimination process, as the dose of drug increases, the plasma concentrations observed and the AUC increase proportionally. That is, if the dose is doubled, the plasma concentration and AUC also double (Figure 10-1).

Because the increase in plasma concentration and AUC is linear with drug dose in first-order processes, this concept is referred to as *linear pharmacokinetics*. When these linear relationships are present, they are used to predict drug dosage. For example, if a 100-mg daily dose of a drug produces a steady-state peak plasma concentration of 10 mg/L, we know that a 200-mg daily dose will result in a steady-state plasma concentration of 20 mg/L. (Note that *linear* does not refer to the plot of natural log of plasma concentration versus time.)

With some drugs (e.g., phenytoin and aspirin), however, the relationships of drug dose to plasma concentrations and AUC are not linear. As the drug dose increases, the peak concentration and the resulting AUC do not increase proportionally (Figure 10-2). Therefore, such drugs are said to follow nonlinear, zero-order, or dose-dependent pharmacokinetics (i.e., the pharmacokinetics change with the dose given). Just as with drugs following linear pharmacokinetics, it is important to predict the plasma drug concentrations resulting from a drug dose. In this lesson, we discuss methods to characterize drugs that follow nonlinear pharmacokinetics.

Nonlinear pharmacokinetics may refer to several different processes, including absorption, distribution, and renal or hepatic elimination (Table 10-1). For example, with nonlinear absorption, the fraction of drug in the GI tract that is absorbed per minute changes with the amount of drug present . Even though absorption and distribution can be nonlinear, the term *nonlinear pharmaco-*

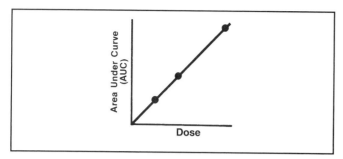

FIGURE 10-1.

Relationship of AUC to drug dose with first-order elimination, where clearance is not influenced by dose.

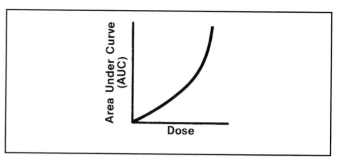

FIGURE 10-2.

Relationship of AUC to drug dose with dose-dependent pharmacokinetics.

kinetics usually refers to the processes of drug elimination.

When a drug exhibits nonlinear pharmacokinetics, usually the processes responsible for drug elimination are saturable at therapeutic concentrations. These elimination processes may include renal tubular secretion (as seen with penicillins) and hepatic enzyme metabolism (as seen with phenytoin). When an elimination process is saturated, any increase in drug dose results in a disproportionate increase in the plasma concentrations achieved because the amount of drug that can be eliminated over time cannot increase. This situation is contrary to first-order linear processes, in which an increase in drug dosage results in an increase in the amount of drug eliminated over any given period.

Of course, most elimination processes are capable of being saturated if enough drug is administered. However, for most drugs, the doses administered do not cause the elimination processes to approach their limitations.

■ CLINICAL CORRELATE

Many drugs exhibit mixed-order pharmacokinetics, displaying first-order pharmacokinetics at low drug concentrations and zero-order pharmacokinetics at high concentrations. It is important to know the drug concentration at which a drug "order" switches from first to zero. Phenytoin is an example of a drug that switches order at therapeutic concentrations, whereas theophylline does not switch until concentrations reach the toxic range.

For a typical drug having dose-dependent pharmacokinetics, with saturable elimination, the plasma drug concentration versus time plot after a dose may appear as shown in Figure 10-3.

After a large dose is administered, an initial slow elimination phase (clearance decreases with higher

TABLE 10-1.

Drugs Having Dose- or Time-Dependent Pharmacokinetics

Process	Agent	Mechanism
Absorption	Riboflavin, methotrexate, gabapentin	Saturable gut wall transport
	Penicillins	Saturable decomposition in GI tract
Distribution	Methotrexate	Saturable transport into and out of tissues
	Salicylates	Saturable protein binding
Renal elimination	Penicillin G	Active tubular secretion
	Ascorbic acid	Active reabsorption
Extrarenal elimination	Carbamazepine	Enzyme induction
	Theophylline, phenytoin	Saturable metabolism

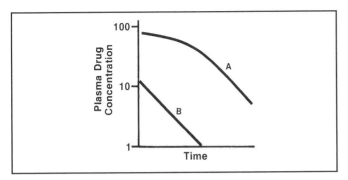

FIGURE 10-3.
Dose-dependent clearance of enzyme-saturable drugs.

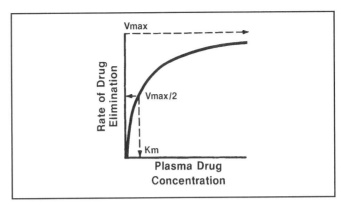

FIGURE 10-4.
Relationship of drug elimination rate to plasma drug concentration with saturable elimination.

plasma concentration) is followed by a much more rapid elimination at lower concentrations (curve A). However, when a small dose is administered (curve B), the capacity of the elimination process is not reached, and the elimination rate remains constant. At high concentrations, the elimination rate approaches that of a zero-order process (i.e., the amount of drug eliminated over a given period remains constant, but the fraction eliminated changes). At low concentrations, the elimination rate approaches that of a first-order process (i.e., the amount of drug eliminated over a given time changes, but the fraction of drug eliminated remains constant).

A model that has been used extensively in biochemistry to describe the kinetics of saturable enzyme systems is known as *Michaelis–Menten kinetics* (for its developers). This system describes the relationship of an enzyme to the substrate (in this case, the drug molecule). In clinical pharmacokinetics, it allows prediction of plasma drug concentrations resulting from administration of drugs with saturable elimination (e.g., phenytoin).

The equation used to describe Michaelis–Menten pharmacokinetics is:

$$\text{drug elimination rate} = \frac{-dC}{dt} = \frac{V_{max}C}{K_m + C}$$

where $-dC/dt$ is the rate of drug concentration decline at time t and is determined by V_{max}, the theoretical maximum rate of the elimination process. K_m is the drug concentration when the rate of elimination is half the maximum rate, and C is the total plasma drug concentration.

V_{max} is expressed in units of amount per unit of time (e.g., milligrams per day) and represents the maximum amount of drug that can be eliminated in the given time period. For drugs metabolized by the liver, V_{max} can be determined by the quantity or efficiency of metabolizing enzymes. This parameter will vary, depending on the drug and individual patient.

K_m, the Michaelis constant, is expressed in units of concentration (e.g., mg/L) and is the drug concentra-

tion at which the rate of elimination is half the maximum rate (V_{max}). In simplified terms, K_m is the concentration above which saturation of drug metabolism is likely.

V_{max} and K_m are related to the plasma drug concentration and the rate of drug elimination as shown in Figure 10-4. When the plasma drug concentration is less than K_m, the rate of drug elimination follows first-order pharmacokinetics. In other words, the amount of drug eliminated per hour directly increases with the plasma drug concentration. When the plasma drug concentration is much less than K_m, the first-order elimination rate constant (K) for drugs with nonlinear pharmacokinetics is approximated by V_{max}; therefore, as V_{max} increases (e.g., by hepatic enzyme induction), K increases.

With drugs having saturable elimination, as plasma drug concentrations increase, drug elimination approaches its maximum rate. When the plasma concentration is much greater than K_m, the rate of drug elimination is approximated by V_{max}, and elimination proceeds at close to a zero-order process.

Next, we consider how V_{max} and K_m can be calculated and how these determinations may be used to predict plasma drug concentrations in patients.

CALCULATION OF V_{MAX}, K_M, AND PLASMA CONCENTRATION AND DOSE

For drugs that have saturable elimination at the plasma concentrations readily achieved with therapeutic doses (e.g., phenytoin), prediction of the plasma concentrations achieved by a given dose is important. For these predictions, it is necessary to estimate V_{max} and K_m. Therefore, we must apply the Michaelis–Menten equation presented earlier in this lesson:

$$\frac{-dC}{dt} = \frac{V_{max}C}{K_m + C}$$

The change in drug concentration over time is related to the Michaelis–Menten parameters V_{max}, K_m, and the plasma drug concentration (C). We know that at steady state (after multiple drug doses) the rate of drug loss from the body (milligrams removed per day) is equal to the amount of drug being administered (daily dose). In the Michaelis–Menten equation, $-dC/dt$ indicates the rate of drug loss from the body; therefore, at steady state:

$$\frac{-dC}{dt} = \text{daily drug dose} = \frac{V_{max}C}{K_m + C}$$

Now we have an equation that relates V_{max}, K_m, plasma drug concentration, and daily dose (at steady state). To use this relationship, it is first helpful to transform the equation to a straight-line form:

⚠
10-1

$$\text{daily dose} = \frac{V_{max}C}{K_m + C}$$

$$\text{daily dose} (K_m + C) = V_{max}C$$

$$\text{daily dose} (K_m) + \text{daily dose} (C) = V_{max}C$$

$$\text{daily dose} (C) = V_{max}C - \text{daily dose} (K_m)$$

Then:

$$\text{daily dose} = -K_m(\text{daily dose}/C) + V_{max}$$

$$Y\,(\text{slope}) \quad = \quad mX \quad + \quad b\,(\text{intercept})$$

So the relationship of the Michaelis–Menten parameters, C, and dose can be expressed as a straight line (Figure 10-5). If the straight line can be defined, then V_{max} and K_m can be determined; if V_{max} and K_m are known, then the plasma concentrations at steady state resulting from any given dose can be estimated.

To define the line, it is necessary to know the steady-state concentrations achieved at a minimum of two different doses. For example, a patient receiving 300 mg of

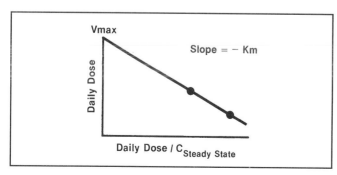

FIGURE 10-5.
Linear plot of the Michaelis–Menten equation.

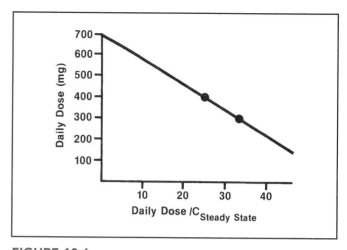

FIGURE 10-6.
Plot of patient data using two steady-state plasma phenytoin concentrations at two dose levels.

phenytoin per day achieved a steady-state concentration (trough) of 9 mg/L; when the daily dose was increased to 400 mg/day, a steady-state concentration of 16 mg/L was achieved. The data for this patient can be plotted as shown in Figure 10-6. Then a line is drawn between the two points, intersecting the y-axis. The y-intercept equals V_{max} (observed to be 700 mg/day), and the slope of the line equals $-K_m$.

Calculating K_m

⚠
10-2

$$\text{slope} = -K_m = \frac{\text{dose}_{initial} - \text{dose}_{increased}}{\text{dose}/C_{initial} - \text{dose}/C_{increased}}$$

$$= \frac{300\ \text{mg/day} - 400\ \text{mg/day}}{\left(\dfrac{300\ \text{mg/day}}{9\ \text{mg/L}} - \dfrac{400\ \text{mg/day}}{16\ \text{mg/L}}\right)}$$

$$= \frac{-100\ \text{mg/day}}{33.3\ \text{L/day} - 25\ \text{L/day}}$$

$$= -12.0\ \text{mg/L}$$

So K_m equals 12 mg/L.

Calculating Dose

Knowing V_{max} and K_m, we can then predict the dose necessary to achieve a given steady-state concentration or the concentration resulting from a given dose. If we wish to increase the steady-state plasma concentration to 20 mg/L, we can use the Michaelis–Menten equation to predict the necessary dose:

$$\text{dose} = \frac{V_{max}C}{K_m + C}$$

$$= \frac{(700\ \text{mg/day})(20\ \text{mg/L})}{12\ \text{mg/L} + 20\ \text{mg/L}}$$

$$= \frac{14{,}000\ \text{mg}^2/(\text{day} \times \text{L})}{32\ \text{mg/L}}$$

$$= 437\ \text{mg/day}$$

Note how units cancel out to yield mg/day.

Calculating Steady-State Concentration from This K_m and Dose

If we wish to predict the steady-state plasma concentration that would result if the dose is increased to 500 mg/day, we can rearrange the Michaelis–Menten equation and solve for C:

⚠️
10-3

$$C = \frac{K_m(\text{daily dose})}{V_{max} - \text{daily dose}}$$

$$= \frac{12\ \text{mg/L}\,(500\ \text{mg/day})}{700\ \text{mg/day} - 500\ \text{mg/day}}$$

$$= \frac{12\ \text{mg/L}\,(500\ \text{mg/day})}{200\ \text{mg/day}}$$

$$= 30\ \text{mg/L}$$

See Lesson 15 for examples of how these calculations are applied.

■ CLINICAL CORRELATE

When performing this calculation using sodium phenytoin or fosphenytoin, be sure to convert doses to their phenytoin free-acid equivalent before substituting these values into the equation. To convert, multiply the daily dose by 0.92 (92% free phenytoin).

The preceding example demonstrates how plasma drug concentrations and drug dose can be predicted. However, it also shows that for drugs like phenytoin, with saturable elimination, when plasma concentrations are above K_m, small dose increases can result in large increases in the steady-state plasma concentration.

When clearance changes with plasma concentration, there is no true half-life as with first-order elimination. As clearance changes, the elimination rate changes, as does

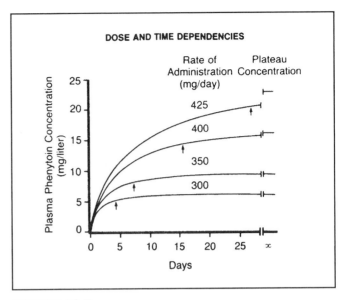

FIGURE 10-7.
Time to reach $t_{90\%}$ (represented by arrows) at different daily dosages.

the time to reach steady state. With high doses and high plasma concentrations (and resulting lower clearance), the time to reach steady state is much longer than with low doses and low plasma concentrations (Figure 10-7). Theoretically, if the dose is greater than V_{max}, steady state will never be reached.

The Michaelis–Menten equation can be rearranged to provide an equation that estimates the time required (in days) for 90% of the steady-state concentration to be reached ($t_{90\%}$), as shown below (where the dose equals the daily dose):

⚠️
10-4

$$t_{90\%} = \frac{K_m(V)}{(V_{max} - \text{daily dose})^2}[2.3V_{max} - 0.9\,\text{dose}]$$

From the previous example, when dose = 300 mg/day, V_{max} = 700 mg/day, K_m = 12 mg/L, and the volume of distribution (V) is estimated to be 50 L:

$$t_{90\%} = \frac{12\ \text{mg/L}(50\ \text{L})}{(700\ \text{mg/day} - 300\ \text{mg/day})^2}[2.3(700\ \text{mg/day}) -$$
$$0.9(300\ \text{mg/day})]$$

$$= \frac{600\ \text{mg}}{(400\ \text{mg/day})^2}\big[1610\ \text{mg/day} - 270\ \text{mg/day}\big]$$

$$= (0.00375\ \text{day}^2/\text{mg})(1340\ \text{mg/day})$$

$$= 5.0\ \text{days}$$

When the dose is increased to 400 mg/day:

$$t_{90\%} = \frac{12\ \text{mg/L}\ (50\ \text{L})}{(700\ \text{mg/day} - 400\ \text{mg/day})^2}[2.3(700\ \text{mg/day}) -$$

$$0.9(400\ \text{mg/day})]$$

$$= \frac{600\ \text{mg}}{(300\ \text{mg/day})^2}[1610\ \text{mg/day} - 360\ \text{mg/day}]$$

$$= (0.0067\ \text{day}^2/\text{mg})(1250\ \text{mg/day})$$

$$= 8.33\ \text{days}$$

We can see that as the dose is increased, it takes a longer time to reach steady state, drug continues to accumulate, and the plasma drug concentration continues to rise. When this occurs with a drug such as phenytoin, toxic effects (e.g., ataxia and nystagmus) probably will be observed if the high dosage is given on a regular basis.

■ CLINICAL CORRELATE

The $t_{90\%}$ equation will only provide a rough estimate of when 90% of steady state has been reached, and its accuracy is dependent on the K_m value used. Other ways to check to see if a patient is at steady state are to examine two levels drawn approximately a week apart. If these levels are ± 10% of each other, then you can assume steady state. Additionally, it is safe to wait at least 2 weeks (and preferably 4 weeks) after beginning or changing a dose before obtaining new steady-state levels.

Review Questions

10-1. Which drug pairs demonstrate nonlinear pharmacokinetics?

    A. phenytoin and salicylate

    B. penicillin G and ascorbic acid

    C. acetaminophen and sulfonamides

    D. A and B

10-2. Linear pharmacokinetics means that the plot of plasma drug concentration versus time after a dose is a straight line.

    A. True

    B. False

10-3. When hepatic metabolism becomes saturated, any increase in drug dose will lead to a proportionate increase in the plasma concentration achieved.

    A. True

    B. False

10-4. When the rate of drug elimination proceeds at half the maximum rate, the drug concentration is known as:

    A. V_{max}.

    B. K_m.

    C. V_{max}.

    D. $(V_{max})(C)$.

10-5. At very high concentrations—concentrations much higher than the drug's K_m—drugs are more likely to exhibit first-order elimination.

    A. True

    B. False

10-6. Which of the equations below describes the form of the Michaelis–Menten equation that relates daily drug dose to V_{max}, K_m, and the steady-state plasma drug concentration?

    A. daily dose = $-K_m$(daily dose/C)(V_{max})

    B. daily dose = $-K_m$(daily dose/C) + V_{max}

    C. daily dose = $-K_m$(daily dose × C) + V_{max}

    D. daily dose = $-K_m$ – (daily dose/C) + V_{max}

The following information is for Questions 10-7 to 10-11. A patient, JH, is administered phenytoin free acid, 300 mg/day, for 2 months (assume steady state is achieved), and a plasma concentration determined just before a dose is 10 mg/L. The phenytoin dose is then changed to 400 mg/day, and 2 months after the dose change the plasma concentration determined just before a dose is 18 mg/L. Assume that the volume of distribution of phenytoin is 45 L.

10-7. Calculate K_m for this patient.

    A. 12.5 mg/L

    B. 25 mg/L

    C. 37.5 mg/L

    D. 10 mg/L

10-8. For the same patient, JH, determine V_{max}.

    A. 123 mg/day

    B. 900 mg/day

    C. 500 mg/day

    D. 678 mg/day

10-9. For the case of JH above, plot both concentrations on a "daily dose/C" versus "V_{max}" plot and then determine this patient's V_{max}.

    A. approximately 550 mg/day

    B. approximately 400 mg/day

    C. approximately 675 mg/day

    D. approximately 800 mg/day

10-10. After the dose of 400 mg/day is begun, how long will it take to reach 90% of the steady-state plasma concentration?

    A. approximately 14 days

    B. approximately 9 days

    C. approximately 30 days

    D. approximately 90 days

10-11. If the patient, JH, misunderstood the dosage instructions and consumed 500 mg/day of phenytoin, what steady-state plasma concentration would result?

    A. 29.4 mg/L

    B. 36.8 mg/L

    C. 27.2 mg/L

    D. 19.6 mg/L

Answers

10-1. A, B, C. Incorrect answers

D. CORRECT ANSWER

10-2. A. Incorrect answer

B. CORRECT ANSWER. *Linear pharmacokinetics* means that the AUC and plasma concentrations achieved are directly related to the size of the dose administered. Drugs with linear pharmacokinetics may exhibit plasma concentrations versus time plots that are not straight lines, as with multiple-compartment drugs.

10-3. A. Incorrect answer

B. CORRECT ANSWER. There will be a disproportionate increase in the plasma concentration achieved because the amount of drug that can be eliminated over time cannot increase.

10-4. A. Incorrect answer. V_{max} is the maximum rate of hepatic metabolism.

B. CORRECT ANSWER

C. Incorrect answer. V_{max} is the rate at which K_m is determined.

D. Incorrect answer. $(V_{max})(C)$ is only the numerator of the Michaelis–Menten equation.

10-5. A. Incorrect answer

B. CORRECT ANSWER. At very low concentrations, drugs are more likely to exhibit first-order kinetics because hepatic enzymes are usually not yet saturated, whereas at higher concentrations, enzymes saturate, making zero-order kinetics more likely.

10-6. A, C, D. Incorrect answers

B. CORRECT ANSWER

10-7. A. CORRECT ANSWER. The K_m is calculated from the slope of the line above:

$$\text{slope} = -K_m = \frac{\text{dose}_1 - \text{dose}_2}{\text{dose}_1/C_1 - \text{dose}_2/C_2}$$

$$= \frac{300 \text{ mg/day} - 400 \text{ mg/day}}{\left(\dfrac{300 \text{ mg/day}}{10 \text{ mg/L}} - \dfrac{400 \text{ mg/day}}{18 \text{ mg/L}} \right)}$$

$$= \frac{-100 \text{ mg/day}}{30 \text{ L/day} - 22 \text{ L/day}}$$

$$= \frac{-100 \text{ mg/day}}{8 \text{ L/day}}$$

$$= -12.5 \text{ mg/L}$$

So K_m equals 12.5 mg/L.

B, C, D. Incorrect answers. Use dose pairs of 300 and 400 and concentration pairs of 10 and 18 to calculate K_m.

10-8. A, C. Incorrect answers. Try again, you probably made a math error.

B. Incorrect answer. Try again, and use either set of dose and concentration pairs (i.e., 300 and 10 or 400 and 18).

D. CORRECT ANSWER.

$$\text{daily dose} = -K_m(\text{daily dose}/C) + V_{max}$$

$$400 = (-12.5)(400/18) + V_{max}$$

$$400 = (-12.5)(22.22) + V_{max}$$

$$400 = -277.77 + V_{max}$$

$$677.77 = V_{max}$$

10-9. A, B, D. Incorrect answers

C. CORRECT ANSWER. See Figure 10-8 for a plot of the daily dose versus daily dose/C.

10-10. A, C, D. Incorrect answers

B. CORRECT ANSWER. The time to reach steady state is calculated by:

$$t_{90\%} = \frac{K_m(V)}{(V_{max} - \text{dose})^2}[2.3V_{max} - 0.9 \text{ dose}]$$

$$= \frac{12.5 \text{ mg/L}(45 \text{ L})}{(670 \text{ mg/day} - 400 \text{ mg/day})^2}[2.3(670 \text{ mg/day}) - 0.9(400 \text{ mg/day})]$$

$$= \frac{562.5 \text{ mg}}{(270 \text{ mg/day})^2}[1541 \text{ mg/day} - 360 \text{ mg/day}]$$

$$= (0.00772 \text{ day}^2/\text{mg})(1181 \text{ mg/day})$$

$$= 9.11 \text{ days}$$

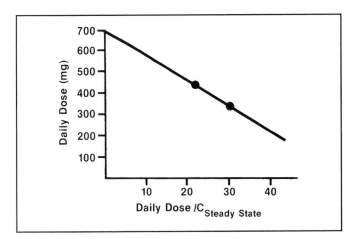

FIGURE 10-8.
Daily dose versus daily dose divided by steady-state concentration.

10-11. A. Incorrect answer. Perhaps you used a 400-mg dose instead of a 500-mg dose.

B. CORRECT ANSWER. The steady-state plasma concentration resulting from a daily dose of 500

mg would be estimated from the line equation as follows:

$$\text{daily dose} = -K_m(\text{dose}/C) + V_{max}$$

$$500 \text{ mg/day} = -12.5 \text{ mg/L}\left(\frac{500 \text{ mg/day}}{C}\right) + 670 \text{ mg/day}$$

Rearranging gives:

$$\frac{-170 \text{ mg/day}}{-12.5 \text{ mg/L}} = \frac{500 \text{ mg/day}}{C}$$

$$13.6 \text{ L/day} = \frac{500 \text{ mg/day}}{C}$$

$$\frac{13.6 \text{ L/day}}{500 \text{ mg/day}} = \frac{1}{C}$$

$$0.0272 \text{ L/mg} = \frac{1}{C}$$

$$C = 36.8 \text{ mg/L}$$

C, D. Incorrect answers. You may have made a simple math error.

Discussion Points

D-1. When using the Michaelis–Menten equation (MME), examine what happens when daily dose is much lower than V_{max}, and when it exceeds V_{max}.

D-2. When using the $t_{90\%}$ equation, examine what happens to $t_{90\%}$ when dose greatly exceeds V_{max}.

D-3. Using two steady-state plasma drug concentrations and two doses to solve for a new K_m, V_{max}, and dose using the MME, examine the values of K_m and V_{max} obtained using this process. Are these values close to the actual patient population parameters? Also, discuss the limitations of these calculations in clinical practice.

D-4. Discuss several practical methods to determine when a nonlinear drug has reached steady state.

D-5. Examine the "time to 90% equation" and note the value of K_m that is used in this equation. Substitute several different phenytoin K_m values based on a range of population values (i.e., from approximately 1 to 15 mg/L) and describe the effect this has on your answer. Based on this observation, what value of K_m would you use when trying to approximate the $t_{90\%}$ for a newly begun dose of phenytoin?

D-6. Discuss the patient variables that can affect the pharmacokinetic calculation of a nonlinear drug when using two plasma drug concentrations obtained from two different doses.

D-7. Write a pharmacy protocol describing an appropriate phenytoin dosing and monitoring service.

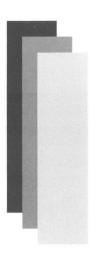

LESSON
11

Pharmacokinetic Variation and Model-Independent Relationships

 OBJECTIVES

After completing Lesson 11, you should be able to:

1. Identify the various sources of pharmacokinetic variation.

2. Explain how the various sources of pharmacokinetic variation affect pharmacokinetic parameters.

3. Describe how to apply pharmacokinetic variation in a clinical setting.

4. Name the potential sources of error in the collection and assay of drug samples.

5. Explain the clinical importance of correct sample collection, storage and assay.

6. Describe ways to avoid or minimize errors in the collection and assay of drug samples.

7. Explain the basic concepts and calculations of the model-independent pharmacokinetic parameters of total body clearance, mean residence time (MRT), volume of distribution at steady state, and formation clearance.

SOURCES OF PHARMACOKINETIC VARIATION

An important reason for pharmacokinetic drug monitoring is that a drug's effect may vary considerably among individuals given the same dose. These differences in drug effect are sometimes related to differences in pharmacokinetics. Some factors that may affect drug pharmacokinetics are discussed below. However, irrespective of pharmacokinetics, drug effects may vary among individuals because of differences in drug sensitivity.

Age

At extremes of age, major organ functions may be considerably reduced compared with those of healthy young adults. In neonates (particularly if premature) and the elderly, renal function and the capacity for renal drug excretion may be greatly reduced. Neonates and the elderly are also more likely to have reduced hepatic function. Renal function declines at a rate of approximately 1 mL/minute/year after the age of 40 years. In the neonate, renal function rapidly progresses in infancy to equal or exceed that of adults. Pediatric patients may have an increased rate of clearance because a child's drug metabolism rate is increased compared to adults. When dosing a drug for a child, the drug may need to be administered more frequently.

Other changes also occur with aging. Compared with adults, the neonate has a higher proportion of body mass made up of water and a lower proportion of body fat. The elderly are likely to have a lower proportion of body water and lean tissue (Figure 11-1) Both of these changes, organ function and body makeup, affect the disposition of drugs and how they are used. Reduced function of the organs of drug elimination generally requires that doses of drugs eliminated by the affected organ be given less frequently. With alterations in body water or fat content, the dose of drugs that distribute into those tissues must be altered. For

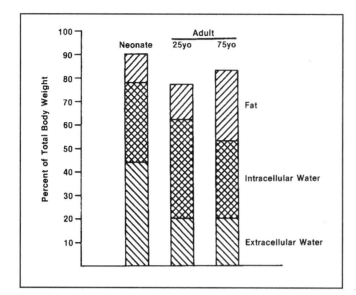

FIGURE 11-1.
Effect of age on body composition.

drugs that distribute into body water, the neonatal dose may be larger per kilogram of body weight than in an adult.

Disease States

Drug disposition is altered in many disease states, but the most common examples involve the kidneys and liver, as they are the major organs of drug elimination. In patients with major organ dysfunction, drug clearance decreases and, subsequently, drug half-life lengthens. Some diseases, such as renal failure or cirrhosis, may even result in fluid retention and an increased volume of drug distribution.

Alterations in drug clearance and volume of distribution require adjustments in the dose administered and/or the dosing interval. For most drugs, when clearance is decreased but the volume of distribution is relatively unchanged, the dose administered may be similar to that in a healthy person but the dosing interval may need to be increased. Alternatively, smaller doses could be administered over a shorter dosing interval. When the volume of distribution is altered, the dosing interval can often remain the same but the dose administered should change in proportion to the change in volume of distribution.

█ CLINICAL CORRELATE

When adjusting a dose of a drug that follows first-order elimination, if you do not change the dosing interval, then the new dose can be calculated using various simple ratio and proportion techniques. For example, if gentamicin peak and trough serum drug concentrations, in a patient receiving 120 mg Q 12 hours), were 9 and 2.3 mcg/mL, respectively, then a new dose can be calculated: "if 120 mg gives a peak

of 9, then X mg will give a desired peak of 6," yielding an answer of 80 mg Q 12 hours. Likewise, one can check to see if this trough would be acceptable with this new dose: "if 120 mg gives a trough of 2.3, then 80 mg will give a trough of X," yielding an answer of 1.5 mcg/mL.

Example

Effect of Volume of Distribution and Impaired Renal/Hepatic Function on Drug Dose

A 23-year-old male experienced a major traumatic injury from a motor vehicle accident. On the third day after injury, his renal function is determined to be good (creatinine clearance = 120 mL/minute), and his weight has increased from 63 kg on admission to 83 kg. Note that fluid accumulation (as evidenced by weight gain) is an expected result of traumatic injury. He is treated with gentamicin for gram-negative bacteremia.

An initial gentamicin dose of 100 mg is given over 1 hour, and a peak concentration of 2.5 mg/L is determined. Four hours after the peak, the plasma concentration is determined to be 0.6 mg/L, and the elimination rate constant and the volume of distribution are determined to be 0.36 hr^{-1} and 33.6 L, respectively. This volume of 33.6 L equals 0.40 L/kg compared to a typical V of 0.2-0.3 L/kg, In this case, the patient's gentamicin elimination rate constant is similar to that found in people with normal renal function, but the volume of distribution is much greater. To maintain a peak plasma gentamicin concentration of 6–8 mg/L, a much larger dose would have to be administered at a dosing interval of 6 or 8 hours. Using the multiple-dose infusion equation from Lesson 5 (see **Equation 5-1**), we would find that a dose as high as 220 mg given every 6 hours would be necessary to achieve the desired plasma concentrations.

On the other hand, we would expect patients with impaired renal function to have a lower creatinine clearance and therefore a smaller elimination rate constant compared to patients with normal renal function. A smaller than normal elimination rate constant would produce a longer half-life and would require an increase in the dosage interval.

In patients with both impaired renal function and abnormal volume of distribution values, the dose and dosing interval should be adjusted accordingly.

Just as renal dysfunction may alter the dosage requirement for drugs eliminated renally, hepatic dysfunction alters the dosage requirement for hepatically metabolized or excreted drugs. For example, the daily dose of theophylline must be reduced in patients with liver dysfunction. With this agent, however, a consistent plasma concentration (as opposed to a large difference in peak and trough plasma concentrations) is desired. Therefore, with liver dysfunction, smaller doses of theophylline than usual are generally administered but at the usual dosage intervals (two to four times daily). For a continuous intravenous infusion, the infusion rate must be reduced.

Genetic Factors and Pharmacogenomics

Pharmacogenomics is the study of how genes affect an individual's response to drugs. Polymorphic expression of abnormal gene sequences (polymorphism) can be a major variable in an individual patient's pharmacokinetic/pharmacodynamic response to drug therapy.

There are many examples of differences in response to drugs and adverse drug reactions due to variation in a patient's genetic sequence. These sequence variations can affect enzymes responsible for drug metabolism, drug targets, and drug transporters, all of which will lead to deviation in absorption, distribution, metabolism, and elimination. With isoniazid, for example, there are two distinct subsets of the population with differences in isoniazid elimination (Figure 11-2) The elimination of isoniazid is said to exhibit a bimodal pattern. This difference in clearance is caused by genetically controlled differences in hepatic microsomal enzyme production. Likewise, genetic differences in drug elimination also have been observed for hydralazine, warfarin, and phenylbutazone. More recently, polymorphism has been observed in some patients associated with decreased expression of P-glycoprotein (a drug transporter in the duodenum). In these patients, the bioavailability of P-glycoprotein substrates, such as digoxin, is greatly increased, and, therefore, a decrease in dose may be required.[1]

Many variants have also been observed in the cytochrome P450 enzyme system. These variations can cause different responses to drugs metabolized by the CYP450 enzyme system. For example, poor CYP2D6 metabolizers have been found to have elevated fluoxetine levels, and poor CYP2C19 metabolizers were found to have an increased incidence of fluoxetine adverse effects.[2]

Pharmacogenomic research is still in progress. Many sequence variations have currently been observed, but there are countless polymorphisms left to be discovered. By applying pharmacogenomic findings to drug therapy, we are able to maximize a patient's response to a drug while minimizing the patient's toxicity.

Obesity

Obesity alters drug pharmacokinetics. Because obesity is common in our society, it is an important source of pharmacokinetic variation. With obesity, the ratio of body fat to lean tissue is greater than in non-obese patients. Fat tissue contains less water than does lean tissue, so the amount of body water per kilogram of total body weight is less in the obese person than in the non-obese person.

For some drugs, alterations in body makeup that accompany obesity require changes in drug dosages. Drugs that are lipophilic (such as thiopental) and distribute well into fat tissues must often be given in larger doses to achieve the desired effects. Drugs that distribute primarily in extracellular fluids (such as the aminoglycosides) may be given in higher absolute doses to the obese person, but the overall milligram per kilogram dose will be lower. The morbidly obese person who is twice ideal body weight will have an aminoglycoside volume of distribution that is approximately 1.4 times greater than a person of ideal body weight.[3]

Other Factors

Many other factors may affect drug pharmacokinetics, including pregnancy and drug interactions. Specific changes in pharmacokinetics during pregnancy include increased renal drug clearance, alterations in volume of distribution, and changes in plasma protein binding. Another example of an effect on pharmacokinetics is the histamine-2 blocker cimetidine, which inhibits the hepatic enzymes that metabolize theophylline, thereby decreasing theophylline clearance. When evaluating drug pharmacokinetics in an individual patient, the clinician must consider the many factors that may cause variations from the expected.

POTENTIAL SOURCES OF ERROR IN THE COLLECTION AND ASSAY OF BIOLOGIC SAMPLES

Pharmacokinetic calculations depend greatly on the validity of the reported drug concentration from a bio-

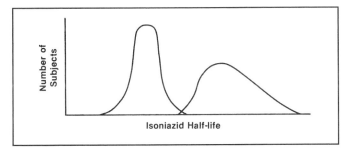

FIGURE 11-2.
Bimodal distribution for isoniazid half-life.

logic sample (e.g., blood, serum, or plasma). Using incorrect concentration values to calculate dosages can result in subtherapeutic or supratherapeutic (i.e., toxic) drug concentrations. Inaccurate concentration values can result from incorrect drug sampling or assay procedures. To ensure that drug concentrations are valid, several factors should be considered:

- proper laboratory sample collection and handling,
- physiochemical factors affecting assay accuracy,
- proper laboratory instrument calibration and controls check, and
- proper drug administration and sample timing.

Sample Collection and Handling

To measure drug concentrations, whole blood is usually collected in a blood collection tube called a *serum separator tube* (SST). The SST contains a gel barrier that separates the fluid portion of blood from the solid portion. After collection, the blood is first allowed to clot, which takes approximately 30 minutes, and is then centrifuged for at least 15 minutes to separate the solid components of the blood (blood cells, fibrin, fibrinogen, etc.) from the fluid component. This fluid component is then called *serum*. If whole blood is centrifuged before it clots, then only the blood cells are separated from the fluid component, which is then called *plasma* (Figure 11-3).

Most assays of therapeutically monitored drugs are performed on serum, hence the term *serum drug concentration*. However, the operations manual of specific assay instruments often indicate whether a particular drug

may be tested using plasma or serum. Most instruments allow the use of either serum or plasma.

The assay should be performed within 24 hours of sample collection. If this is not possible, refrigerate the sample (at 2–6°C) until the assay can be performed.

If plastic or glass SSTs are used, it is important to ensure that the drug to be assayed is not affected (i.e., absorbed or adsorbed) by the polymeric gel barrier used to separate the plasma from the cells. The composition of this barrier depends on the brand of SST used. The barriers are usually made of acrylic, silicon, or polyester polymers, and though they are generally chemically inert, they can absorb or adsorb to the drug being tested.

The degree of absorption or adsorption depends on the hydrophilicity of the drug, the type of barrier used in the SST, the amount of contact time, and the volume of the plasma sample. For example, decreases ranging from 6 to 64% were reported in measured concentrations of phenytoin, phenobarbital, lidocaine, quinidine, and carbamazepine when plasma was stored in Vacutainer SST collection tubes.[4] Adsorption or absorption of drug to the SST barrier is of particular concern when small sample volumes are used (e.g., in pediatric patients) or prolonged storage times are required.

Physicochemical Factors Affecting Assay Accuracy

Most commercially available drug assay methods are immunoassays that use an antibody specific for binding sites only on the drug to be assayed. Various detection methods, such as fluorescence polarization with instruments such as Abbott Diagnostics' TDX/FLEX/ADX and other instruments, are used to quantitate the amount of drug present. These assays can detect the presence of drug at very low concentrations (i.e., microgram or nanogram amounts).

Several assay-specific factors, listed in the assay kit package insert, can aid in the clinical interpretation of a plasma drug concentration.

Lower Limit of Drug Detection

The lower limit of drug detection indicates the lowest drug concentration that the assay can reliably report. This is a function of the particular assay instrument and is called *assay sensitivity*. Assay sensitivity is the lowest measurable drug concentration that can be distinguished from zero with 95% confidence. Plasma drug concentrations lower than this concentration should be reported as less than this value.

Upper Limit of Drug Detection

The upper limit of drug detection indicates the highest drug concentration that can be accurately measured.

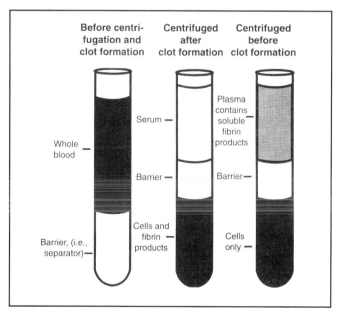

FIGURE 11-3.
Blood products.

Plasma drug concentrations above the upper limit will often be reported as higher than this value. If this occurs, assay parameters can be adjusted to increase the dilution volume of the plasma sample, thus allowing higher drug concentrations to be measured.

Assay Interference

Assay interferences are generally categorized as *cross-reactivity* and *physiologic interferences*. The degree of cross-reactivity with other structurally similar compounds is called *assay specificity*. Cross-reactivity is a function of the specificity of the antibody used to bind to the drug. Often, this antibody will also at least partially bind to other compounds that are structurally related to the desired analyte, such as metabolites and chemical analogues of the analyte.

For example, gentamicin assays cross-react with netilmicin, and amikacin assays cross-react with kanamycin; however, gentamicin and tobramycin assays do not generally cross-react. In addition, patients with impaired renal function that are receiving vancomycin have been shown to accumulate a vancomycin metabolite called *vancomycin crystalline degradation product 1* (CDP-1). CDP-1 cross-reacts with vancomycin when assayed using the TDx/TDxFLx instruments from Abbott Diagnostics. According to the TDx/TDxFLx package insert, a method to overcome the cross-reactivity of vancomycin and CDP-1 has not been discovered; therefore, clinicians must be aware of this potential for cross-reactivity. Physiologic substances in the patient's sample may also interfere with the assay. Examples include excess amounts of bilirubin, hemoglobin (i.e., hemolyzed sample), protein, and triglycerides. Plasma drug concentrations are usually not affected by such interferences.

■ CLINICAL CORRELATE

Ask your laboratory's clinical chemistry department for copies of the assay kit package inserts for all drugs that they assay in-house. These inserts will provide useful information, such as the upper and lower limits of assay sensitivity, as well as interfering and cross-reacting substances.

Instrument Calibration and Controls Check

Each drug assay should be calibrated to establish a linear relationship between drug concentration and the instrument's detection method. Calibration of the assay is an automatic process of measuring and plotting different known drug concentrations (i.e., calibrators) based on the instrument's method of detection and measurement. Most assay instruments use some type of spectro-

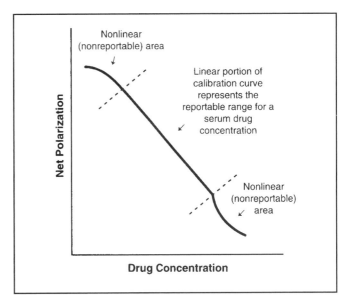

FIGURE 11-4.
Drug concentration versus net polarization.

photometric measurement unit, such as fluorescence polarization with Abbott's TDX instrument. Figure 11-4 is a plot of drug concentration versus the instrument's detection measure (polarization), showing the linear relationship between concentration and polarization. Note that the calibration curve is not linear at very high and very low drug concentrations.

Once this calibration plot or curve is stored in the instrument's software, other unknown drug concentrations (i.e., patient samples) can be accurately determined from this plot. As a quality control check, at least two different known concentrations (control values) should be tested for each drug assay per working shift. If these control values are out of range, as defined per individual laboratory standards, then this assay should be recalibrated and measurement of the patient's plasma drug concentration repeated.

Drug Administration and Sample Timing

To accurately assess drug concentration data and make dosing recommendations, it is important to be aware of administration and sampling factors that may affect the reported drug concentrations. First, drug administration times should be documented, noting any deviations from the recommended dosing schedule. Second, sampling times should be carefully noted so that adjustments can be made in dosage calculations if necessary. Third, it is important to note any other medications the patient is receiving. Occasionally, a patient's sample will contain two drugs, one of which can inactivate the other, particularly if both drugs are infused concomitantly, the sample is taken while the interfering drug is infusing, or a sample containing both drugs is stored at room temperature for a prolonged period.

A good example is the *in vitro* inactivation of the aminoglycosides by penicillins. Cephalosporins have not been shown to inactivate aminoglycosides.[5] Penicillins and aminoglycosides form a chemical complex that is not detected by commercially available drug assays.[6] This *in vitro* inactivation results in a falsely low plasma drug concentration report, which can in turn result in an unnecessary dosage increase. Quantitatively, the aminoglycoside concentration can decline to less than 10% of its original concentration within 24 hours of the beginning of this reaction. These reactions are time and temperature dependent. Refrigerating the sample slows the inactivation process, and freezing the sample stops it completely. To avoid the inactivation process, it is important to adjust the administration times to avoid concomitant infusions of aminoglycosides and penicillins. Drawing a plasma aminoglycoside concentration during infusion of the penicillin should be avoided as well.

 ## CLINICAL CORRELATE

When assaying the concentration of an aminoglycoside from a patient who is concomitantly receiving a penicillin, the laboratory must perform the assay immediately or freeze the sample. Freezing the sample instantly stops the *in vitro* inactivation of the aminoglycoside by the penicillin, whereas refrigerating the sample only slows down this degradation reaction. If the assay is not performed immediately the aminoglycoside level from the assay will be lower than the patient's actual serum aminoglycoside level.

MODEL-INDEPENDENT RELATIONSHIPS

Until now, we have used a major assumption in constructing models for drug pharmacokinetics: that drug clearance remains constant with any size dose. Drug clearance remains constant for small or large doses when drug elimination processes are first order (as described in previous lessons). With a first-order elimination process, as the dose of drug increases the plasma concentrations observed and the area under the plasma drug concentration versus time curve (AUC) increase proportionally. That is, if the dose is doubled, the plasma concentration and AUC also double.

Throughout this self-instructional course, we have emphasized the mathematical relationships of specific pharmacokinetic compartmental models (e.g., one- or two-compartment model after an intravenous bolus or oral dose administration). This lesson reviews several pharmacokinetic parameters that are derived without the assumption of a specific model.

The primary purpose of rigorous pharmacokinetic data analysis, compartmental or model-independent, is to determine the pharmacokinetic parameters useful in dosing drugs for patients. Consequently, multiple plasma drug concentrations are obtained at specific time points in healthy and diseased persons to assess a drug's population pharmacokinetic parameters. In clinical practice, it may be difficult to obtain multiple plasma samples after the first dose to determine a patient's pharmacokinetic parameters. Consequently, clinicians use population parameters from the literature to make individual patient dosage calculations.

Model-independent pharmacokinetic data analysis provides the opportunity to obtain pharmacokinetic values that do not depend on a compartmental model. Total body clearance, mean residence time (MRT), volume of distribution at steady state, and formation clearance are four of the most frequently used model-independent parameters and are the focus of this section.

The use of model-independent data analysis techniques to generate model-independent parameters offers several advantages over traditional compartmental approaches. First, it is not necessary to assume a compartmental model. Many drugs possess complex distribution patterns requiring two, three, or more exponential terms to describe their elimination. As the number of exponential terms increases, a compartmental analysis requires more intensive blood sampling and rigorous data calculations. Second, several drugs (e.g., gentamicin) can be described by one, two, or more distribution compartments, depending on the characteristics of the patients evaluated or the aggressiveness of the blood sampling. Therefore, a compartmental approach would require that pharmacokinetic parameters be obtained for each distribution pattern, making it difficult to compare one data set to another. Third, calculations are generally easier with model-independent relationships and do not require a computer with sophisticated software.

One drawback of using model-independent parameters is the inability to visualize or predict plasma concentration versus time profiles. This may result in the loss of specific information that provides important insight regarding drug disposition.

Like compartmental pharmacokinetic data analysis, the main purpose of assessing plasma concentration versus time data with model-independent relationships is to determine useful pharmacokinetic parameters. These parameters are usually, but not always, obtained from serial plasma concentration determinations after a single intravenous bolus or oral dose of a drug.

In practice, total body clearance and apparent volume of distribution are the two most important pharmacokinetic parameters because they facilitate the calculation of maintenance and loading dose regimens, respectively.

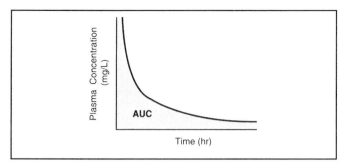

FIGURE 11-5.
Concentration versus time profile after a single intravenous dose. AUC = area under the plasma drug concentration versus time curve.

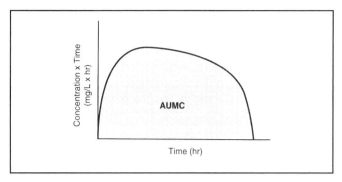

FIGURE 11-6.
Concentration × time versus time curve. AUMC = area under the first moment curve.

Understanding the effect that disease, altered physiologic state, or drug–drug interaction may have on these pharmacokinetic parameters is important in applying these principles to clinical practice. AUC and area under the first moment curve (AUMC) are two tools used to calculate most model-independent parameters. AUC and AUMC are discussed in the next section.

Total Body Clearance

Total body clearance (Cl_t) is the most important pharmacokinetic parameter because it relates the dosing rate of a drug to its steady-state concentration. It is usually used to calculate a maintenance-dosing regimen. An estimate of Cl_t for a drug is usually obtained after a single intravenous bolus dose (Figure 11-5). Total body clearance is calculated with the following equation:

$$Cl_t = \frac{X_0}{AUC_{0 \to \infty}}$$

(See **Equation 3-5**.)
where:
X_0 = drug dose, and
$AUC_{\to \infty}$ = area under the concentration versus time curve from time zero to infinity.

This is a model-independent relationship because calculations do not depend on a specific compartmental model. In other words, we only need the dose and the $AUC_{0 \to \infty}$ to calculate total body clearance. Because the dose is known, a determination of the $AUC_{\to \infty}$ is all that is needed.

As you can see from Figure 11-6, the trapezoidal rule applies only to drugs whose clearance is constant with respect to dose and does not apply to drugs whose clearance is nonlinear. Remember, the trapezoidal rule is a model-independent approach used to directly calculate the AUC of the drug from time zero

to the time point that coincides with the last measured plasma concentration value (t_{last}). However, because AUC must include all of the area from zero to infinity after a single intravenous bolus dose, an estimate of the area between t_{last} and infinity is needed. This terminal area can be easily obtained by the following equation:

$$\text{terminal area} = \frac{C_{last}}{\lambda}$$

where:
C_{last} = last measured plasma concentration, and
λ = terminal elimination rate constant.

Two key assumptions in estimating this terminal AUC are that you have a reliable estimate of the terminal elimination rate constant (i.e., slope) and that this value remains constant between t_{last} and infinity.

To determine several model-independent relationships, such as MRT and volume of distribution at steady state, it is important to understand how to calculate the AUMC. The AUMC is the "area under the drug concentration versus time" versus "time" curve. The AUMC is generated with the AUC data from the concentration versus time profile for a single intravenous bolus dose (see Figure 11-5).

To calculate AUMC after a single intravenous bolus dose of a drug, it is necessary to collect serial drug plasma concentrations over time, determine concentration × time for each plasma concentration, and plot these values versus time on graph paper (see Figure 11-6).

As you can see from Figure 11-6, the shape of the [concentration × time] versus time curve is very different from the drug plasma concentration (C) versus time (t) plot used to calculate AUC. The trapezoidal rule can be used to calculate AUMC. Following a plot as in Figure 11-6, a series of straight lines can be drawn from the concentration × time point to its accompanying time value on the x-axis, forming individual trapezoids (Fig-

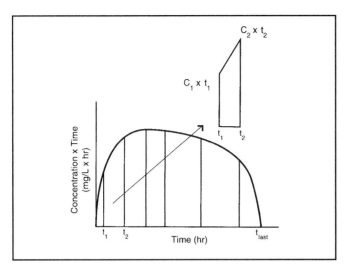

FIGURE 11-7.
Concentration × time versus time curve with trapezoids.

ure 11-7). The area of each trapezoid is calculated with the following equation:

$$\text{area of trapezoid} = \frac{(C_2 \times t_2) + (C_1 \times t_1)}{2}(t_2 - t_1)$$

The sum of all the trapezoidal areas yields an estimate of the AUMC from time zero to the last observed time point. As in calculating AUC, it is important to obtain AUMC from time zero to infinity. Consequently, the terminal area, which includes the portion of the curve from t_{last} to infinity, must be estimated. Assuming the terminal elimination slope remains constant over this time period, the terminal area is calculated with the following equation:

$$\text{terminal area} = \frac{(C_{\text{last}} \times t_{\text{last}})}{\lambda} + \frac{C_{\text{last}}}{\lambda^2}$$

where:
  C_{last} = last observed plasma concentration,
  t_{last} = time of the last observed plasma concentration, and
  λ = terminal elimination rate constant from the concentration versus time curve. λ is used here (instead of K) to indicate that this represents elimination in a model-independent or noncompartmental analysis.

Mean Residence Time

MRT is defined as the average time intact drug molecules transit or reside in the body. For a population of drug molecules, individual molecules spend different times within the body. Following the principles of statistical probability, specific drug molecules may be eliminated quickly whereas others may remain in the body

much longer. Consequently, a distribution of transit times can be characterized by a mean value. In other words, elimination of a drug can be thought of as a random process. Residence time reflects how long a particular drug molecule remains or resides in the body. The MRT reflects the overall behavior of a large number of drug molecules. This parameter is not used frequently in clinical practice to monitor patients. However, it is useful when comparing the effect of disease, altered physiologic state, or drug–drug interaction on the pharmacokinetics of a specific drug. MRT can be calculated with the following equation:

$$\text{MRT} = \frac{\text{AUMC}_{0 \to \infty}}{\text{AUC}_{0 \to \infty}}$$

Volume of Distribution at Steady State

Volume of distribution at steady state (V_{ss}) is a parameter that relates total amount of drug in the body to a particular plasma concentration after a single dose. This parameter is not affected by changes in drug elimination or clearance, making it a useful tool in assessing the effect disease, altered physiologic state, or drug–drug interaction may have on the volume of distribution of a drug. V_{ss} was calculated previously but was only applicable to a drug fitting a two-compartment model. The following equation for V_{ss} does not depend on the model used to describe drug distribution or elimination from the body:

$$V_{ss} = \text{MRT} \times Cl_t$$

And since:

$$\text{MRT} = \frac{\text{AUMC}_{0 \to \infty}}{\text{AUC}_{0 \to \infty}} \quad \text{and} \quad Cl_t = \frac{X_0}{\text{AUC}_{0 \to \infty}}$$

then:

$$V_{ss} = \frac{X_0 \times \text{AUMC}_{0 \to \infty}}{(\text{AUC}_{0 \to \infty})^2}$$

Formation Clearance

Formation clearance ($Cl_{P \to mX}$) is a model-independent parameter that provides a meaningful estimate of the portion of the total body clearance that is accounted for by production of a specific metabolite. Formation clearance is analogous to systemic and renal clearance of a drug and refers to the formation of metabolites in the course of drug elimination. This parameter is not used to individualize a patient's drug dosing regimen but is useful when assessing the impact that a specific drug treatment, disease, or altered physiologic state may have on a specific metabolic pathway of a drug. The following equations are used to calculate the formation clearance of a drug:

$$Cl_{P \to m1} = F_{m1} Cl_t$$

where:

$Cl_{P \to m1}$ = fractional clearance of the parent drug (P) to form metabolite 1 (m_1),

F_{m1} = fraction of metabolite m_1 formed from a single dose of the parent drug, and

Cl_t = total body clearance.

Or:

$$Cl_{P \to m1} = \frac{m_{1,u}}{X_0} \times \frac{X_0}{AUC_{0 \to \infty}}$$

$$= \frac{m_{1,u}}{AUC_{0 \to \infty}}$$

where:

$m_{1,u}$ = amount of metabolite m_1 excreted in the urine.

For example, if a drug is metabolized by three separate enzyme systems, each producing a unique metabolite, what effect would the addition of a known hepatic enzyme inducer have on the individual metabolic pathways? Figure 11-8 provides a visual perspective of this situation.

To simplify this example, we will assume that systemic clearance equals hepatic clearance, these three metabolic pathways account for 100% of the hepatic clearance of the drug, the metabolite is rapidly secreted unchanged in the urine, and the dose is equal to 100 mg. Table 11-1 shows the effect of an enzyme inducer on each metabolic pathway portrayed in Figure 11-8 as shown by changes in the percentage of drug dose excreted in the urine for each metabolite and formation clearance.

As Table 11-1 shows, the administration of an enzyme inducer substantially increased the systemic clearance of this drug, from 25 to 75 mL/minute. However, the change in the percentage of the dose excreted as a spe-

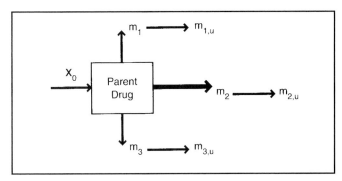

FIGURE 11-8.

Metabolic pathways for a parent drug, where m_1 = metabolite 1, $m_{1,u}$ = amount of m_1 excreted in the urine, m_2 = metabolite 2, $m_{2,u}$ = amount of m_2 excreted in the urine, and m_3 = metabolite 3, $m_{3,u}$ = amount of m_3 excreted in the urine.

cific metabolite does not exactly reflect the change in formation clearance values. The percentage of dose excreted in the urine for m_1 was reduced threefold, but no change in the formation clearance was observed. This means that the enzyme inducer had no effect on the enzyme responsible for producing m_1.

On the other hand, treatment with the enzyme inducer produced only a 1.3-fold increase in the percentage of the dose excreted in the urine for m_2 but a fourfold increase in its formation clearance. Finally, the percentage of dose excreted in urine for m_3 was unchanged despite a threefold increase in its formation clearance. Because the formation clearance of a drug to a metabolite reflects more accurately the activity of that specific enzyme, the data would suggest that the enzyme(s) responsible for the formation of m_2 and m_3 are significantly increased by the enzyme inducer, whereas the enzyme(s) responsible for the formation of m_1 was unaffected. The preceding example demonstrates the value of formation clearance versus the more traditional approach of calculating the percentage of a drug dose excreted as a specific metabolite.

TABLE 11-1.
Changes in Formation Clearance of Three Metabolites as a Result of Enzyme Induction

	Metabolite	Percentage of Dose Excreted in Urine	Formation Clearance (mL/minute)
Control (Cl_t = 25 mL/minute)	m_1	20.0	5.0
	m_2	50.0	12.5
	m_3	30.0	7.5
Enzyme induction (Cl_t = 75 mL/minute)	m_1	6.7	5.0
	m_2	63.3	47.5
	m_3	30.0	22.5

REFERENCES

1. Evans WE, McLeod HL. Pharamacogenomics—Drug disposition, drug targets, and side effects. *N Engl J Med* 2003;348 (6):538–47.

2. Mancana D, Kerewin RW. Role of pharmacogenomics in individualising treatment with SSRIs. *CNS Drugs* 2003: 17(3):143–51.

3. Bauer LA, Blouin RA, Griffin WO, et al. Amikacin pharmacokinetics in morbidly obese patients. *Am J Hosp Pharm* 1980;37:519–22.

4. Dasgupta A, Dean R, Saldana S, et al. Absorption of therapeutic drugs by barrier gels in serum separator blood collection devices. *Am J Clin Pathol* 1994;101:456–61.

5. Spruill WJ, McCall CY, Francisco GE. In vitro inactivation of tobramycin by cephalosporins. *Am J Hosp Pharm* 1985;42:2506–9.

6. Riff LF, Jackson GG. Laboratory and clinical conditions for gentamicin inactivation by carbenicillin. *Arch Intern Med* 1972;130:887–91.

■ Review Questions

11-1. The proportion of total body weight that is water is lowest in:

A. healthy adults.

B. neonates.

C. elderly.

D. teenagers.

11-2. With dysfunction of the major organs of drug elimination (kidneys and liver), drug clearance, volume of distribution, and drug plasma protein binding may be affected.

A. True

B. False

11-3. For drugs that distribute primarily in extracellular fluid, a dose for an obese person should be calculated using total body weight.

A. True

B. False

11-4. The fluid portion of a sample of whole blood allowed to clot for 30 minutes before centrifugation is called:

A. serum.

B. plasma.

C. serous fluid.

D. citrated blood.

11-5. The fluid portion of whole blood centrifuged before clot formation is called:

A. serum.

B. plasma.

C. serous fluid.

D. citrated blood.

11-6. *Assay cross-reactivity* refers to diminished assay performance caused by:

A. physiologic substances found in some patients' plasma that directly affect the assay itself.

B. structurally related drug compounds or metabolites for which the assay method measures as if they were the desired assay compound.

C. an *in vitro* inactivation of one drug by another drug that is also present in the patient's plasma.

D. none of the above.

Indicate *Yes* or *No* for questions 11-7 through 11-10:

Yes = the accuracy of the drug concentrations is of concern and should be redrawn.

No = the accuracy of the drug concentrations is not of particular concern.

11-7. A gentamicin concentration from a sample stored at controlled room temperature and assayed 24 hours after it was collected from a patient receiving both ampicillin and gentamicin.

A. Yes

B. No

11-8. A plasma tobramycin concentration from a sample stored at controlled room temperature and assayed 24 hours after it was collected from a patient receiving both tobramycin and ceftazidime.

A. Yes

B. No

11-9. A plasma gentamicin concentration from a sample stored in a freezer until assayed 12 hours after it was collected from a patient receiving both ampicillin and gentamicin.

A. Yes

B. No

11-10. A plasma gentamicin concentration from a sample assayed immediately after it was collected from a patient receiving both piperacillin and gentamicin.

A. Yes

B. No

11-11. The trapezoidal rule can be used to calculate AUC for model-independent relationships.

A. True

B. False

11-12. The ratio of $AUMC_{\to\infty}$ to $AUC_{\to\infty}$ is called:

A. trapezoidal rule.

B. total body clearance.

C. mean residence time.

D. formation clearance.

11-13. Which statement(s) is/are *false* about the calculation of formation clearance ($Cl_{P \to mX}$)? Formation clearance can be used to calculate the

    A. clearance rate of individual metabolites of a drug.

    B. mean residence time

    C. total body clearance of a drug that has multiple metabolites.

    D. A and C.

Answers

11-1. A, B, D. Incorrect answers

    C. CORRECT ANSWER. The proportion of the body that is water is greatest in the neonate and lowest in the elderly.

11-2. A. CORRECT ANSWER. Major organ dysfunction can affect most pharmacokinetic parameters

    B. Incorrect answer

11-3. A. Incorrect answer

    B. CORRECT ANSWER. The proportion of fat tissue that is extracellular fluid is less than in lean tissue, but the drug will still distribute somewhat in the adipose extracellular fluid.

11-4. A. CORRECT ANSWER

    B. Incorrect answer. Plasma contains clotting factors.

    C. Incorrect answer. Serous fluid is a natural body fluid and is not centrifuged to remove cellular components.

    D. Incorrect answer. Citrated blood contains citrate additives that keep the blood from clotting.

11-5. A. Incorrect answer. Serum does not contain clotting factors.

    B. CORRECT ANSWER.

    C. Incorrect answer. Serous fluid is a natural body fluid and is not centrifuged to remove cellular components.

    D. Incorrect answer. Citrated blood contains citrate additives that keep the blood from clotting.

11-6. A. Incorrect answer. This is assay interference.

    B. CORRECT ANSWER

    C. Incorrect answer. Assay cross-reactivity does not involve assay measurement of inactivated products that result from some physiochemical process.

    D. Incorrect answer

11-7. A. CORRECT ANSWER. Ampicillin will inactivate gentamicin *in vitro*.

    B. Incorrect answer

11-8. A. Incorrect answer

    B. CORRECT ANSWER. Aminoglycosides are not inactivated by cephalosporins, just penicillins.

11-9. A. Incorrect answer

    B. CORRECT ANSWER. Freezing this sample will stop inactivation from occurring.

11-10. A. Incorrect answer

    B. CORRECT ANSWER. Inactivation does not have time to occur if you assay the sample immediately.

11-11. A. CORRECT ANSWER. The trapezoidal rule is a model independent method for AUC calculation.

    B. Incorrect answer

11-12. A. Incorrect answer. Trapezoidal rule is a method to calculate AUC.

    B. Incorrect answer. Total body clearance is $X_0/AUC_{0 \to \infty}$.

    C. CORRECT ANSWER

    D. Incorrect answer. Formation clearance is a calculation of metabolite clearance.

11-13. A, C, and D are all incorrect.

    B. CORRECT ANSWER. MRT is calculated using AUC and AUMC.

Discussion Points

D-1. Write a pharmacy protocol to ensure proper serum drug concentration collection and assay.

D-2. Try to get a package insert from your laboratory on any therapeutically monitored drug. Describe the type of information found. Specifically, how are the issues of assay sensitivity, specificity, and cross-reactivity noted?

Practice Set 3

Definitions of symbols and key equations are:

AUC = area under plasma concentration versus time curve

F = fraction of drug reaching systemic circulation

Cl_t = total drug clearance from body = dose/AUC

K_a = absorption rate constant

The following applies to questions PS3-1 to 3-4. The relative bioavailabilities of two dosage forms (a sustained-release tablet and an oral solution) of oral morphine sulfate are being compared. The following plasma drug concentrations were obtained after 30 mg of each was administered:

Concentration (mg/L)

Time after Dose (hours)	Sustained-Release Tablet	Oral Solution
0	0	0
0.5	2.26	19.80
1.0	4.57	18.31
1.5	5.27	15.49
2.0	6.73	12.37
3.0	7.36	9.62
4.0	7.40	6.85
5.0	7.50	5.52
6.0	6.24	3.10
8.0	4.70	1.79
12.0	2.76	1.58

Before proceeding to the questions below, on graph paper (linear), plot the plasma drug concentration versus time data for the two formulations.

QUESTIONS

PS3-1. What is the $AUC_{0-12\ hr}$ for the oral tablet formulation (using the trapezoidal method)?

A. 7.25 (mg/L) × hour

B. 71.25 (mg/L) × hour

C. 62.34 (mg/L) × hour

D. 64.51 (mg/L) × hour

PS3-2. What is the $AUC_{0-12\ hr}$ for the oral solution formulation (using the trapezoidal method)?

A. 6.25 (mg/L) × hour

B. 71.25 (mg/L) × hour

C. 47.42 (mg/L) × hour

D. 64.51 (mg/L) × hour

PS3-3. What are the peak plasma drug concentrations for the oral tablet and oral suspension, respectively?

A. 7.5 and 19.8 mg/L

B. 6.5 and 18.9 mg/L

C. 4.5 and 12.5 mg/L

D. 19.5 and 7.9 mg/L

PS3-4. Which product has greater bioavailability?

A. Oral solution

B. Oral tablet

The following applies to question PS3-5. A single oral dose (500 mg) of a sustained-release procainamide tablet was given, and the following plasma drug concentrations were determined:

Time after Dose (hours)	Plasma Drug Concentration (mg/L)
0	0
0.1	0.60
0.25	1.35
0.5	2.34
0.75	3.05
1.0	3.55
2.0	4.33
4.0	3.89
8.0	2.41
12.0	1.49

Before proceeding to question PS3-5, plot the concentration versus time data on semilog graph paper.

PS3-5. What is the absorption rate constant (K_a) of this formulation (using the method of residuals)?

    A. 2.1 hr^{-1}

    B. 1.2 hr^{-1}

    C. 2.5 hr^{-1}

    D. 3.2 hr^{-1}

ANSWERS

PS3-1. A, B, D. Incorrect answers

C. CORRECT ANSWER. Using the equation found in Figure 3-10,

$$\frac{(2.26+0)(0.5-0)}{2} = 0.56$$

$$\frac{(4.57+2.26)(1-0.5)}{2} = 1.71$$

$$\frac{(5.27+4.57)(1.5-1)}{2} = 2.46$$

$$\frac{(6.73+5.27)(2-1.5)}{2} = 3.00$$

$$\frac{(7.36+6.73)(3-2)}{2} = 7.05$$

$$\frac{(7.40+7.36)(4-3)}{2} = 7.38$$

$$\frac{(7.50+7.40)(5-4)}{2} = 7.45$$

$$\frac{(6.24+7.50)(6-5)}{2} = 6.87$$

$$\frac{(4.70+6.24)(8-6)}{2} = 10.94$$

$$\frac{(2.76+4.70)(12-8)}{2} = 14.92$$

$$+ \underline{}$$

$$= 62.34 \text{ (mg/L)} \times \text{hr}$$

PS3-2. A, C, D. Incorrect answers

B. CORRECT ANSWER. Using the equation found in Figure 3-10,

$$\frac{(0+19.80)(0.5-0)}{2} = 4.95$$

$$\frac{(18.31+19.80)(1-0.5)}{2} = 9.53$$

$$\frac{(15.49+18.31)(1.5-1)}{2} = 8.45$$

$$\frac{(12.37+15.49)(2-1.5)}{2} = 6.97$$

$$\frac{(9.62+12.37)(3-2)}{2} = 10.99$$

$$\frac{(6.85+9.62)(4-3)}{2} = 8.24$$

$$\frac{(5.52+6.85)(5-4)}{2} = 6.18$$

$$\frac{(3.10+5.52)(6-5)}{2} = 4.31$$

$$\frac{(1.79+3.10)(8-6)}{2} = 4.89$$

$$\frac{(1.59+1.79)(12-8)}{2} = 6.74$$

$$+ \underline{}$$

$$= 71.25 \text{ (mg/L)} \times \text{hr}$$

PS3-3. A. CORRECT ANSWER. Observe peak concentration from AUC plot.

B, C, D. Incorrect answers

PS3-4. A. CORRECT ANSWER. The oral tablet has a smaller AUC and therefore has a lower bioavailability than the oral solution.

B. Incorrect answer

PS3-5. A, C, D. Incorrect answers

B. CORRECT ANSWER. First, the data points at 4, 8, and 12 hours are on the straight-line terminal portion of the plot and therefore are not used to calculate the residual line. Next, the terminal, straight-line portion of the graph is back-extrapolated to the y-axis. For each time at which a concentration was actually determined, the concentration corresponding to the back-extrapolated line is noted (extrapolated concentration). The residual is the remainder of the actual concentration subtracted from the extrapolated concentration. The K_a is the negative slope of the natural log of the residual concentration versus time curve. We can choose any two residual points to determine the

slope, but it is usually best to select the points most widely separated by time. Therefore,

$$K_a = -\left(\frac{\Delta y}{\Delta x}\right) = \frac{\ln 5.57 - \ln 0.5}{0.1 \text{ hr} - 2.0 \text{ h}}$$

$$= -\left(\frac{1.72 - (-0.56)}{-1.9 \text{ hr}}\right)$$

$$= 1.20 \text{ hr}^{-1}$$

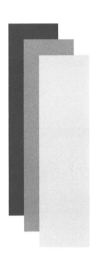

LESSON

12

Aminoglycosides

In this lesson, Cases 1–5 focus on the safe and appropriate dosing of aminoglycosides. Individualization of aminoglycoside dosing regimens is important to optimize efficacy while minimizing potential toxicity. Cases 1–4 outline traditional dosing methods of individualized dosing, and Case 5 focuses on the extended interval administration of aminoglycosides.

Because the currently available intravenous aminoglycosides (gentamicin, tobramycin, and amikacin) exhibit similar pharmacokinetics, case discussions of one aminoglycoside can be extrapolated to any other. Although amikacin has the same pharmacokinetic profile as other aminoglycosides, it requires doses and target concentrations approximately four times as high as the other aminoglycosides.

Several key points should be reviewed before beginning these cases. Aminoglycosides are excreted unchanged by renal glomerular filtration. Their elimination, therefore, is proportional to a patient's glomerular filtration rate (GFR), which can be estimated by determining creatinine clearance (CrCl). That is, we assume:

$$GFR = CrCl$$

CALCULATION OF MEASURED CREATININE CLEARANCE

To calculate aminoglycoside doses, we must measure or estimate the patient's creatinine clearance. The most accurate way to determine creatinine clearance is by direct measurement. Therefore, it is necessary to collect a 24-hour urine specimen. Then creatinine clearance is calculated:

$$CrCl = \frac{UV}{P \times 1440}$$

where:
 U = urinary creatinine concentration,

V = volume of urine collected,
P = plasma creatinine concentration (taken at midpoint of urine collection), and
1440 = number of minutes in 24 hours.

CALCULATION OF ESTIMATED CREATININE CLEARANCE

Sometimes it is impractical or impossible to collect a 24-hour urine specimen; creatinine clearance must then be estimated from serum creatinine. Although there are several formulas for estimating creatinine clearance, we use the Cockcroft–Gault equation[1]:

$$CrCl_{male} = \frac{(140 - age)IBW}{72 \times SCr} \text{ per } 1.73 \text{ m}^2 \text{ BSA}$$

(See **Equation 9-1**.)
or

$$CrCl_{female} = \frac{(0.85)(140 - age)IBW}{72 \times SCr} \text{ per } 1.73 \text{ m}^2 \text{ BSA}$$

where:
 CrCl = creatinine clearance (milliliters per minute per 1.73 m^2 body surface area [BSA]),
 age = patient's age (years),
 IBW = ideal body weight (kilograms) or adjusted body weight (AdjBW) in obese patients, and
 SCr = serum creatinine concentration (milligrams per deciliter).

■ CLINICAL CORRELATE

Note that in this formula creatinine clearance is expressed per 1.73 m^2 of BSA. However, this factor of 1.73 m^2 is commonly omitted when dosing aminoglycosides. Therefore, one should not divide the creatinine clearance value from either equation above by 1.73 m² to obtain a proper estimation of CrCl when dosing aminoglycosides.

This formula also requires the following patient data:

- IBW (lean body weight) or AdjBW,
- age,
- sex, and
- steady-state serum creatinine concentration.

Calculation of Ideal Body Weight or Adjusted Body Weight

Because creatinine is produced by muscle metabolism (and not by fat), we must use the patient's IBW or AdjBW when estimating creatinine clearance. The IBW for adult males can be estimated by:

IBW = 50 kg + 2.3 kg for each inch over 5 feet in height
(See **Equation 9-2**.)

The IBW for adult females is:

IBW = 45.5 kg + 2.3 kg for each inch over 5 feet in height (See **Equation 9-2**.)

In obese patients, the use of total body weight (TBW) overestimates creatinine clearance, and the use of IBW underestimates creatinine clearance. Consequently, AdjBW should be used. If a patient's TBW is more than 20% over IBW, then the AdjBW must be used to calculate creatinine clearance:

AdjBW = IBW + 0.4 (TBW − IBW) (See **Equation 9-3**.)

For a patient who weighs less than IBW, the actual body weight would be used.

■ *CLINICAL CORRELATE*

Close examination of the Cockcroft–Gault equation reveals that serum creatinine values less than 1 mg/dL greatly elevates the calculated creatinine clearance value. This is especially true for elderly patients, for whom unrealistically high creatinine clearance values may be calculated using this equation. The elderly often have reduced muscle mass as a fraction of TBW and so may generate less creatinine than a younger patient of similar weight. In this population, the serum creatinine value may not be an appropriate indicator of the patient's true renal function. It has been recommended to either round the low serum creatinine values up to 1 mg/dL before calculating creatinine clearance or round the final calculated creatinine clearance value down to 100 to 120 mL/minute or less. Although these recommended adjustments yield more accurate estimations, they still add error to the original creatinine clearance calculation.

ESTIMATING ELIMINATION RATE AND VOLUME OF DISTRIBUTION

To calculate an initial maintenance dose and dosing interval using traditional dosing methods, we must use population estimates for the elimination rate constant (K) and the volume of distribution (V). Population estimates of K are derived from small studies that correlate an aminoglycoside's clearance (and hence K) to the patient's creatinine clearance (Figure 12-1). Creatinine clearance and aminoglycoside clearance are not equal; some aminoglycoside is eliminated by organs other than the kidneys. When creatinine clearance is zero, the aminoglycoside clearance is still approximately 0.014 mL/minute, reflecting this nonrenal clearance and perhaps some active tubular secretion.

The equation for the line of best fit through these points can be used to estimate an elimination rate constant (K) for this sample of patients, as follows:

$$Y = mX + b$$

Or, for example, one commonly used regression equation is:

$$slope (K) = 0.00293 (CrCl) + 0.014$$

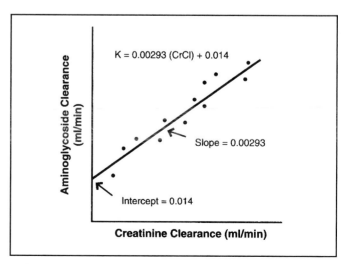

FIGURE 12-1.
Aminoglycoside clearance versus creatinine clearance.

where K is the elimination rate constant for aminoglycosides (population estimate). This equation will be used throughout the lesson for all aminoglycosides. These estimates also involve the appropriate calculations of creatinine clearance and IBW. Because many small-sample studies have been done to estimate K and V, there are many different estimates for both. We shall use:

⚠ $K = 0.00293 \, (CrCl) + 0.014$
12-1

⚠ $V = 0.24 \, L/kg \, (IBW)$
12-2

Approximately 10% of a given aminoglycoside dose distributes into adipose tissue. When calculating aminoglycoside volume of distribution, one can use either IBW or an $AdjBW_{AG}$ formula that reflects this 10% of distribution into adipose tissue as follows:

⚠ $AdjBW_{AG} = IBW + 0.1(TBW - IBW)$
12-3

Note that this adjustment is less than that used when calculating AdjBW for use in the creatinine clearance formula and is therefore rarely used.

▮ CLINICAL CORRELATE

These initial population estimates for K and V only represent a statistical best average estimate to begin with, and individual patient values can vary widely. Consequently, these estimated values should only be used to initiate a dose, and serum drug concentrations should be obtained as soon as possible to calculate patient-specific (i.e., actual) values for K and V.

▮ CLINICAL CORRELATE

Some clinicians would use the above K and V equations as initial population estimates for all aminoglycosides; however, other clinicians may use similar equations with slightly different numbers based on regression equations from other similar studies. Additionally, most clinicians will use the same estimates for all aminoglycosides; however, some will use slightly different equations for each aminoglycoside. We will use the above equation for all aminoglycosides as they are all excreted renally via the exact same mechanism.

▮ CLINICAL CORRELATE

The values for K and V represent population estimates of the elimination rate and volume of distribution, respectively, based on statistical averages with relatively large standard deviations. For this reason, it is important to obtain peaks and troughs after the initial dosing regimen is established to properly adjust the dosage and dosing interval based on the individual patient's specific pharmacokinetic data.

EXTENDED-INTERVAL AMINOGLYCOSIDE DOSING

Administering the total daily dose of aminoglycoside once daily, rather than in divided doses, is being used in attempts to improve efficacy and possibly reduce toxicity.[2] This type of dosing is referred to as *extended-interval* aminoglycoside dosing. Aminoglycosides have concentration-dependent bactericidal action—that is, larger doses can result in lower bacterial counts in the residual population and longer intervals before significant regrowth occurs.[3,4] Aminoglycosides also exhibit a relatively long post-antibiotic effect (PAE), defined as persistent suppression of bacterial growth despite residual drug concentrations below the minimal inhibitory concentration (MIC). The duration of the PAE is directly proportional to the maximum concentration (C_{peak}) of the aminoglycoside (i.e., the higher the C_{peak}, the longer the PAE).[5-7] In addition, the PAE lasts longer *in vivo* than *in vitro*,[8,9] is dependent on the bacterium studied, and increases in the presence of neutrophils.[10,11]

If consecutive doses of aminoglycosides are given before significant regrowth of bacteria occurs, the bactericidal effect of each dose accumulates, and the tissue is eventually cleared of the organism. If the dosing interval is too long, however, the bacterial count may rise in the latter portion of each dosing interval, and the effectiveness of the agent is diminished. The ability to prolong the dosing interval of antibiotics without loss of efficacy depends on several factors, including:

- effectiveness of host defenses;
- pharmacokinetics, such as the elimination rate of the drug; and
- pharmacodynamic effects of the drug.

The pharmacodynamic characteristics of aminoglycosides favor the use of large, single daily doses of aminoglycoside rather than equivalent dosage spread over the day.

Clinical studies of extended-interval dosing of aminoglycosides have shown little difference in efficacy or toxicity between the single and multiple daily dose regimens.[12-15] However, several questions about extended-interval dosing of aminoglycosides remain unanswered, and this dosing regimen may not be appropriate for all patients or for treatment of all infections.[16]

▇ CLINICAL CORRELATE

Extended-interval dosing of aminoglycosides has not been adequately studied in the elderly, obese, or pregnant populations. Moreover, this type of dosing has not been evaluated in patients with a creatinine clearance less than 20 mL/minute. Limited data are available for patients with certain diseases, such as endocarditis, osteomyelitis, and meningitis.

Traditional monitoring of peak and trough values in this type of dosing may have limited value because the optimal plasma concentrations have not yet been determined. Several alternatives for plasma concentration assessment have been used by investigators. The distribution phase of high-dose aminoglycoside therapy also has not been adequately studied, so the sampling and interpretation of peak concentrations may have limited clinical value. It has been postulated that higher extended-interval dosing may exhibit a longer distribution phase than smaller extended-interval doses. If the peak plasma concentration is drawn during this longer distribution phase, then the level may be inaccurate. Although peak plasma concentrations are not routinely monitored with extended-interval aminoglycoside dosing, trough levels or levels 18–20 hours after a dose may be measured to assure an aminoglycoside-free interval. The reader is referred to several literature reviews.[1-3,17-20]

Desired Aminoglycoside Plasma Concentrations

The traditional ranges for desired aminoglycoside plasma concentrations are a peak of 4–10 mg/L for gentamicin and tobramycin and 15–30 mg/L for amikacin, and a trough of less than 2 mg/L for gentamicin and tobramycin and less than 8 mg/L for amikacin. For extended-interval administration, the dose is typically 4–7 mg/kg actual body weight for gentamicin and tobramycin, and peak concentrations will usually be above these ranges. Attainment of adequate peak concentrations is related to efficacy for some infections, and a low trough concentration may minimize the risk of nephrotoxicity and ototoxicity. For extended-interval dosing, the goal is to provide a higher ratio of the peak concentration to the MIC of the bacteria (C_{peak}: MIC). These desired concentrations are often modified based on patient-specific variables or pathogen susceptibility.

CASE 1

A 59-year-old white man, TM, is hospitalized for a ruptured colonic diverticulum that was surgically repaired. Before surgery, you are asked to begin this patient on an aminoglycoside. Other pertinent patient data include: height, 5 feet, 1 inch; weight, 55 kg; and serum creatinine, 1.3 mg/dL.

Problem 1A. Calculate an appropriate aminoglycoside maintenance dose, including the most appropriate dosing interval, for patient TM. Assume a desired C_{peak} of 6 mg/L and a C_{trough} of 1 mg/L.

Population values of K and V for the aminoglycosides should be used to estimate maintenance doses. A patient usually will receive a loading dose over 1 hour when therapy is initiated because a loading dose quickly brings aminoglycoside plasma concentration close to the desired therapeutic concentration. If a loading dose is not given, the patient's aminoglycoside concentration will not reach the desired concentration until steady state is achieved—in five drug half-lives.

Lessons 4 and 5 describe the mathematical models used for various multiple dose, intravenous, drug dosing situations. For aminoglycosides, which are usually given intravenously over 30–60 minutes at regular (i.e., intermittent) intervals, Lesson 5 describes the appropriate dosing equation. A quick review of Lessons 4 and 5 may help you understand the derivation of these equations.

Briefly, this equation is arrived at by taking the equation from Lesson 4 for a single intravenous bolus dose and adding the appropriate factors for the following:
- multiple doses,
- simultaneous drug administration and drug elimination,
- drug administration over 30–60 minutes instead of an intravenous bolus, and
- attainment of steady state (for simplicity, 1 hour is assumed for the drug administration time).

The equation is:

$$C_{peak(steady\ state)} = \frac{K_0(1-e^{-Kt})}{VK(1-e^{-K\tau})}$$

(See **Equation 5-1**.)

where:

$C_{peak(steady\ state)}$ = desired peak concentration at steady state (milligrams per liter),

K_0 = drug infusion rate (also maintenance dose you are trying to calculate, in milligrams per hour),

V = volume of distribution (population estimate for aminoglycoside in liters),

K = elimination rate constant (population estimate for aminoglycosides, in reciprocal hours),

t = infusion time (hours), and

τ = desired or most appropriate dosing interval (hours).

To solve this equation, we must:

1. Determine creatinine clearance (Cl_{Cr})
2. Insert population estimates for V and K.
3. Choose a desired C_{peak}, based on clinical and microbiologic data.
4. Determine our infusion time in hours.
5. Calculate an appropriate dosing interval (τ), as shown below.
6. Determine K_0 (maintenance dose in mg/hour)

To calculate an initial maintenance dose and dosing interval, we use the population estimates of K and V calculated from **Equations 12-1 and 12-2**:

$$K = 0.00293\ hr^{-1} \times creatinine\ clearance\ (in\ mL/minute) + 0.014$$

$$V = 0.24\ L/kg \times IBW$$

For patient TM, we can calculate the IBW:

$$IBW = 50 + 2.3\ kg\ per\ inch\ over\ 60\ inches$$

$$= 50 + 2.3\ (1) = 52.3\ kg$$

Estimated creatinine clearance (via the Cockcroft–Gault equation) is:

$$\begin{aligned} CrCl_{male} &= \frac{(140 - age)IBW}{72 \times SCr} \\ &= \frac{(140 - 59)\ 52}{72 \times 1.3} \\ &= 45\ mL/min \end{aligned}$$

Furthermore:

$$\begin{aligned} estimated\ K &= 0.00293\ (CrCl) + 0.014 \\ &= 0.00293\ (45) + 0.014 \\ &= 0.146\ hr^{-1} \end{aligned}$$

$$\begin{aligned} estimated\ T\tfrac{1}{2} &= 0.693\ /\ K\ (See\ \textbf{Equation 3-3}.) \\ &= 0.693\ /\ 0.146\ hr^{-1} \\ &= 4.75\ hours \end{aligned}$$

$$\begin{aligned} estimated\ V &= 0.24\ L/kg\ (IBW) \\ &= (0.24)\ (52) \\ &= 12.48\ L,\ rounded\ to\ 12.5\ L \end{aligned}$$

$$C_{peak(desired)} = 6\ mg/L$$

$$C_{trough(desired)} = 1\ mg/L$$

ESTIMATION OF BEST DOSING INTERVAL (τ)

The choice of dosing interval influences the C_{peak} and C_{trough} eventually obtained as well as the magnitude of the fluctuations in C_{peak} and C_{trough}. The equation below is used to determine the most appropriate dosing interval (τ) that will yield the desired C_{peak} and C_{trough}. As can be seen, this calculation is driven by the patient's elimination rate constant (K) and the C_{peak} and C_{trough} desired:

⚠ 12-4
$$\tau = \frac{1}{-K}(\ln C_{trough(desired)} - \ln C_{peak(desired)}) + t$$

where t is the duration of the infusion in hours. This equation can be used to evaluate several different C_{peak} and C_{trough} combinations to find an appropriate dosing interval.

DERIVATION OF ABOVE DOSING INTERVAL EQUATION

The above dosing interval equation comes from a simple rearrangement of the equation for K as shown below.

For a concentration versus time curve (following first-order elimination), the terminal slope equals $-K$ and:

$$-K = \frac{Y_2 - Y_1}{X_2 - X_1} = \frac{\ln C_{trough} - \ln C_{peak}}{\tau - t}$$

(See **Equation 3-1**.)

This equation can be rearranged to easily calculate τ as shown below:

Step 1. Rearrange the above equation and then solve for τ:

$$(-K)(\tau - t) = \ln C_{trough} - \ln C_{peak}$$

Step 2. Divide both sides by $-K$:

$$\tau - t = \frac{\ln C_{trough} - \ln C_{peak}}{-K}$$

Step 3. Transpose t to the right-hand side of the equation:

$$\tau = \frac{\ln C_{trough} - \ln C_{peak}}{-K} + t$$

Step 4. Rearrange:

$$\tau = \frac{1}{-K}(\ln C_{trough} - \ln C_{peak}) + t$$

Step 5. Further rearrange Step 4 by considering the rule of logarithms:

$$\log a - \log b = \log (a/b)$$

Therefore:

$$\tau = \frac{1}{-K}\ln\left[\frac{\text{trough}}{\text{peak}}\right] + t$$

The equation in either Steps 4 or 5 can be used to calculate the dosing interval (τ). You may find the equation in Step 5 easier to enter into a hand-held calculator.

Calculating the dosing interval with both equations (Steps 4 and 5) will serve as an added arithmetic check, because both methods should give the same answer.

CALCULATION OF BEST DOSING INTERVAL (τ) FOR PATIENT TM

For patient TM, the calculation of the dosing interval (τ, in hours) proceeds as follows if we want a C_{peak} of 6 mg/L and a C_{trough} of 1 mg/L:

$$\tau = \frac{1}{-K}(\ln C_{\text{trough(desired)}} - \ln C_{\text{peak(desired)}}) + t$$

$$= \frac{1}{-0.146}(\ln 1\text{ mg/L} - \ln 6\text{mg/L}) + 1\text{ hr}$$

$$= (-6.849)(0 - 1.79) + 1\text{ hr}$$

$$= (-6.849)(-1.79) + 1\text{ hr}$$

$$= 13.26\text{ hr}$$

At this point, we know that the best dosing interval to obtain our desired C_{peak} and C_{trough} concentrations is 13.26 hours. In practice, this number would be rounded down to 12 hours.

CALCULATION OF MAINTENANCE DOSE FOR TM

Next, we must determine the maintenance dose to be given at our desired interval of 12 hours. Note that in this example we are calculating the maintenance dose first and will use it to calculate the proper loading dose.

Once K and V have been estimated, the desired C_{peak} and C_{trough} concentrations determined, and τ calculated, these values can be substituted in our general equation and solved for K_0 (maintenance dose):

$$C_{\text{peak(steady state)}} = \frac{K_0(1-e^{-Kt})}{VK(1-e^{-K\tau})}$$

(See **Equation 5-1**.)
where:
$C_{\text{peak(steady state)}}$ = desired peak drug concentration at steady state (milligrams per liter),

K_0 = drug infusion rate (also maintenance dose you are trying to calculate, in milligrams per hour),
V = volume of distribution (population estimate for aminoglycosides, in liters),
K = elimination rate constant (population estimate for aminoglycosides, in reciprocal hours),
t = duration of infusion (hours), and
τ = desired or most appropriate dosing interval (hours).

Then:

$$6\text{ mg/L} = \frac{K_0(1 - e^{-0.146\text{ hr}^{-1}(1\text{ hr})})}{0.146\text{ hr}^{-1}(12.5)(1 - e^{-0.146\text{ hr}^{-1}(12\text{ hr})})}$$

$$= \frac{K_0(0.1358)}{(1.825)(0.8265)}$$

$$= K_0(0.0898)$$

$$66.7\text{ mg} = K_0$$

which would be given over 1 hour for an infusion rate (K_0) of 66.7 mg/hour.

Therefore, patient TM should receive 66.7 mg every 12 hours. In practice, the dose would be rounded to 70 mg every 12 hours. This amount is the initial estimated maintenance dose until C_{peak} and C_{trough} results are obtained. Because we have rounded the dose up from the calculated value of 66.7 to 70 mg, the actual $C_{\text{peak(steady state)}}$ will be slightly higher than our desired value of 6 mg/L. This actual $C_{\text{peak(steady state)}}$ can be determined via a simple ratio:

$$\text{desired level} \times \frac{\text{actual (rounded) dose}}{\text{calculated dose}} = \text{actual peak}$$

For this patient, the actual $C_{\text{peak(steady state)}}$ is calculated as follows:

$$6\text{ mg/L} \times \frac{70\text{ mg}}{66.7\text{ mg}} = 6.3\text{ mg/L}$$

Problem 1B. Calculate the C_{trough} concentration expected from the dose of 70 mg every 12 hours for patient TM.

The answer to this problem requires the use of another equation:

$$C = C_0e^{-Kt} \quad \text{(See **Equation 3-2**.)}$$

where:
C = drug concentration at time t,
C_0 = drug concentration at time zero or some earlier time, and

e^{-Kt} = fraction of original or previous concentration remaining at time t.

This general equation can be rewritten to show the calculation of patient TM's C_{trough} concentration after he receives his dose of 70 mg every 12 hours:

$$C_{trough(steady state)} = C_{peak(steady state)}\, e^{-Kt'}$$
(See **Equation 3-2**.)

where $t' = \tau$ – time of infusion (t), or the change in time from the first concentration to the second.

In this case, we are saying that C_{trough} equals C_{peak} multiplied by the fraction of C_{peak} remaining (as described by $e^{-Kt'}$) after elimination has occurred for t hours (i.e., 11 hours). As shown in Figure 12-2, because the peak concentration occurs at the end of the 1-hour infusion, t' in this equation is always (dosing interval) minus t (duration of infusion).

You should understand how t, τ, and t' differ.

In patient TM's case, the estimated C_{trough} would be:

$$
\begin{aligned}
C_{trough(steady state)} &= C_{peak(steady state)}\, e^{-Kt'} \\
&= (6.3\ \text{mg/L})e^{-(0.146\ \text{hr}^{-1})(12\ \text{hr} - 1\ \text{hr})} \\
&= (6.3\ \text{mg/L})e^{-(0.146\ \text{hr}^{-1})(11\ \text{hr})} \\
&= (6.3\ \text{mg/L})e^{-1.606} \\
&= (6.3\ \text{mg/L})(0.200) \\
&= 1.26\ \text{mg/L; round to 1.3 mg/L}
\end{aligned}
$$

This calculation tells us that 70 mg every 12 hours will give an estimated C_{peak} of 6.3 mg/L and an estimated C_{trough} of 1.3 mg/L. Remember that we actually picked a desired C_{trough} of 1 mg/L, but we also shortened the desired dosing interval from 13.2 to 12 hours, making the estimated C_{trough} higher than the initial desired C_{trough}. If, based on clinical judgment, a lower C_{trough} is desired, the dose can be recalculated with a longer dosing interval, such as 16 hours.

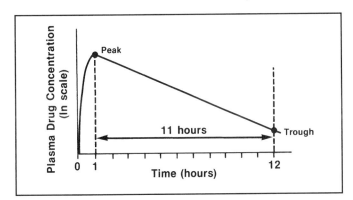

FIGURE 12-2.
Hours of elimination after drug peaks.

In patient TM's case, if a C_{trough} close to 2 mg/L had been attained, it would have been because we chose a dosing interval shorter than that recommended by our dosing interval calculation. Therefore, we would need to reexamine the rounding of our dosing interval and would probably round it up from 13.2 to 16 or 18 hours.

CASE 2

In Case 1, we showed how to calculate an appropriate maintenance dose and dosing interval. For this case, we use the data presented in Case 1 and continue treating patient TM.

Problem 2A. Calculate an appropriate loading dose to approximate a plasma concentration of 6 mg/L.

There are several methods to calculate a loading dose, and two are presented. Because one method requires estimation of the maintenance dose first, the loading dose is determined after the maintenance dose and dosing interval are calculated. In clinical practice, the loading and maintenance doses would be calculated at the same time.

Like all drugs given at the same maintenance dose via intermittent administration, aminoglycosides will not reach the desired steady-state therapeutic concentration for three (87.5% of steady state) to five (96.9% of steady state) drug half-lives. Therefore, subtherapeutic concentrations may exist for 1–2 days of therapy in patients with renal dysfunction.

Figure 12-3a shows a plasma drug concentration versus time simulation for an aminoglycoside given at the same dose six times. We saw in Lesson 4 that it takes three to five drug half-lives to reach steady-state concentrations. A patient's drug half-life is dependent on the elimination rate constant (K), as described in Lesson 3. Mathematically, $T^{1/2}$ equals $0.693/K$ and, vice versa, K equals $0.693/T^{1/2}$. Thus, time to reach steady state is dependent on the elimination rate constant (K) for a given patient.

■ *CLINICAL CORRELATE*

This is an interesting and conflicting concept. Reaching a steady-state drug concentration depends only on the patient's elimination rate (K). Steady state occurs in three to five drug half-lives. The time to steady state cannot be shortened with a loading dose infusion. However, a loading dose infusion can produce a plasma drug concentration approximately

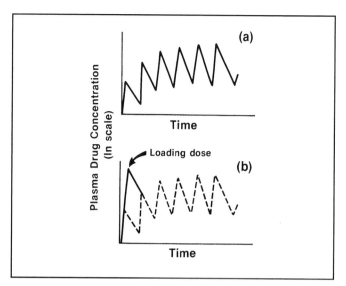

FIGURE 12-3.
(a) Drug accumulation to steady state without a loading dose.
(b) Concentration versus time simulation for the same aminoglycoside dose preceded by a loading dose.

equal to the eventual steady-state concentration (see Figure 12-3b). That is, a loading dose infusion will quickly bring the patient's drug concentration to a concentration that approximates the concentration at steady state. In addition, any time the dose or dosing interval is changed it will take another three to five half-lives to reach a new steady-state concentration. After changing a dosing regimen, remember to allow enough time to reach a new steady-state concentration before repeating plasma drug concentrations.

CALCULATING A LOADING DOSE

The loading dose infusion can be calculated from the formula for an intermittent infusion not at steady state as shown in Lesson 5:

$$C_{peak(steady\ state)} = \frac{K_0}{VK}(1-e^{-Kt})$$

where:

$C_{peak(steady\ state)}$ = desired peak drug concentration at steady state,
K_0 = loading dose (in mg) to be infused ÷ duration of infusion (in hours),
V = volume of distribution (population estimate, in liters),
K = elimination rate constant (population estimate, in reciprocal hours), and
t = duration of infusion (1 hour).

CLINICAL CORRELATE

In Lesson 5, we calculated the loading dose of a drug administered by intravenous push, $X_0 = C_{0(desired)}V$. This equation assumes a rapid infusion of a drug. Because aminoglycosides are infused over 30 minutes to an hour, the equation below must be used to calculate a loading dose to account for the amount of drug eliminated over the infusion period. The term $(1 - e^{-Kt})$ represents the fraction remaining after (t), the time of infusion.

This equation can be rearranged to isolate K_0 on one side of the equation:

$$K_0 = \frac{C_{peak(steady\ state)}(VK)}{(1-e^{-Kt})}$$

Patient TM's loading dose infusion can then be calculated:

$$\text{loading dose} = \frac{(6\ mg/L)(12.5\ L)(0.146\ hr^{-1})}{(1-e^{-(0.146\ hr^{-1})(1\ hr)})}$$

$$= \frac{10.95}{0.1358}$$

$$= 80.6\ mg$$

By this method, the loading dose infusion can be determined before the maintenance dose is calculated, but only with a complicated equation.

Another, easier loading dose formula that requires calculation of the maintenance dose first is shown below:

12-5 $$\text{loading dose} = \frac{K_0}{(1-e^{-K\tau})}$$

where:

K_0 = estimated maintenance dose,
$1/(1 - e^{-K\tau})$ = accumulation factor at steady state (see **Equation 4-2**), and
τ = dosing interval at which estimated maintenance dose is given.

With this loading dose formula, you are, in essence, multiplying the desired maintenance dose by a factor (the accumulation factor) representing the sum of the "fraction of doses" that have accumulated at steady state. This factor describes how much the concentration will be increased at steady state.

These two formulas are derivations of each other, as shown below. Begin with our general formula and rearrange it to solve for K_0:

$$C_{peak(steady\ state)} = \frac{K_0(1-e^{-Kt})}{VK(1-e^{-K\tau})}$$

$$K_0 = \frac{C_{peak(steady\ state)}(VK)(1-e^{-K\tau})}{(1-e^{-Kt})}$$

The first numerator/denominator combination in the above equation is also found in the equation for the loading dose:

$$loading\ dose = \frac{C_{peak(steady\ state)}(VK)}{(1-e^{-Kt})}$$

Therefore, the right-hand term of this loading dose equation can be substituted into the general equation for K_0 (Step 1 below) and then rearranged (Step 2 below) to then yield our other loading dose formula:

Step 1: $K_0 = (loading\ dose)\dfrac{1-e^{-K\tau}}{t}$

Step 2: $loading\ dose = \dfrac{K_0}{1-e^{-K\tau}}$

For patient TM, the loading dose should be:

$$\begin{aligned}
loading\ dose &= \frac{K_0}{1-e^{-K\tau}}\\[6pt]
&= \frac{66.7\ mg/hr}{1-e^{-(0.146\ hr^{-1})(12\ hr)}}\\[6pt]
&= \frac{66.7\ mg/hr}{0.826}\\[6pt]
&= 80.8\ mg
\end{aligned}$$

Both loading dose formulas will give approximately the same number. However, some prefer the loading dose equation that requires the maintenance dose to be calculated first because it is simple. Patient TM should receive a loading dose of 80 mg (rounded) followed by a maintenance dose of 70 mg every 12 hours. The 80-mg loading dose should give an approximate C_p of 6 mg/L. Based on the estimated parameters, steady state should be attained in three to five half-lives (3 × 4.75 = 14.25 hours; 5 × 4.75 = 23.75 hours). (See **Equation 3-3**.)

CASE 3

To continue with patient TM from Cases 1 and 2, blood was drawn for drug concentration assessment "around" the fourth dose (i.e., approximately 5 minutes before dose was due and immediately after the 1-hour dose infusion). C_{peak} and C_{trough} were determined as follows:

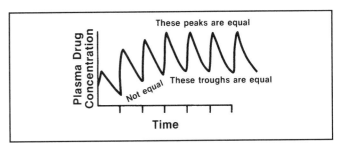

FIGURE 12-4.
Peak and trough concentrations at steady state.

- 7:55 a.m.: C_{trough} was 0.4 mg/L.
- 8–9 a.m.: 70-mg dose was infused over 1 hour.
- 9 a.m.: C_{peak} was 4.6 mg/L.

Although a "peak and trough" was ordered, a "trough and peak" was actually drawn. In this example, the trough level was taken just before the fourth dose was given, and the peak level was obtained just after the fourth dose was given. This procedure is normal and appropriate if the concentrations are at steady state. Figure 12-4 illustrates that, at steady state, C_{trough} from a "trough and peak" is equal to the C_{trough} from a "peak and trough" because all C_{trough} and all C_{peak} values are the same. We know that if we measured a C_{trough} after the C_{peak}, it would equal the C_{trough} before the C_{peak}. This is not true before steady state is reached. In this case, therefore, when a "peak and trough" is ordered, the literal interpretation would be:

1. Give the infusion from 8 to 9 a.m.
2. Draw a sample to determine C_{peak} at approximately 9 a.m.
3. Wait until the end of TM's 12-hour dosing interval (approximately 7:55 p.m.) to draw a sample to determine C_{trough}.

In practice, this method is too cumbersome for pharmacy, nursing, and laboratory staff, so usually a "trough and peak" is drawn if steady state has been attained.

It is recommended that C_{peak} be measured either at the end of a 1-hour infusion, 30 minutes after the end of a 30-minute infusion, or 1 hour after an intramuscular injection. Infusing aminoglycosides over 1 hour allows simpler pharmacokinetic calculations in that the duration of infusion (t) is 1 hour and the infusion rate (K_0) is simply the dose given. Remember that K_0 is expressed as mg/hour. So, if the drug is infused over 30 minutes (0.5 hour), then K_0 = Dose (mg) / 0.5 (hour).

Problem 3A. Are patient TM's concentrations of 4.6 mg/L (peak) and 0.4 mg/L (trough) at steady state?

Patient TM's concentrations were determined around the fourth dose, meaning 36 hours after his first dose. Lesson 4 explains that it takes three to five drug half-lives to reach steady state. To determine whether the drug is at steady state, we must use C_{peak} and C_{trough} to calculate TM's actual K and $T\frac{1}{2}$. These calculations are done in Problem 3C, and the results are 0.222 hr^{-1} for K and 3.12 hours for $T\frac{1}{2}$. Five half-lives would equal 15.6 hours (3.12 × 5), which is less than the 36 hours elapsed. Therefore, these concentrations are considered to be at steady state. If the drug is not at steady state, the pre-dose C_{trough} would be less than the post-dose C_{trough} and would overestimate K.

Problem 3B. How can you determine when to order drug concentration samples so they are likely to be at steady state?

You want to determine C_{peak} and C_{trough} after the patient is at steady state. Therefore, you must draw blood samples three to five drug half-lives after the first dose. You must estimate the patient's K and $T\frac{1}{2}$ using population estimates as in Case 1 and then multiply the $T\frac{1}{2}$ by three to five. As shown in Lesson 4, after three half-lives, concentrations are 87.5% of steady state, whereas after five half-lives, they are 96.9% of steady state. Use judgment when choosing three, four, or five half-lives to calculate time to steady state. Plasma concentration sampling should be scheduled to follow the dose that achieves steady state.

For patient TM, the estimated K and $T\frac{1}{2}$ (from Case 1, Problem 1A) were 0.146 hr^{-1} and 4.75 hours, respectively. Therefore, steady state would be reached in 23.75 (5 × 4.75) hour. You could then schedule C_{peak} and C_{trough} determinations at the next dose after 24 hours has elapsed.

■ CLINICAL CORRELATE

By calculating the patient's actual elimination rate (K) and volume of distribution (V), pharmacists can more accurately predict patient-specific pharmacokinetic data, thereby optimizing patient care. Once patient-specific parameters are known, it is important not to continue to use population estimates to adjust dosages or dosage intervals.

Problem 3C. Adjust patient TM's dosing regimen, based on C_{peak} and C_{trough} concentrations, to obtain the desired C_{peak} of 6 mg/L and C_{trough} of 1 mg/L.

Adjustment of patient TM's dose involves using the measured drug concentrations to calculate an actual K and V and then substituting these new values for our initial estimates of K and V in **Equations 3-2, 5-1,** and **12-4**, used in Case 1. The formula for K below comes from a rearrangement of the general equation used to calculate the slope of the natural log of plasma drug concentration versus time line as described in Case 1.

Remember that because concentration decreases with time, the slope (and hence $-K$) is a negative number.

CALCULATION OF TM'S ACTUAL ELIMINATION RATE (K)

To calculate K, the equation is:

$$K = -\frac{\ln C_{trough} - \ln C_{peak}}{\tau - t}$$

(See **Equation 3-1**.)
where:

  K = elimination rate constant (in reciprocal hours),
  C_{trough} = measured trough concentration (0.4 mg/L),
  C_{peak} = measured peak concentration (4.6 mg/L),
  τ = dosing interval at the time concentrations are obtained (12 hours), and
  t = duration of infusion (1 hour).

Again, remembering a rule of logarithms:

$$\ln a - \ln b = \ln (a/b)$$

we can simplify this equation for hand-held calculators:

$$K = -\frac{\ln\left(\dfrac{C_{trough}}{C_{peak}}\right)}{\tau - t}$$

Either form of this equation may be used to calculate K, as follows:

$$K = -\frac{\ln 0.4 \text{ mg/L} - \ln 4.6 \text{ mg/L}}{12 \text{ hr} - 1 \text{ hr}}$$

$$= -\frac{-0.916 - 1.52}{11}$$

$$= -\frac{-2.44}{11}$$

$$= 0.222$$

Therefore, K = 0.222 hr^{-1}, compared to 0.146 hr^{-1}, which was our estimate.

Or:

$$K = -\frac{\ln\left(\dfrac{0.4 \text{ mg/L}}{4.6 \text{ mg/L}}\right)}{12 \text{ hr} - 1 \text{ hr}}$$

$$= -\frac{\ln (0.0869)}{11 \text{ hr}}$$

$$= -\frac{-2.442}{11 \text{ hr}}$$

$$= 0.222 \text{ hr}^{-1}$$

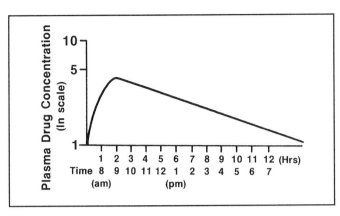

FIGURE 12-5.
K from any two points.

Patient TM's actual K of 0.222 hr^{-1} is greater than the estimated value of 0.146 hr^{-1}, so his elimination probably was greater than estimated. His actual drug half-life ($T\frac{1}{2}$) is 3.12 hours, shorter than the population-estimated $T\frac{1}{2}$ of 4.75 hours:

$$T\frac{1}{2} = 0.693/K \text{ (See \textbf{Equation 3-3}.)}$$

$$= 0.693/0.222 \text{ hr}^{-1}$$

$$= 3.12 \text{ hours}$$

The formula for K above can also be used to calculate the slope, $-K$, for any two points on the natural log of plasma drug concentration versus time line. For instance, suppose that instead of a C_{peak}, patient TM had a concentration measured at 11 a.m. (2 hours after C_{peak}). This concentration was 2.95 mg/L. You can still calculate his K value as follows (Figure 12-5):

$$K = -\frac{\ln 0.4 \text{ mg/L} - \ln 2.95 \text{ mg/L}}{12 \text{ hr} - 1 \text{ hr} - 2 \text{ hr}}$$

$$= -\frac{-0.916 - 1.0818}{9}$$

$$= -\frac{-1.9978}{9}$$

$$= 0.222$$

Note that this K value is the same as the one calculated with the measured C_{peak} and C_{trough} concentrations.

CALCULATION OF TM'S ACTUAL VOLUME OF DISTRIBUTION (V)

Patient TM's actual volume of distribution (V) is calculated with the equation from Case 1. Use the actual C_{peak} and C_{trough} values, dose, and dosing interval.

$$C_{peak(steady state)} = \frac{K_0(1 - e^{-Kt})}{VK(1 - e^{-K\tau})}$$

(See **Equation 5-1**.)
where:

   t = the duration of the infusion, and

   τ = dosing interval at the time concentrations are obtained.

In this case, some of the variables substituted in this equation are different from those used when initially estimating a dose. The changes from Case 1 are shown here in bold type:

   $C_{peak(steady state)}$ = C_{peak} **measured at steady state**,

   K_0 = **maintenance dose infused at time C_{peak} and C_{trough} were measured**,

   V = **patient's actual** volume of distribution **that you are trying to determine based on C_{peak} and C_{trough} values**,

   K = elimination rate constant **calculated from patient's C_{peak} and C_{trough} values**,

   t = duration of infusion (hours), and

   τ = **patient's** dosing interval **at time C_{peak} and C_{trough} were measured**.

In patient TM's case, he received a maintenance dose of 70 mg every 12 hours, with subsequent C_{peak} and C_{trough} concentrations of 4.6 and 0.4 mg/L, respectively. His K value from these concentrations was 0.222 hr^{-1}.

If we substitute these values into the previous equation, we can solve for patient TM's actual V:

$$4.6 \text{mg/L} = \frac{(70 \text{ mg/hr})(1 - e^{-(0.222 \text{ hr}^{-1})(1 \text{ hr})})}{(V)(0.222 \text{ hr}^{-1})(1 - e^{-(0.222 \text{ hr}^{-1})(12 \text{ hr})})}$$

$$4.6 \text{mg/L} = \frac{(315)(0.199)}{(V)(0.930)}$$

$$V = 14.7 \text{ L}$$

Compared to 12.5 L that we estimated.

Patient TM's V value of 14.7 L (which equals 0.28 L/kg IBW) is larger than estimated and would tend to make his real C_{peak} and C_{trough} lower than estimated.

Now that we have calculated the patient's actual K and V, we need to recalculate the dose and dosing interval. As when we estimated the first dose, we must first calculate the new dosing interval (τ) and then calculate the new dose.

$$\tau = \frac{1}{-K}(\ln C_{trough \text{ (desired)}} - \ln C_{peak \text{ (desired)}}) + t$$

where t is the duration of infusion in hours and K is the actual elimination rate calculated from patient's peak and trough values and *not* the estimated value of 0.146 hr^{-1}. Then:

⚠️
12-4 $\tau = \dfrac{1}{-0.222\ hr^{-1}}(\ln 1\ mg/L - \ln 6\ mg/L) + 1 hr$

$= (-4.5)(0 - 1.79) + 1 hr$

$= (-4.5)(-1.79) + 1 hr$

$= 9.06\ hr$

This adjusted τ should be compared with our initial τ estimate of 13.26 hours from Case 1, Problem 1A. Because our real τ is shorter than previously estimated, C_{peak} and C_{trough} values less than those predicted also would be expected. In other words, we initially administered a dose every 12 hours when, in actuality, the patient needed a dose every 9 hours.

This calculated dosing interval of 9 hours may be rounded down to 8 hours for ease in scheduling.

Problem 3D. How is patient TM's adjusted maintenance dose now calculated?

Once again, we shall use the general equation from Case 1 and solve for K_0. This time, we shall replace the estimates of K and V with the calculated (actual) values and use the adjusted τ value of 8 hours:

$$C_{peak(steady\ state)} = \frac{K_0(1 - e^{-Kt})}{VK(1 - e^{-K\tau})}$$

(See **Equation 5-1**.)
where:

$C_{peak(steady\ state)}$ = desired steady-state C_{peak} (6 mg/L);
K_0 = drug infusion rate (also adjusted maintenance dose you are trying to calculate, in milligrams per hour);
V = actual volume of distribution determined from patient's measured C_{peak} and C_{trough} values, in liters;
K = actual elimination rate constant calculated from patient's measured C_{peak} and C_{trough} values, in reciprocal hours;
t = infusion time, in hours; and
τ = adjusted dosing interval rounded to a practical number.

Strikeovers in the following equation show differences from initial estimated maintenance dose calculations (see Case 1):

6 mg/L $= \dfrac{K_0}{(\cancel{12.5}\ \ 14.7\ L)(\cancel{0.146}\ \ 0.222\ hr^{-1})\left[\dfrac{(1 - e^{-\cancel{0.146}\ \ 0.222\ hr^{-1}(1\ hr)})}{(1 - e^{-\cancel{0.146}\ \ 0.222\ hr^{-1}(\cancel{12}\ \ 8\ hr)})}\right]}$

$= \dfrac{K_0}{(3.263)}\dfrac{0.199}{0.831}$

$= K_0(0.0732)$

$K_0 = 81.9$, rounded to 80 mg

If 81.9 mg gives a peak of 6 mg/L, then our rounded dose of 80 mg will give a peak of 5.86 mg/L.

Problem 3E. If we give 80 mg every 8 hours, what will be our steady-state C_{trough}?

If we give 81.9 mg "exactly" every 9 hours, our C_{trough} would be precisely as desired: 1 mg/L. But because we rounded our dosing interval and adjusted the maintenance dose down to practical numbers, we must calculate the steady-state C_{trough} that will result. Our roundings could make our C_{trough} too high.

This C_{trough} calculation is performed similarly to the one in Case 1, Problem 1B (strikeovers show differences from our initial calculations):

$$C_{trough(steady\ state)} = C_{peak(steady\ state)}e^{-Kt'}$$
(See **Equation 3-2**.)

$= 5.86\ mg/L\ [e^{-(\cancel{0.146})(0.222\ hr^{-1})(\tau - 1\ hour)}]$

$= 5.86\ mg/L\ [e^{-(\cancel{0.146})(0.222)(\cancel{11}\ 7)}]$

$= 5.86\ (e^{-1.554})$

$= 5.86\ (0.211)$

$= 1.24\ mg/L$

So, in this case, a dose of 80 mg every 8 hours will give a steady-state C_{trough} of 1.24 mg/L, still well below the usual maximum acceptable trough concentration of 2 mg/L.

CASE 4

Four days later, another set of peak and trough concentrations are obtained. Patient TM has been receiving 80 mg every 8 hours. However, his renal function has declined, as seen by an increase in serum creatinine from 1.3 mg/dL at baseline to 1.7 mg/dL today. C_{peak} and C_{trough} were determined as follows:

- 7:55 a.m.: C_{trough} was 3.2 mg/L.
- 8–9 a.m.: an 80-mg dose was infused over 1 hour.
- 9:00 a.m.: C_{peak} was 9.2 mg/L.

A new adjusted K, τ, V, and maintenance dose (K_0) were calculated using the methods described in Case 3. These values are shown below; see if you obtain the same numbers:

new $K = 0.151\ hr^{-1}$,
new $T\frac{1}{2} = 4.6$ hours,
new $V = 11.1\ L$,

new τ = 12.6 (rounded to 12 hours),
new maintenance dose (K_0) = 60 mg every 12 hours,
and
new trough concentration = 1.1 mg/L.

Problem 4A. Because patient TM's C_{trough} on 80 mg every 8 hours is now too high (3.2 mg/L), how long would you wait before beginning the new dose of 60 mg every 12 hours?

Before switching, you must wait for the patient's C_{trough} to decrease to approximately 1 mg/L. Therefore, the dose should be held for some time before you begin a new lower dose. The formula for calculating the number of hours to hold the dose is:

$$C_{trough(steady\ state)(desired)} = C_{trough(steady\ state)}\ e^{-Kt'}$$
(See **Equation 3-2**.)

where t' is the amount of time to hold the dose after the end of the 8-hour dosing interval.

This formula is an application of the general formula described in Case 1:

$$C = C_0 e^{-Kt}\quad \text{(See Equation 3-2.)}$$

which means:

concentration at a time = previous concentration × fraction of dose remaining

In patient TM's case:

$$1\ mg/L = (3.2\ mg/L)\ e^{-0.151\ hr^{-1}\ (t')}$$

$$0.312\ mg/L = e^{-0.151(t')}$$

Next, take the natural log of both sides:

$$\ln 0.312 = \ln (e^{-0.151(t')})$$

$$-1.163 = -0.151\ (t')$$

$$7.70\ hours = t'$$

Thus, we should hold patient TM's dose for an additional 7.7 (round to 8) hours after the next C_{trough} time and then begin his new dose. The next C_{trough} time for this patient would be 3:45 p.m., 7.75 hours after his last (8 a.m.) dose. The C_{trough} at this time, at steady state, would also be expected to be approximately 3.2 mg/L. We would need to hold the regularly scheduled 4 p.m. dose for 8 hours, until 12 midnight, at which time we would then begin his new dose of 60 mg every 12 hours.

The calculation of the time to hold a dose can be illustrated (Figure 12-6) by plotting patient TM's C_{peak}

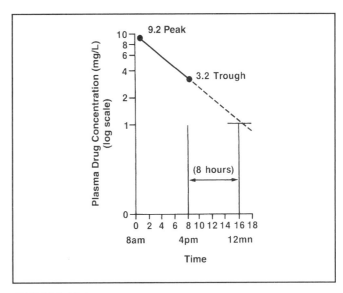

FIGURE 12-6.
Calculation of the time to hold a dose.

and C_{trough} values on semilog graph paper and then extending the line connecting them until it reaches our desired C_{trough} of 1 mg/L. You can then count the hours needed to reach this 1-mg/L concentration and hold the dose accordingly.

Another, and often more practical, way to estimate the time to hold a patient's dose is by examining the half-life. By definition, the drug concentration decreases by one-half over each half-life. Therefore, we can estimate how many drug half-lives to wait for the concentration to approach our desired 1 mg/L as follows.

For patient TM (trough of 3.2 mg/L and $T\frac{1}{2}$ of 4.6 hours), the concentration will drop to 1.6 mg/L (half of 3.2) in one half-life of 4.6 hours and then drop to 0.8 mg/L (half of 1.6) in another 4.6 hours. Therefore, we can hold patient TM's doses for approximately two half-lives (4.6 × 2 = 9.2 hours) before beginning our new dose.

In patient TM's case, another dose was given from 8 to 9 a.m., after the C_{trough} of 3.2 was obtained at 7:55 a.m. Therefore, his next C_{trough} will occur at approximately 3:45 p.m. (shortly before the next scheduled dose). We need to hold this dose for an additional 9.2 (round to 9) hours and then begin our new regimen of 60 mg every 12 hours.

CASE 5

A 48-year-old white woman, patient CS, is admitted to the intensive care unit with a presumptive diagnosis of bilateral pneumonia. Other pertinent patient data include: height, 5 feet, 4 inches; weight, 52 kg; and serum creatinine, 0.9 mg/dL; white blood cell count of 16,000/mm³ and 80% neutrophils.

Problem 5A. Recommend a dose of gentamicin to be given as an extended interval dose to patient CS.

The average dose for gentamicin when given once daily is 4–7 mg/kg based on **actual** body weight.

The dose should depend on the immunologic status of the patient and the site of infection. For patient CS, a recommended dose (X_0) would be:

⚠️
12-6

$$X_0 = 4\text{--}7 \text{ mg/kg actual body weight}$$

$$= 6 \text{ mg/kg} \times 52 \text{ kg}$$

$$= 312 \text{ mg}$$

which should be rounded to 300 mg and administered every 24 hours.

To ensure that once-daily aminoglycoside dosing is appropriate in patient CS, an assessment of renal function is necessary to ensure that the doses can be eliminated adequately over the dosing interval:

$$\text{CrCl} = 0.85 \frac{(140 - \text{age})(\text{IBW})}{72 \times \text{SCr}}$$

$$= 0.85 \frac{(140 - 48)(52)}{72 \times 0.9}$$

$$= 63 \text{ mL/min}$$

Notice in this situation that we used patient CS's actual body weight to perform this calculation because her actual body weight is less than her IBW.

Estimated K:

$$K = 0.00293 \text{ hr}^{-1} (\text{CrCl}) + 0.014$$

$$= 0.00293 \text{ hr}^{-1} (63) + 0.014$$

$$= 0.199 \text{ hr}^{-1}$$

Estimated $T^{1/2}$:

$$T^{1/2} = 0.693 / K$$

$$= 0.693 / 0.199 \text{ hr}^{-1}$$

$$= 3.48 \text{ hours}$$

Therefore, with a $T^{1/2}$ of approximately 3.5 hours, this patient's renal function is adequate to receive extended interval dosing of gentamicin. Five half-lives would be 17.5 hours, so, the dose would be almost totally eliminated within 24 hours.

The calculated dose may be infused over 30–60 minutes, and blood samples for C_{peak} should be taken at some point after the end of the infusion. Recent evidence has indicated that higher doses of aminoglyco-sides (gentamicin – 7 mg/kg) may take up to 2 hours to distribute; therefore, sampling for plasma levels before 2 hours may provide erroneous estimations of C_{max}. Intermediate and low doses (≤4–5 mg/kg) are thought to distribute completely in 1 hour, so sampling 1 hour after the infusion is completed may be adequate.[19] From population data, C_{peak} would be expected to be 15–20 mg/L and C_{trough} less than 0.5 mg/L. Steady-state plasma concentrations may be measured, and if the dose needs to be adjusted to achieve the target plasma concentration, individualized pharmacokinetic dosing as previously reviewed may be applied. However, a target peak concentration for extended-interval aminoglycosides has not been clearly established.

REFERENCES

1. Cockcroft DW, Gault MH. Prediction of creatinine clearance from serum creatinine. *Nephron* 1976;15:31–41.
2. Gilbert DW. Once daily aminoglycoside therapy. *Antimicrob Agents Chemother* 1991;35:399–405.
3. Moore RD, Leitman P, Smith CR. Clinical response to aminoglycoside therapy: importance of the ratio of peak concentration to minimum inhibitory concentration. *J Infect Dis* 1987;155:93–7.
4. Noone P, Parsons TM, Pattison JR, et al. Experience in monitoring gentamicin therapy during treatment of serious gram-negative sepsis. *Br Med J* 1974;1:477–81.
5. Bundtzen RW, Berber AU, Cohn DL, et al. Post-antibiotic suppression of bacterial growth. *Rev Infect Dis* 1981;3:28–37.
6. Isaksson B, Nilsson L, Maller R, et al. Postantibiotic effect of aminoglycosides on gram-negative bacteria evaluated by a new method. *J Antimicrob Chemother* 1988;22:23–33.
7. Kapsunik JE, Hackbarth CJ, Chambers HF, et al. Single large daily dosing versus intermittent dosing of tobramycin in experimental pseudomonas pneumonia. *J Infect Dis* 1988;158:7–12.
8. Vogelman B, Gudmundsson S, Turnidge J, et al. In vivo postantibiotic effect in a thigh infection in mice. *J Infect Dis* 1988;157:287–98.
9. Zhanel GG, Hoban DJ, Harding GK. The postantibiotic effect: a review of in vitro and in vivo data. *Ann Pharmacother* 1991;25:153–63.
10. Craig WA, Vogelman BS. Postantibiotic effects. *Ann Intern Med* 1987;106:900–2.
11. Fantin B, Ebert S, Leggett J, et al. Factors affecting duration of in vivo postantibiotic effect for aminoglycosides against gram-negative bacilli. *J Antimicrob Chemother* 1990;27:829–36.
12. Gilbert DN, Lee BL, Dworkin RJ, et al. A randomized comparison of the safety and efficacy of once daily gentamicin or thrice-daily gentamicin in combination with ticarcillin-clavulanate. *Am J Med* 1998;105:182–91.
13. Mitra AG, Whitten MK, Laurent SL, et al. A randomized, prospective study comparing once-daily gentamicin ver-

sus thrice-daily gentamicin in the treatment of puerperal infection. *Am J Obstet Gynecol* 1997;177:786–92.

14. Nordstrom L, Ringberg H, Cronberg S, et al. Does administration of an aminoglycoside in a single daily dose affect its efficacy and toxicity? *J Antimicrob Chemother* 1990;25:159–73.

15. Prins JM, Buller HR, Kuijper EJ, et al. Once versus thrice daily gentamicin in patients with serious infections. *Lancet* 1993;341:335–9.

16. Rotschafer JC, Rybak MJ. Single daily dosing of aminoglycosides: a commentary. *Ann Pharmacother* 1994;28:797–801.

17. Preston SL, Briceland LL. Single daily dosing of aminoglycosides. *Pharmacotherapy* 1995;15(3):297–316.

18. Tam VH, Preston SL, Briceland LL. Once-daily aminoglycosides in the treatment of gram-positive endocarditis. *Ann Pharmacother* 1999;33:600–6.

19. Wallace AW, Jones M, Bertino JS. Evaluation of four once-daily aminoglycoside dosing intervals. *Pharacotherapy* 2002;22(9):1077–83.

20. Winston L, Benowitz N. Once-daily dosing of aminoglycosides: How much monitoring is truly required? *Am J Med* 2003;114:239–40.

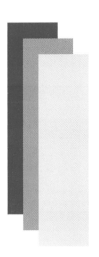

LESSON

13

Vancomycin

In this lesson, Cases 1–4 focus on the antibiotic vancomycin. Before beginning, however, a few key points about vancomycin should be reviewed. Vancomycin is usually administered via intermittent intravenous infusions. For systemic infections, vancomycin is only given by the intravenous route; only this route is considered in this lesson. To minimize the occurrence of an adverse reaction called *red-man syndrome*, vancomycin doses >1000 mg should be diluted in a larger volume of fluid and infused over 2 hours. Vancomycin is the drug of first choice for serious methicillin-resistant staphylococci infections and enterococci (group D streptococcus). Because these organisms have begun to also become resistant to vancomycin, the Centers for Disease Control and Prevention periodically releases recommendations for prudent use of vancomycin.[1]

The average volume of distribution for vancomycin is approximately:

13-1 0.9 L/kg total body weight (TBW)

(Note that, unlike the aminoglycosides, it is recommended that TBW be used to calculate the volume of distribution.) Pharmacokinetically, vancomycin is an example of a two-compartment model, a concept that is discussed in Lesson 6. After intravenous administration, vancomycin displays a pronounced distribution phase (α phase) (Figure 13-1) while the drug equilibrates between plasma and tissues. During this initial distribution phase (1–3 hours), plasma drug concentrations are quite high. As the drug distributes throughout the body, the plasma drug concentration declines rapidly over a short period. This biexponential elimination curve for vancomycin is an important consideration when evaluating plasma vancomycin concentration determinations. It is important not to

obtain plasma drug concentrations during this initial distribution phase, as inaccurate pharmacokinetic calculations may result.

Vancomycin is eliminated almost entirely by glomerular filtration. Therefore, a reduction in renal function results in a decreased vancomycin clearance and an increased half-life. The average vancomycin half-life for a patient with normal renal function is approximately 6 hours ($K = 0.116$ hr^{-1}). One method of determining population estimates for the elimination rate constant (K) based on creatinine clearance (CrCl) is:

13-2 $K = 0.00083$ hr^{-1} [CrCl (in mL/minute)] + 0.0044

This equation, developed by Gary Matzke from regression analysis of vancomycin clearance versus creatinine clearance, has units of reciprocal hours, not milliliters per minute. In this type of equation, units are not supposed to cancel out; rather, they assume the units of the correlated value, K.

Because of vancomycin's strange initial distribution phase, there is some confusion about the "therapeutic" values for peak and trough concentrations. Older data that suggested peak concentrations of 30–40 mg/L are wrong because they were sampled during this initially high distribution phase. It is now thought that peak concentrations should be in the range of 18–26 mg/L, whereas trough concentrations should be between 5 and 10 mg/L, except in certain enterococcal infections, for which vancomycin is only bacteriostatic, such as in enterococcal endocarditis. In these cases, trough concentrations should be between 10 and 15 mg/L.

Finally, there is some controversy about the amount of nephrotoxicity and ototoxicity associated with vancomycin. Most documentation of toxicity was reported in the

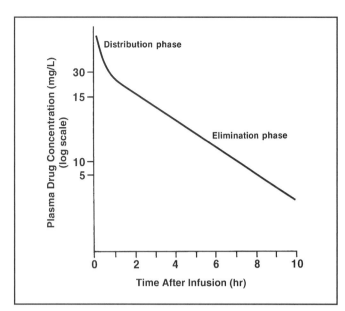

FIGURE 13-1.

Typical plasma concentration versus time curve for vancomycin, demonstrating distribution and elimination phases.

1960s, when the available intravenous product contained many impurities. It now appears that vancomycin is much less toxic than originally thought due to removal of impurities.

Serum drug concentration monitoring is still important, especially for patients with significant degrees of renal insufficiency, such as the elderly. In addition, vancomycin should be monitored from an efficacy and cost standpoint. Subtherapeutic dosing of vancomycin promotes the selection of resistant organisms, and excess use of vancomycin is a pharmacoeconomic waste.

CASE 1

WM, a 34-year-old man, 5 feet 5 inches tall, weighing 63 kg, is admitted to the hospital for a right colectomy because of colon cancer. Initially, he has normal renal function: serum creatinine concentration of 0.7 mg/dL, with an estimated creatinine clearance of 134 mL/minute. The patient develops a postoperative wound infection, which is treated with surgical drainage and an intravenous cephalosporin.

Culture of the wound fluid reveals *Staphylococcus aureus*, which is found to be resistant to penicillins and cephalosporins. Patient WM is then started on intravenous vancomycin. The desired steady-state plasma concentrations are 20 mg/L (2 hours after completion of the vancomycin infusion) and 5–10 mg/L at the end of the dosing interval.

Problem 1A. Determine an appropriate dosing regimen of vancomycin to achieve the desired steady-state plasma concentrations of 20 mg/L for the peak (drawn 2 hours after the end of a 2-hour infusion) and approximately 7 mg/L for the trough. How many doses are required to reach steady state?

Several approaches are recommended for the calculation of vancomycin dosage; one relatively simple method is presented here. With this method, we assume that the plasma concentrations during the elimination phase are more valuable for therapeutic drug monitoring than the relatively high, transient vancomycin concentrations of the distribution phase (the first 1–2 hours after the infusion). With this assumption, a one-compartment model can be used to predict vancomycin dosage or plasma concentrations (Figure 13-2). We ignore the distribution phase.

To predict the appropriate dosage given the desired plasma concentrations, we need to know the approximate volume of distribution and the elimination rate constant. These parameters are used in the multiple-dose infusion equation for steady state also shown in Lesson 5. Because we do not have patient-specific plasma concentration data, the values used for the volume of distribu-

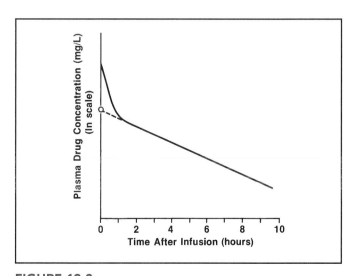

FIGURE 13-2.

Plasma concentration versus time curve for vancomycin, showing simplification with one-compartment model (*dashed line*).

tion and elimination rate constant are the population estimates given in the introduction. Note that this equation is similar to those used to determine aminoglycoside dosages:

⚠
13-3
$$C_{peak(steady\ state)} = \frac{K_0(1-e^{-Kt})}{VK(1-e^{-K\tau})}e^{-Kt'}$$
(See **Equation 5-1**.)

where:

$C_{peak(steady\ state)}$ = desired peak concentration 2 hours after infusion;

K_0 = drug infusion rate (dose/infusion time);

t = duration of infusion (usually 2 hours for vancomycin);

K = estimated elimination rate constant (0.116 hr^{-1});

V = volume of distribution (population estimate of 0.9 L/kg × 63 kg = 56.7 L);

t' = time between end of infusion and collection of blood sample (2 hours; inclusion of t' is different from the calculation for aminoglycosides [see Lesson 12] because sampling time for vancomycin is actually at least 4 hours after the beginning of the infusion); and

τ = desired dosing interval, determined as follows:

⚠
13-4
$$\tau = \frac{1}{-K}\left[\ln C_{trough\ (desired)} - \ln C_{peak\ (desired)}\right] + t + t'$$

$$= \frac{1}{-0.116\ hr^{-1}}\left[\ln 7\,mg/L - \ln 20\,mg/L\right] + 2\,hr + 2\,hr$$

$$= 13.05\ hr,\ rounded\ down\ to\ 12\ hr$$

(See **Equation 12-4**.)

These values are then put into the equation:

$$C_{peak(steady\ state)} = \frac{K_0(1-e^{-0.116\ hr^{-1}(2\ hr)})}{(56.7\ L)(0.116\ hr^{-1})(1-e^{-0.116\ hr^{-1}(12\ hr)})}e^{-0.116\ hr^{-1}(2\ hr)}$$

$$20\,mg/L = \frac{K_0(0.21)}{(56.7\ L)(0.116\ hr^{-1})(0.751)}(0.79)$$

$$K_0 = \frac{(20\,mg/L)(56.7\ L)(0.116\ hr^{-1})(0.751)}{(0.21)(0.79)}$$

$$= 595\ mg\ vancomycin\ per\ 1\ hr$$

Because vancomycin is infused over 2 hours,

Total dose = (595 mg/hr)(2 hr)

= 1190 mg vancomycin over 2 hr

With this regimen, we can then predict the vancomycin plasma concentration at the end of the dosing interval (trough):

⚠
13-5
$$C_{trough} = C_{peak(steady\ state)}e^{-Kt''}$$
(See **Equation 3-2**.)

where t'' is the difference in time between the two plasma concentrations. In this case, t'' equals τ (12 hours) – t (2 hours) – t'(2 hours), or 8 hours.

$$C_{trough} = 20\ mg/L\ e^{(-0.116\ hr^{-1})(8\ hr)}$$

$$= 20\ mg/L\ (0.395)$$

$$= 7.9\ mg/L$$

So the regimen should result in the desired plasma concentrations.

Note that the dose of 1190 mg could have been rounded to 1000 or 1100 mg or rounded up to 1200 mg for ease of dose preparation. If so, the desired peak would not be 20 mg/L. The resultant peak from any such dose rounding can easily be calculated with the general equation:

(rounded dose)/(actual calculated dose) × (desired peak concentration)

In this case, if we rounded our dose down to 1000 mg, the resultant peak calculation is as follows:

(1000 mg/1190 mg) × 20 mg/L = 16.8 mg/L

When rounding a dose, the trough concentration would also need to be recalculated. For example, if we used 1000 mg, giving a peak of only 16.8 mg/L, the trough concentration would be only 6.6 mg/L.

The number of doses required to attain steady state can be calculated from the estimated half-life and the dosing interval. Steady state is attained in three to five half-lives. In patient WM's case, we will use five half-lives and our estimated K of 0.116 hr^{-1} in our calculations as follows:

time to steady state = 5 × $T\frac{1}{2}$

$$T\frac{1}{2} = \frac{0.693}{K}$$

time to steady state = 5 × $T\frac{1}{2}$

$$= 5 \times \frac{0.693}{0.116\ hr^{-1}}$$

$$= 5(5.97\ hr)$$

$$= 29.85\ hr,\ or\ about\ 30\ hr$$

If doses are given every 12 hours, then steady state should be achieved by administration of the fourth dose

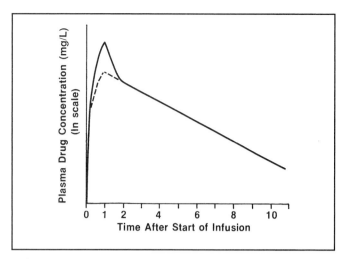

FIGURE 13-3.
Plasma concentrations over time for a loading dose. Dashed lines represent simplification to one-compartment model.

(by the end of the third dosing interval). Remember that doses would be given at 0, 12, 24, and 36 hours.

Problem 1B. To achieve the desired concentrations rapidly, a loading dose can be given. Determine an appropriate loading dose for patient WM. Assume that the loading dose will be a 2-hour intravenous infusion.
To estimate a loading dose, we need to know the volume of distribution and the elimination rate constant. Because we do not know the patient-specific pharmacokinetic values, the population estimates can be used (volume of distribution of 0.9 L/kg TBW [see **Equation 13-1**] and elimination rate constant of 0.116 hr^{-1}) (see **Equation 13-2**). Then the equation as shown in Lesson 5 describing plasma concentration over time with an intravenous infusion is applied. Note that again we ignore the distribution phase and assume that a one-compartment model is adequate (Figure 13-3):

$$C_{peak(steady\ state)} = \frac{X_0/t}{VK}(1-e^{-Kt})e^{-Kt'}$$

(See **Equation 13-3**.)
where:

$C_{peak(steady\ state)}$ = desired peak plasma concentration 2 hours after infusion,
X_0 = dose (note: $X_0/t = K_0$),
t = duration of infusion (2 hours),
K = 0.116 hr^{-1},
V = 56.7 L, and
t' = time after end of infusion (2 hours).

Note that the term $e^{-Kt'}$ describes the decline in plasma concentration from the end of the infusion to some later time (2 hours in this example). Then, insertion of the known values gives:

$$20\ mg/L = \frac{(X_0/2\ hr)(1-e^{-0.116\ hr^{-1}(2\ hr)})}{(56.7\ L)(0.116\ hr^{-1})}e^{-0.116\ hr^{-1}(2\ hr)}$$

$$= \frac{(X_0/2\ hr)(0.21)}{(6.58\ L/hr)}(0.79)$$

$$X_0 = \frac{(20\ mg/L)(6.58\ L/hr)(2\ hr)}{(0.79)(0.11)}$$
$$= 1586\ mg\ vancomycin,\ rounded\ to\ 1500\ mg$$
given over 2 hr

In this case, the loading dose is not much larger than the maintenance dose.

■ CLINICAL CORRELATE

Close observation of Figure 13-3 confirms that we are not actually measuring a true peak concentration, as we did for aminoglycosides. We are, rather, measuring a 2-hour postpeak concentration that places this point on the straight-line portion of the terminal elimination phase.

Problem 1C. After administration of the loading dose (1500 mg) and seven doses (1000 mg each) at 12-hour intervals, plasma vancomycin concentrations are determined to be 29 mg/L (2 hours after the end of the 2-hour infusion) and 15 mg/L at the end of the dosing interval. Although these plasma concentrations are not necessarily harmful, we want to decrease the dosage to attain the original target peak and trough concentrations (20 and 5–10 mg/L, respectively). Therefore, determine a modified dosing regimen for patient WM using the new information.
The information needed to determine a new dosing regimen is the same as described in Problem 1A. However, because we now have data about this specific patient, we no longer have to rely on population estimates. To begin, we should calculate the patient's vancomycin elimination rate constant, half-life, and volume of distribution from the plasma concentrations determined.

Calculation of K

First, the elimination rate constant (K) is easily calculated from the slope of the plasma drug concentration versus time curve during the elimination phase (Figure 13-4) (see Lesson 3):

$$K = -\frac{\ln C_2 - \ln C_1}{t_2 - t_1}$$
$$= -\frac{\ln 15\ mg/L - \ln 29\ mg/L}{10\ hr - 2\ hr}$$
$$= -\frac{2.71 - 3.37}{8\ hr}$$

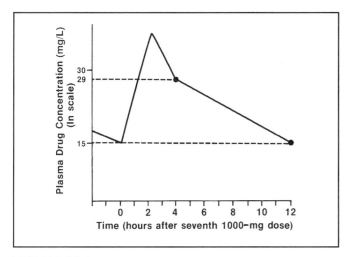

FIGURE 13-4.
Calculation of elimination rate constant given two plasma concentrations (29 mg/L at 2 hours after the infusion and 15 mg/L at 10 hours after the end of a 2-hour infusion).

$$= 0.083 \text{ hr}^{-1}$$

(See **Equation 3-1**.)

 CLINICAL CORRELATE

Be careful when selecting t_2 and t_1. In the above example, if dose one is begun at 8 a.m. and infused for 2 hours, then the patient would receive the entire dose by 10 a.m. The peak plasma level would then be drawn 2 hours later, or 12 noon. Given that the trough concentration will be attained immediately before dose two (given at 8 p.m.), the total time elapsed between the plasma readings is 8 hours, or $(t_2 - t_1)$.

The half-life $(T\frac{1}{2})$ can then be calculated:

$$T\frac{1}{2} = \frac{0.693}{K}$$
$$= \frac{0.693}{0.083 \text{ hr}^{-1}}$$
$$= 8.35 \text{ hr}$$

(See **Equation 3-3**.)

Calculation of V

Note that the elimination rate constant is lower and the half-life greater than originally estimated. Now the volume of distribution (V) can be estimated with the multiple-dose infusion equation for steady state:

$$C_{\text{peak(steady state)}} = \frac{K_0(1 - e^{-Kt})}{VK(1 - e^{-K\tau})}e^{-Kt'}$$

(See **Equation 13-3**.)

where:

$C_{\text{peak(steady state)}}$ = peak concentration 2 hours after infusion = 29 mg/L,
K_0 = maintenance dose (1000 mg over 2 hours),
t = duration of infusion (2 hours),
t' = time between end of infusion and collection of blood sample (2 hours),
K = elimination rate constant (0.083 hr^{-1}),
V = volume of distribution (to be determined), and
τ = dosing interval (12 hours).

These values are then put into the equation:

$$C_{\text{peak(steady state)}} = \frac{(1000 \text{ mg/2 hr})(1 - e^{-0.083 \text{ hr}^{-1}(2 \text{ hr})})}{V(0.083 \text{ hr}^{-1})(1 - e^{-0.083 \text{ hr}^{-1}(12 \text{ hr})})}e^{-0.083 \text{ hr}^{-1}(2 \text{ hr})}$$

$$29 \text{ mg/L} = \frac{(1000 \text{ mg/2 hr})(0.153)}{V(0.083 \text{ hr}^{-1})(0.631)}(0.847)$$

Rearranging gives:

$$V = \frac{(1000 \text{ mg/2 hr})(0.153)(0.847)}{(0.083 \text{ hr}^{-1})(0.631)(29 \text{ mg/L})}$$
$$= 42.67 \text{ L or } 0.7 \text{ L/kg}$$

So the original estimate for the volume of distribution was close to the volume determined with the plasma concentrations.

Calculation of New τ

Before calculating a new maintenance dose, we can first check to see if we need to use a new dosing interval, as follows:

$$\tau_{\text{desired}} = \frac{1}{-K}\Big[\ln C_{\text{trough (desired)}} - \ln C_{\text{peak (desired)}}\Big] + t + t'$$

(See **Equation 13-4**.)
where:
t = duration of infusion (2 hours);
t' = time after end of infusion (2 hours); and
τ = dosing interval, calculated as follows:

$$\tau = \frac{1}{-0.083 \text{ hr}^{-1}}(\ln 7 \text{ mg/L} - \ln 20 \text{ mg/L}) + 2 \text{ hr} + 2 \text{ hr}$$

$$= \frac{1}{-0.083 \text{ hr}^{-1}}(1.95 - 3.0) + 4 \text{ hr}$$

$$= 16.65 \text{ hr, round to 18 hr}$$

Therefore, we can change our dosing interval to 18 hours. This every-18-hour dosing interval is a nonstandard interval and can result in administration time errors. Only use intervals such as every 18 or 16 hours when a more standard interval of every 12 or 24 hours does not yield acceptable plasma drug concentrations.

Calculation of New K_0

Now with the calculated elimination rate constant, volume of distribution, and dosing interval, a revised dosing regimen can be reapplied to solve for the dose. For the concentration at 2 hours after the infusion, we would use the desired concentration of 20 mg/L:

$$C_{peak(steady\ state)} = \frac{K_0(1-e^{-Kt})}{VK(1-e^{-K\tau})}e^{-Kt'}$$

$$20\ mg/L = \frac{K_0(1-e^{-0.083\ hr^{-1}(2\ hr)})}{(0.083\ hr^{-1})(42.67\ L)(1-e^{-0.083\ hr^{-1}(18\ hr)})}e^{-0.083\ hr^{-1}(2\ hr)}$$

$$= \frac{K_0(0.153)}{(0.083\ hr^{-1})(42.67\ L)(0.776)}(0.847)$$

Rearranging gives:

$$K_0 = \frac{(20\ mg/L)(0.083\ hr^{-1})(42.67\ L)(0.776)}{(0.153)(0.847)}$$

$$= (423\ mg/hr)(2\ hr\ infusion)$$

$$= 846\ mg,\ round\ to\ 800\ mg\ or\ 900\ mg$$

(See **Equation 13-3**.)
If this dose of 846 mg is rounded up to 900 mg, it will yield a desired peak of 21.3 mg/L. If the dose is rounded down to 800, then the peak will be 18.9 mg/L. In this instance, a peak of more than 20 mg/L is more desirable than a peak less than 20 mg/L, so we would use the dose of 900 mg. The resulting concentration at the end of the dosing interval (trough) can be estimated:

$$C_{trough} = C_{peak(steady\ state)}e^{(-0.083\ hr^{-1})(14\ hr)}$$

(See **Equation 13-5**.)

$$= 21.3\ mg/L\ (0.313)$$

$$= 6.67\ mg/L$$

In summary, a dose of 900 mg every 18 hours should give patient WM a peak of approximately 20 mg/L and a trough of about 7 mg/L.

CASE 2

A 24-year-old woman, patient JH (weighing 72 kg), is admitted to the hospital after sustaining multiple traumatic injuries in a motor vehicle accident. Her recovery is complicated by the onset of acute renal failure 1 week

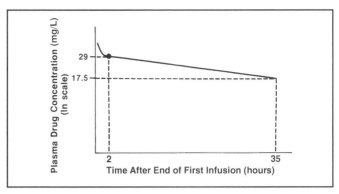

FIGURE 13-5.
Plasma concentrations after loading dose of vancomycin in patient with renal impairment (29 mg/L at 2 hours and 17.5 mg/L at 35 hours after the end of the infusion).

after admission. During the second week, she experiences a spiking fever; gram-positive bacilli, resistant to methicillin but susceptible to vancomycin, are subsequently cultured from her blood. Her physicians decide to begin a course of vancomycin.

Problem 2A. Two hours after the end of a 1000-mg loading dose administered over 1 hour, the vancomycin plasma concentration was 29 mg/L; it is 17.5 mg/L at 35 hours after the end of this infusion (Figure 13-5). Calculate the vancomycin elimination rate constant, half-life, and volume of distribution in this patient.

Note that there are two opportunities to calculate patient-specific pharmacokinetic values—after the first dose or after steady state has been achieved. In this case, because the patient has such a long half-life, it is decided to calculate these parameters after the first dose, which allows for subsequent dose adjustments without waiting the many days necessary for steady state to be reached. The reason for calculating this patient's elimination rate constant and volume of distribution is to predict how often a vancomycin dose will be needed, when the next dose should be given, and the size of the next dose. First, we calculate the elimination rate constant (K) and half-life ($T^{1/2}$):

$$K = -slope\ of\ natural\ log\ of\ vancomycin\ concentration\ versus\ time\ plot$$

$$= -\frac{\ln C_2 - \ln C_1}{t_2 - t_1}$$

$$= -\frac{\ln 17.5\ mg/L - \ln 29\ mg/L}{35\ hr - 2\ hr}$$

$$= 0.015\ hr^{-1}$$

(See **Equation 3-1**.)

■ CLINICAL CORRELATE

Remember that the second plasma level was taken 35 hours after the end of the infusion, not 35 hours after the first plasma level. Therefore, we must account for the 2 hours that lapsed between the end of the infusion and first plasma level.

When calculating the elimination rate constant from two different plasma concentrations, the concentrations should be at least one half-life apart to determine a reasonably accurate slope of the line. Drug concentrations less than one half-life apart can incur great errors in the estimate of the elimination rate constant (K).

The half-life in this case can be calculated:

$$T \tfrac{1}{2} = \frac{0.693}{K}$$
$$= \frac{0.693}{0.015 \text{ hr}^{-1}}$$
$$= 46.2 \text{ hr}$$

(See **Equation 3-3**.)

Now the volume of distribution (V) can be estimated, using the simple relationship given below:

loading dose = plasma concentration achieved × volume of distribution

By rearranging, we get:

$$V = \frac{\text{loading dose}}{\text{plasma concentration achieved}}$$
$$= \frac{1000 \text{ mg}}{29 \text{ mg/L}}$$
$$= 34.5 \text{ L}$$

Note that the patient's calculated V is much less than the estimated V of 64.8 L; consequently, the loading dose gave us a peak concentration much higher than 20 mg/L.

Problem 2B. With the information just determined, calculate when the next vancomycin dose should be given and what it should be. Assume that the plasma vancomycin concentration should decline to 10 mg/L before another dose is given and that the plasma concentration desired 2 hours after the infusion is complete is 20 mg/L.

First, we must know the time needed for the plasma concentration to decline to 10 mg/L. It can easily be calculated from the known plasma concentrations, the

elimination rate constant, and the desired trough plasma concentration:

$$C_{\text{trough}} = C_{\text{peak(steady state)}} e^{-Kt}$$

where:

$C_{\text{peak(steady state)}}$ = observed concentration of 29 mg/L,
K = elimination rate constant (0.015 hr^{-1}), and
t = time between observed concentration of 29 mg/L and trough concentration of 10 mg (unknown).

Then:

$$10 \text{ mg/L} = (29 \text{ mg/L})(e^{-0.015 \text{ hr}^{-1})t})$$

To solve for t, we can first take the natural log of each side of the equation:

$$\ln 10 \text{ mg/L} = \ln 29 \text{ mg/L } (-0.015 \text{ hr}^{-1})(t)$$

Rearranging gives:

$$t = \frac{\ln 10 \text{ mg/L} - \ln 29 \text{ mg/L}}{-0.015 \text{ hr}^{-1}}$$
$$= 71 \text{ hr}$$

Therefore, at approximately 71 hours after the plasma concentration of 29 mg/L is observed (or 73 hours after the end of the infusion), the next vancomycin dose can be given.

Next, we determine dosing interval and maintenance dose as follows:

$$\tau_{\text{desired}} = \frac{1}{-K} [\ln C_{\text{trough (desired)}} - \ln C_{\text{peak (desired)}}] + t + t'$$
$$= \frac{1}{-0.015 \text{ hr}^{-1}} [\ln 10 \text{mg/L} - \ln 20 \text{mg/L}] + 1 \text{ hr} + 2 \text{ hr}$$
$$= \frac{1}{-0.015 \text{ hr}^{-1}} [2.30 - 3.00] + 3 \text{ hr}$$
$$= 49.6 \text{ hr, rounded to 48 hr}$$

(See **Equation 13-4**.)

The maintenance dose can then be calculated as follows:

$$C_{\text{peak(steady state)}} = \frac{K_0 (1 - e^{-Kt})}{VK(1 - e^{-K\tau})} e^{-Kt'}$$

(See **Equation 13-3**.)
where:

$C_{\text{peak(steady state)}}$ = concentration 2 hours after end of infusion,
τ = 48 hours,
t = duration of infusion (1 hour),
t' = time after end of infusion (2 hours),
V = 34.5 L, and
K = 0.015 hr^{-1}.

Rearranging to solve for K_0:

$$K_0 = \frac{VK(C_{peak(steady\ state)})(1-e^{-K\tau})}{(1-e^{-Kt})(e^{-Kt'})}$$

$$= \frac{(34.5\ L)(0.015\ hr^{-1})(20\ mg/L)(1-e^{-0.015\ hr^{-1}(48\ hr)})}{(1-e^{-0.015\ hr^{-1}(1\ hr)})(e^{-0.015\ hr^{-1}(2\ hr)})}$$

$$= \frac{5.31\ mg/hr}{(0.015)(0.970)}$$

= 366 mg, rounded down to 350 mg because we rounded our dosing interval down to 48 hr

Because 350 mg is used instead of 366 mg, the peak will be 19.1 mg instead of 20 mg.

Finally, we must check to see what our trough concentration will be after rounding both dose and dosing interval.

$$C_{trough} = C_{peak}e^{-Kt''} \quad (\text{See } \textbf{Equation 13-5}.)$$

where:

$$t'' = \text{time between } C_{trough} \text{ and } C_{peak}$$

$$= \tau - t - t'$$

$$= 48 - 1 - 2 = 45\ hr$$

and:

$$C_{trough} = (19.1\ mg/L)e^{(-0.015\ hr^{-1})45\ hr}$$

$$= 9.7\ mg/L$$

If we decided to give 400 mg every 48 hours, our respective peak and trough values would be 21.9 and 11.2 mg/L.

CASE 3

A 60-year-old woman, patient BA (weighing 70 kg), is being treated for a hospital-acquired, methicillin-resistant, *Staphylococcus aureus* bacteremia seeding from an infected sacral decubitus ulcer. Her estimated CrCl is 30 mL/minute. She was given a 1000-mg vancomycin loading dose and is now receiving 500 mg (infused over 1 hour) every 12 hours.

Problem 3A. Predict the steady-state C_{peak} and C_{trough} from this dose, using population average values for K and V. How do they compare to the recommended C_{peak} of 18–26 mg/L and C_{trough} of 5–10 mg/L?

The equation for a one-compartment, intermittent-infusion drug can be used to solve for $C_{peak(steady\ state)}$ and $C_{trough(steady\ state)}$:

$$C_{peak(steady\ state)} = \frac{K_0(1-e^{-Kt})}{VK(1-e^{-K\tau})}e^{-Kt'}$$

(See **Equation 13-3**.)

where:

$C_{peak(steady\ state)}$ = desired peak plasma concentration at steady state,

K_0 = drug infusion rate (also maintenance dose given over 1 hour),

V = volume of distribution (population estimate for vancomycin of 0.9 L/kg TBW),

K = elimination rate constant (population estimate for vancomycin),

t = infusion time (1 hour in this case),

τ = patient's current dosing interval, and

t' = time between end of infusion and collection of blood sample (2 hours).

First, we must calculate patient BA's K and V values for use in this equation. The estimated K would be:

$$K = 0.00083\ hr^{-1}\ (CrCl) + 0.0044 \quad (\text{See } \textbf{Equation 13-2}.)$$

$$= 0.00083\ (30) + 0.0044$$

$$= 0.029\ hr^{-1}$$

which we shall round to 0.03 hr^{-1} for ease of calculation.

Patient BA's estimated volume of distribution (V) is calculated from the population estimate of 0.9 L/kg TBW:

$$0.9\ L/kg \times 70\ kg = 63\ L \quad (\text{See } \textbf{Equation 13-1}.)$$

Now that we have these estimates of K and V, we can calculate the C_{peak} and C_{trough} values that would be obtained with this dose of 500 mg every 12 hours. By application of the general equation for a one-compartment, first-order, intermittently infused drug, we get:

$$C_{peak(steady\ state)} = \frac{K_0(1-e^{-Kt})}{VK(1-e^{-K\tau})}e^{-Kt'}$$

(See **Equation 13-3**.)

where:

$C_{peak(steady\ state)}$ = desired peak plasma concentration at steady state,

K_0 = drug infusion rate (maintenance dose per hour),

V = volume of distribution (population estimate for vancomycin),

K = elimination rate constant (population estimate for vancomycin),

t = duration of infusion,

t' = time from end of infusion until concentration is determined (2 hours for peak), and

τ = desired or most appropriate dosing interval.

Therefore:

$$C_{peak(steady\ state)} = \frac{(500\ mg/1\ hr)(1-e^{-0.03\ hr^{-1}(1\ hr)})}{(63\ L)(0.03\ hr^{-1})(1-e^{-0.03\ hr^{-1}(12\ hr)})}e^{-0.03\ hr^{-1}(2\ hr)}$$

$$= \frac{(500 \text{ mg/hr})(0.029)}{(1.89 \text{ L/hr})(0.302)}(0.94)$$

$$= (264.5 \text{ mg/L})(0.096)(0.94)$$

$$= 23.9 \text{ mg/L}$$

This value is within the desired C_{peak} range of 18–26 mg/L for this patient. Patient BA's $C_{trough(steady\ state)}$ can be estimated with the following equation:

$$C_{trough(steady\ state)} = C_{peak(steady\ state)}e^{-Kt}$$

In this case, patient BA's C_{trough} will equal the C_{peak} (drawn 2 hours after the 1-hour infusion began) multiplied by the fraction of this C_{peak} remaining after elimination has occurred for t' hours, which in this case is 9 hours (12-hour dosing interval minus 3 hours).

The patient's estimated $C_{trough(steady\ state)}$ is calculated as follows:

$$C_{trough(steady\ state)} = (23.9 \text{ mg/L})e^{(-0.03 \text{ hr}^{-1})9 \text{ hr}}$$

$$= (23.9)(0.76)$$

$$= 18.2 \text{ mg/L}$$

This C_{trough} value is much greater than the desired range of 5–10 mg/L, so a dosing adjustment is needed.

Problem 3B. What vancomycin dose would you recommend for patient BA to attain a C_{peak} of 25 mg/L (drawn 2 hours after the end of a 1-hour infusion) and a C_{trough} of 7 mg/L?

Using the estimates of K (0.03 hr^{-1}) and V (63 L), we should first determine the best dosing interval (τ) for patient BA:

$$\tau = \frac{1}{-K}[\ln C_{trough\ (desired)} - \ln C_{peak\ (desired)}] + t + t'$$

(See **Equation 13-4**.)
where t is the time of infusion and t' is the time after the end of the infusion. Then:

$$\tau = \frac{1}{-0.03 \text{ hr}^{-1}}(\ln 7 \text{mg/L} - \ln 25 \text{mg/L}) + 1 \text{ hr} + 2 \text{ hr}$$

$$= -33.33 \text{ hr} (1.945 - 3.218) + 3 \text{ hr}$$

$$= 45.42 \text{ hr, rounded to } 48 \text{ hr}$$

Using this new dosing interval of 48 hours, we can solve for the maintenance dose that gives our desired C_{peak} and C_{trough} of 25 and 5–10 mg/L, respectively:

$$C_{peak(steady\ state)} = \frac{K_0(1 - e^{-Kt})}{VK(1 - e^{-K\tau})}e^{-Kt'}$$

(See **Equation 13-3**.)

where:

$C_{peak(steady\ state)}$ = desired peak concentration at steady state,

K_0 = drug infusion rate (also maintenance dose you are trying to calculate),

V = volume of distribution (population estimate for vancomycin),

K = elimination rate constant (population estimate for vancomycin),

t = duration of infusion,

t' = time from end of infusion until concentration is determined (2 hours for peak), and

τ = desired or most appropriate dosing interval.

Then:

$$C_{peak(desired)} = \frac{K_0(1 - e^{-0.03 \text{ hr}^{-1}(1 \text{ hr})})}{(63 \text{ L})(0.03 \text{ hr}^{-1})(1 - e^{-0.03 \text{ hr}^{-1}(48 \text{ hr})})}e^{-0.03 \text{ hr}^{-1}(2 \text{ hr})}$$

$$25 \text{ mg/L} = \frac{K_0(0.03)}{(1.89)(0.76)}(0.94)$$

$$= \frac{K_0}{(1.89)}(0.039)(0.94)$$

$$= (0.020)K_0(0.94)$$

$$K_0 = 1316 \text{ mg, rounded to } 1300 \text{ mg}$$

Note that this answer can range from 1245 to 1345 mg, depending on the amount of rounding used in this complex calculation.

If patient BA is given 1300 mg every 48 hours, her corresponding C_{trough} value can be determined with the following equation:

$$C_{trough(steady\ state)} = C_{peak(steady\ state)}e^{-Kt}$$

(See **Equation 13-5**.)
In this case, C_{trough} will equal the C_{peak} (drawn 2 hours after the 1-hour infusion is complete) multiplied by the fraction of this C_{peak} remaining after elimination has occurred for t hours, which in this case is 45 hours (48-hour dosing interval minus 2 hours minus 1 hour). So:

$$C_{trough(steady\ state)} = (25 \text{ mg/L})e^{(-0.03 \text{ hr}^{-1})45 \text{ hr}}$$

$$= 25 (0.26)$$

$$= 6.5 \text{ mg/L}$$

Thus, we would give patient BA 1300 mg every 48 hours for an estimated C_{peak} of 25 mg/L and an estimated C_{trough} of 6.5 mg/L.

CLINICAL CORRELATE

Don't let these equations intimidate you. Try to develop a step-by-step model to walk you through the calculations, such as:

1. Determine patient-specific K and V values. If these values are not known, use population estimates.
2. Determine the dosing interval.
3. Determine the drug infusion rate (K_0).
4. Check the trough to make sure it is within normal limits.

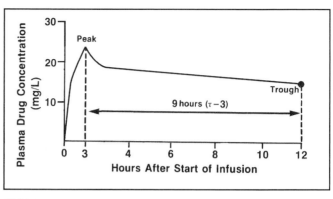

FIGURE 13-6.
Time between peak and trough.

Problem 3C. Patient BA received a vancomycin dose of 500 mg every 12 hours before her pharmacokinetic assessment. While she was on this dose, plasma concentrations from the laboratory were out of the desired range, confirming that this dose was wrong. C_{peak} (drawn 2 hours after the end of a 1-hour infusion) was 23 mg/L, and C_{trough} was 14 mg/L (Figure 13-6). Adjust patient BA's dose to give a C_{peak} of 25 mg/L and a $C_{trough(steady\ state)}$ of approximately 7 mg/L.

To adjust this patient's dose, we must first determine her real K and V values, then calculate a new dosing interval, and finally solve for a new maintenance dose.

To calculate K, we can use:

$$K = -\frac{\ln C_{trough} - \ln C_{peak}}{\tau - t - t'}$$

$$= -\frac{\ln 14\ mg/L - \ln 23\ mg/L}{9\ hr}$$

$$= -\frac{2.64 - 3.13}{9\ hr}$$

$$= \frac{0.49}{9\ hr}$$

$$= 0.054\ hr^{-1}$$

(See **Equation 3-1**.)

To calculate V, we can use:

$$C_{peak(steady\ state)} = \frac{K_0(1 - e^{-Kt})}{VK(1 - e^{-K\tau})}e^{-Kt'}$$

(See **Equation 13-3**.)
where:

$C_{peak(steady\ state)}$ = measured steady-state peak plasma concentration (23 mg/L) drawn 2 hours after end of a 1-hour infusion,
K_0 = drug infusion rate (maintenance dose of 500 mg over 1 hour),
V = volume of distribution (unknown),
K = elimination rate constant calculated from C_{peak} and C_{trough} (0.054 hr^{-1}),
t = infusion time (1 hour),

t' = time from end of infusion until concentration is determined (2 hours for peak), and
τ = dosing interval at time concentrations are obtained (12 hours).

By substituting the above values, we obtain:

$$23\ mg/L = \frac{(500\ mg\ /\ 1\ hr)(1 - e^{-0.054\ hr^{-1}(1\ hr)})}{V(0.054\ hr^{-1})(1 - e^{-0.054\ hr^{-1}(12\ hr)})}e^{-0.054\ hr^{-1}(2\ hr)}$$

$$= \frac{(500\ mg/hr)(0.053)}{V(0.054\ hr^{-1})(0.48)}(0.90)$$

$$V = 40\ L$$

Note the differences between the previously estimated K and V of 0.03 hr^{-1} and 63 L and the calculated values of 0.054 hr^{-1} and 40 L. Because our measured K of 0.054 hr^{-1} is larger than the estimated value, the half-life would be shorter (23.1 vs. 12.8 hours), indicating the need for a smaller dosing interval.

Now, to calculate the best dosing interval to get a C_{peak} of 25 mg/L and a $C_{trough(steady\ state)}$ of approximately 7 mg/L, we would use:

$$\tau = \frac{1}{-K}[\ln C_{trough\ (desired)} - \ln C_{peak\ (desired)}] + t + t'$$

$$= \frac{1}{-0.054\ hr^{-1}}[\ln 7\ mg/L - \ln 25\ mg/L] + 1\ hr + 2\ hr$$

$$= \frac{1}{-0.054\ hr^{-1}}[1.945 - 3.218] + 3\ hr$$

$$= 26.6\ hr,\ rounded\ to\ 24\ hr$$

(See **Equation 13-4**.)

The new maintenance dose now can be calculated:

$$C_{peak(steady\ state)} = \frac{K_0(1 - e^{-Kt})}{VK(1 - e^{-K\tau})}e^{-Kt'}$$

(See **Equation 13-3**.)

where:

$C_{peak(steady\ state)}$ = desired peak concentration at steady state (25 mg/L),

K_0 = drug infusion rate (also maintenance dose you are trying to calculate, in milligrams per hour),

V = volume of distribution (40 L),

K = elimination rate constant calculated from C_{peak} and C_{trough} (0.054 hr^{-1}),

t = infusion time (1 hour),

t' = time from end of infusion until concentration is determined (2 hours for peak), and

τ = desired or most appropriate dosing interval (24 hours).

Then:

$$C_{peak(steady\ state)} = \frac{K_0(1-e^{-0.054\ hr^{-1}(1\ hr)})}{(40\ L)(0.054\ hr^{-1})(1-e^{-0.054\ hr^{-1}(24\ hr)})}e^{-0.054\ hr^{-1}(2\ hr)}$$

$$25\ mg/L = \frac{K_0(0.053)}{(2.16)(0.73)}(0.90)$$

$$= \frac{K_0}{2.16}(0.073)(0.90)$$

$$K_0 = 883\ mg$$

Being conservative, we would round this dose to 800 mg, which would slightly lower the actual peak value from 25 to approximately 24 mg/L. This calculation is shown below:

$$(800\ mg/833\ mg) \times 25\ mg/L = 24\ mg/L$$

Problem 3D. Calculate the $C_{trough(steady\ state)}$ for patient BA if she receives the new dose of 800 mg every 24 hours.

We can use the following equation, where t'' is now the number of hours between the peak and trough ($t'' = \tau - t - t'$). Therefore, $t'' = 21$ hours.

$$C_{trough(steady\ state)} = C_{peak(steady\ state)}e^{-t''}$$
(See **Equation 13-5**.)

$$= (24\ mg/L)e^{(-0.054\ hr^{-1})21\ hr}$$

$$= 7.7\ mg/L$$

The new dose of 800 mg every 24 hours will give a C_{peak} of approximately 24 mg/L and a C_{trough} of about 8 mg/L.

Problem 3E. Patient BA's C_{trough} is too high after the regimen of 500 mg every 12 hours. How long will you hold this dose before beginning the new regimen of 800 mg every 24 hours?

Before changing to 800 mg every 24 hours, you must wait for patient BA's C_{trough} of 14 mg/L to decrease to the desired C_{trough} of approximately 7 mg/L. The for-

mula for calculating the number of hours to hold the dose is:

$$C_{trough(desired)} = C_{trough(actual)}e^{-Kt}\ \text{(See Equation 3-2.)}$$

where t is the amount of time to hold the dose. This formula is an application of the general formula (see Lesson 3) that the concentration at any time equals a previous concentration multiplied by the fraction remaining:

$$C = C_0e^{-Kt}$$

where:

C = drug concentration at time t,

C_0 = drug concentration at some earlier time or time zero, and

e^{-Kt} = fraction of original or previous concentration remaining.

In patient BA's case:

$$7\ mg/L = (14\ mg/L)e^{(-0.054\ hr^{-1})(t)}$$

$$0.50\ mg/L = e^{(-0.054\ hr^{-1})(t)}$$

Next, take the natural logarithm of both sides:

$$\ln 0.50 = \ln (e^{(-0.054\ hr-1)(t)})$$

$$-0.693 = -0.054(t)$$

$$t = 12.83\ hr$$

We should hold this patient's dose for an additional 13 hours after the next C_{trough} and then begin her new dose. The same equation can be used to determine the amount of time to hold the dose from the last C_{peak} of 23 mg/L. Again, the general equation is:

$$C = C_0e^{-Kt}\ \text{(See Equation 3-2.)}$$

where:

C = drug concentration at time t (representing here the desired C_{trough} of 7 mg/L),

C_0 = drug concentration at some earlier time (representing here C_{peak} of 23 mg/L), and

e^{-Kt} = fraction of previous concentration remaining.

In patient BA's case:

$$7\ mg/L = (23\ mg/L)e^{(-0.054\ hr^{-1})(t)}$$

$$0.30\ mg/L = e^{(-0.054\ hr^{-1})(t)}$$

Next, take the natural logarithm of both sides:

$$\ln 0.30 = \ln (e^{(-0.054 \text{ hr}^{-1})(t)})$$

$$-1.203 = -0.054(t)$$

$$22.28 \text{ hr} = t$$

We should hold this patient's dose for an additional 22 hours after the C_{peak} and then begin her new dose. Note that you can calculate time to hold using either C_{peak} or C_{trough}; both methods give the correct answer.

A more intuitive method for estimating the time to hold patient BA's dose is by examination of the vancomycin half-life. We know that the drug concentration decreases by half over each half-life. We can estimate how many drug half-lives to wait for her concentration to approach our desired amount of 7 mg/L as follows. For patient BA (C_{trough} of 14 mg/L and $T\frac{1}{2}$ of 12.83 hours [0.693/0.054]), the concentration will drop from 14 to 7 mg/L in one half-life of 13 hours. Because a concentration of 7 mg/L is acceptable, we only need to hold the next scheduled dose for an additional 13 hours before beginning the new dose of 800 mg every 24 hours.

CASE 4

A 65-year-old man, patient MT, has a history of subacute bacterial endocarditis secondary to a mitral valve replacement 5 years ago. He is currently hospitalized for *Staphylococcus aureus* bacteremia. He has been treated with 750 mg of vancomycin every 16 hours for the last 10 days. His most recent C_{peak} was 26 mg/L (drawn 2 hours after a 1-hour vancomycin infusion), and his most recent C_{trough} was 9 mg/L.

Problem 4A. Patient MT's physician wants to discharge him and allow a local home infusion company to administer his vancomycin on a once-a-day basis. You are asked to determine if it is possible to obtain a C_{peak} of approximately 25 mg/L and a C_{trough} of around 5 mg/L with a once-a-day dose. What is your response?
Before answering this question, we must be sure we know what the question is asking. Basically, this question is asking whether, based on the patient's pharmacokinetic parameters, a dose can be given to obtain a satisfactory C_{peak} and C_{trough} given a dosing interval of 24 hours.

First, we must determine patient MT's pharmacokinetic parameters based on his C_{peak} of 26 mg/L and C_{trough} of 9 mg/L. To calculate K, we can use:

$$-K = \frac{\ln C_{trough(measured)} - \ln C_{peak(measured)}}{\tau - t - t'}$$

(See **Equation 3-1**.)

where t' represents 2 hours, the number of hours after the infusion that the C_{peak} was drawn. Then:

$$K = -\frac{\ln 9 \text{mg/L} - \ln 26 \text{mg/L}}{13 \text{ hr}}$$

$$= -\frac{2.20 - 3.26}{13 \text{ hr}}$$

$$= 0.082 \text{ hr}^{-1}$$

To calculate V, we can use:

$$C_{peak(steady\ state)} = \frac{K_0(1-e^{-Kt})}{VK(1-e^{-K\tau})}e^{-Kt'}$$

(See **Equation 13-3**.)
where:
$C_{peak(steady\ state)}$ = measured peak plasma concentration (26 mg/L),
K_0 = drug infusion rate (also maintenance dose of 750 mg),
V = volume of distribution (unknown),
K = elimination rate constant calculated from C_{peak} and C_{trough} (0.082 hr^{-1}),
t = duration of infusion (1 hour),
t' = time from end of infusion until concentration is determined (2 hours for peak), and
τ = dosing interval at time concentrations are obtained (16 hours).

By substituting the above values, we obtain:

$$26 \text{ mg/L} = \frac{(750 \text{ mg})(1-e^{-0.082 \text{ hr}^{-1}(1 \text{ hr})})}{V(0.082 \text{ hr}^{-1})(1-e^{-0.082 \text{ hr}^{-1}(16 \text{ hr})})}e^{-0.082 \text{ hr}^{-1}(2 \text{ hr})}$$

$$= \frac{(750 \text{ mg})(0.079)}{V(0.082 \text{ hr}^{-1})(0.731)}(0.848)$$

$$V = 32.2 \text{ L}$$

Next, we use our general equation to solve for K_0 (maintenance dose) with our predetermined 24-hour dosing interval:

$$C_{peak(steady\ state)} = \frac{K_0(1 - e^{-Kt})}{VK(1 - e^{-K\tau})}e^{-Kt'}$$

where:
$C_{peak(steady\ state)}$ = desired peak concentration at steady state (25 mg/L),
K_0 = drug infusion rate (also maintenance dose you are trying to calculate, in milligrams per hour),
V = calculated volume of distribution (33.5 L),
K = elimination rate constant calculated from C_{peak} and C_{trough} (0.082 hr^{-1}),
t = duration of infusion time,
t' = time from end of infusion until concentration is determined (2 hours for peak), and
τ = dosing interval desired (24 hours).

By substituting the above values, we obtain:

$$26 \text{ mg/L} = \frac{K_0(1 - e^{-0.082 \text{ hr}^{-1}(1 \text{ hr})})}{(32.2 \text{ L})(0.082 \text{ hr}^{-1})(1 - e^{-0.082 \text{ hr}^{-1}(24 \text{ hr})})} \, e^{-0.082 \text{ hr}^{-1}(2 \text{ hr})}$$

$$26 \text{ mg/L} = \frac{K_0(0.079)}{(2.64)(0.860)}(0.848)$$

$$K_0 = 847 \text{ mg}$$

This dose could be rounded up or down to 800 or 900 mg given every 24 hours. Remember that the desired peak concentration of 25 mg/L will be slightly higher or lower if the dose is rounded up or down, and the adjusted desired peak can be calculated as shown in previous cases. If the dose is rounded up to 900 mg, C_{peak} will become 26.6 mg/L; if the dose is rounded down to 800 mg, C_{peak} will become 23.6 mg/L.

Finally, we must check to see that our C_{trough} concentration with this dose is acceptable (assume a dose of 900 mg was given for a desired peak of 26.6 mg/L):

$$C_{trough(steady state)} = C_{peak(steady state)}e^{-Kt''}$$

(See **Equation 13-5**.)

In this case, patient MT's C_{trough} will be equal to his C_{peak} of 26.6 mg/L multiplied by the fraction of the C_{peak} remaining after elimination has occurred for t'' hours, which in this case is 21 hours (24-hour dosing interval minus t [1 hour] minus t' [2 hours]).

Therefore:

$$C_{trough(steady state)} = (26.6 \text{ mg/L})e^{(-0.082 \text{ hr}^{-1})21 \text{ hr}}$$

$$= 26.6(0.179)$$

$$= 4.75 \text{ mg/L}$$

A dose of 900 mg every 24 hours will give acceptable concentrations, thus allowing for a more convenient once-daily outpatient administration of patient MT's vancomycin.

If the trough concentration of 4.75 mg/L is too low, a slightly higher dose, such as 1000 mg, can be used. Corresponding peak and trough values are 29.5 and 5.3 mg/L, respectively, for 1000 mg every 24 hours. Even though once-daily dosing is convenient for this patient, we need to consider whether the trough concentration will be adequate for this patient with endocarditis.

REFERENCE

1. Examples of such recommendations can be found in *Morbidity and Mortality Weekly Report* (e.g., *MMWR* 1995;44:1–13) and at the Centers for Disease Control and Prevention Web site: http://www.cdc.gov.

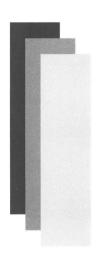

LESSON
14

Theophylline

In this lesson, Cases 1–4 focus on dosing of theophylline. Individualization of theophylline dosage maximizes therapeutic benefit while minimizing adverse effects. Theophylline is used less frequently in the treatment of asthma as beta-2 agonists and anti-inflammatory agents (corticosteroids) have become the first-line therapies. However, theophylline is still occasionally used for treatment of nocturnal or mild persistent asthma, and dosage individualization is necessary.[1] Theophylline may also be useful to decrease inhaled corticosteroid requirements.[2] Although theophylline was once thought to have primarily a bronchodilator effect, it is now recognized to have anti-inflammatory effects as well. These effects may be the primary benefit to asthma patients.[3] The therapeutic range is now generally accepted to be 5–15 mg/L, a decrease from the previously accepted range of 10–20 mg/L. This newer range is probably more relevant to bronchodilator effects; anti-inflammatory effects may be achieved at lower concentrations.

Theophylline is eliminated from circulation through hepatic oxidative metabolism (cytochrome P450) and has a low intrinsic clearance (see Lesson 9). Therefore, total hepatic clearance of theophylline is determined by the intrinsic clearance of the liver and is not dependent on liver blood flow. Theophylline may undergo nonlinear, or Michaelis–Menten, pharmacokinetics (see Lesson 10) even within the therapeutic range, but this is more likely to occur at concentrations above the therapeutic range.[4] Diseases that affect liver blood flow, such as cirrhosis and heart failure, may reduce theophylline clearance. Drugs that alter hepatic oxidative metabolism can also dramatically affect theophylline clearance. Some drugs, such as cimetidine[5] and erythromycin,[6] will decrease theophylline clearance and cause increased plasma theophylline concentrations (Table 14-1).

Theophylline may be administered intravenously or orally. Suppository and rectal solution forms of the drug are available but are not commonly used. Intravenous infusion involves administration of theophylline itself or in a salt form (such as aminophylline). When theophylline derivatives are used, the theophylline dose equivalent should be calculated. For example, aminophylline is 80% theophylline. Therefore, to obtain the theophylline dose equivalent, the aminophylline dose should be multiplied by 0.8.

Many different oral formulations of theophylline are available. Some of these are rapidly absorbed after administration. Others are designed to slowly release drug in the gastrointestinal tract for up to 24 hours after administration. The type of oral product used directly affects the pharmacokinetic calculations.

CASE 1

JM is a 34-year-old, 70-kg, black man seen in the emergency room with status asthmaticus refractory to epinephrine and corticosteroid therapy. A serum theophylline level at this time was zero, indicating JM had not been on theophylline recently.

Problem 1A. Determine an appropriate loading dose of aminophylline to produce a theophylline concentration of 15 mcg/mL.

To calculate a loading dose of aminophylline requires that we know the desired plasma concentration we want the loading dose to achieve, the patient's theophylline volume of distribution, the aminophylline salt equivalent for theophylline, and the fraction of drug administered that reaches the systemic circulation.

In this case, the desired plasma theophylline concentration is 15 mcg/mL, the aminophylline salt equivalent (S) is 0.8, and the fraction of drug administered reaching systemic circulation (F) is 1.

TABLE 14-1.
Factors and Drugs That Alter Theophylline Clearance

Factors	Total Body Clearance (L/kg/hour)	Clearance Adjustment (× 0.04 L/kg/hour)
Hepatic disease	0.02	0.5
Acute pulmonary edema	0.02	0.5
Severe COPD	0.03	0.8
HF	0.016	0.5
Cor pulmonale	0.028	0.7
Cigarette smoking	0.063	1.6
Ex cigarette smoking (quit >2 years)	0.051	1.2
Marijuana smoking	0.072	1.7
Marijuana and cigarettes	0.09	2.2
Elderly cigarette smokers	0.045	1.1

Drug	Clearance Adjustment (× 0.04 L/kg/hour)
Cimetidine (after 2 or more days)	0.5–0.7
Oral contraceptives	0.7
Interferon	0.15
Ciprofloxacin	0.7–0.75
Diltiazem	0.8–0.9
Norfloxacin	0.85
Phenytoin	1.35–1.5
Phenobarbital	1.35–1.5
Erythromycin	0.75–0.8
Propranolol	0.5–0.7
Verapamil	0.8–0.9
Rifampin	1.35–1.5
Phenytoin + smoking	1.9

The patient's volume of distribution (V) is calculated from the patient's weight and the expected volume (in liters per kilogram) from published literature:

$$V \text{ (L)} = \text{weight (kg)} \times 0.5 \text{ L/kg}$$

14-1

$$= 70 \text{ kg } (0.5 \text{ L/kg})$$

$$= 35 \text{ L}$$

▮ CLINICAL CORRELATE

For theophylline, the patient's actual body weight should be used to calculate the volume of distribution unless the patient is more than 50% above ideal body weight. In patients more than 50% above ideal body weight, volume of distribution should be calculated using ideal body weight.[7]

Based on the information we now have, we can calculate an aminophylline loading dose for JM.

The basic loading dose equation can be derived from the plasma concentration equation we learned in Lesson 1.

$$\text{concentration} = \frac{\text{amount of drug in body}}{\text{volume in which drug is distributed}}$$

$$C = \frac{X}{V}$$

(See **Equation 1-1.**)

We can rewrite this equation to:

$$D = C \times V$$

Taking into consideration the S and F values for aminophylline, we can rewrite the above variation of Equation 1-1 as follows:

14-2

$$D = \frac{CpdV}{SF}$$

where:

D = the loading dose (mg);
Cpd = the desired concentration (mg/L);
V = the volume of distribution (L);
S = salt form; and
F = bioavailability, which is equal to 1 for drugs given intravenously.

$$D = \frac{15 \text{ mg/L} \times (35 \text{ L})}{0.8}$$

$$= 656.3 \text{ mg}$$

$$\sim 650 \text{ mg}$$

This 650-mg aminophylline loading dose will produce a serum concentration slightly less than 15 mcg/mL.

Note: Remember, aminophylline is a salt form of theophylline and contains approximately 80% theophylline equivalents.

Problem 1B. It appears the laboratory had mixed up JM's profile with another patient, and JM actually has a theophylline concentration of 4.3 mcg/mL. Recalculate the desired loading dose to achieve a concentration of 15 mcg/mL.

In this situation, we will slightly modify the loading dose Equation 14-2 to the following:

$$D = \frac{(Cpd-Cpi)V}{SF}$$

(See **Equation 14-2**.)
where:
  D = the loading dose;
  Cpd = the desired concentration (mg/L);
  Cpi = the initial concentration (mg/L);
  V = the volume of distribution (L);
  S = salt form; and
  F = bioavailability, which is equal to 1 for drugs administered intravenously.

$$D = \frac{(15 \text{ mg/L} - 4.3 \text{ mg/L})35 \text{ L}}{0.8}$$

$$= 468.1 \text{ mg}$$

$$\sim 450 \text{ mg}$$

This 450-mg aminophylline loading dose will result in a serum concentration slightly less than 15 mg/L.

Problem 1C. The loading dose is to be given over 30 minutes, and a maintenance infusion is to be started immediately. Suggest an aminophylline infusion rate to achieve a plasma theophylline concentration of 13 mcg/mL.

STEP A
The first step in solving this problem is to estimate JM's theophylline clearance by using the following equation:

⚠ 14-3   Cl = (0.04 L/kg/hr) × weight (kg)

= (0.04 L/kg/hr) × 70 kg

= 2.8 L/hr

where:
  Cl = clearance (L/hour; clearance is based on the patient's actual body weight), and
  0.04 L/kg/hour = population estimate found in literature.

STEP B
To solve for a maintenance dose (mg/hour), we can rearrange Equation 4-3, insert the Cl calculated in Step A, insert S and F values, and solve for $\bar{C}$.

$$\bar{C} = \frac{\text{dose}}{Cl_t \times \tau}$$

(See **Equation 4-3**.)

⚠ 14-4 $$D = \frac{\bar{C}p_{ss} \, Cl \, \tau}{SF}$$

(See **Equation 4-3**.)
where:
  D = the maintenance dose (mg/hour);
  $\bar{C}p_{ss}$ = average steady state concentration desired (mcg/mL);
  Cl = clearance (L/hour);
  S = salt form;
  F = bioavailability; and
  τ = dosing interval, which is 1 hour for continuous intravenous infusion.

$$D = \frac{13 \text{ mcg/mL} \times 2.8 \text{ L/hr} \times 1 \text{ hr}}{0.8}$$

$$= 45.5 \text{ mg/hr}$$

$$\sim 45 \text{ mg/hr}$$

Figure 14-1 demonstrates the relationship between serum levels achieved with the loading and maintenance doses of theophylline or aminophylline.

Problem 1D. JM starts to experience headaches, nausea, and vomiting. A theophylline level is ordered immediately and is reported by the

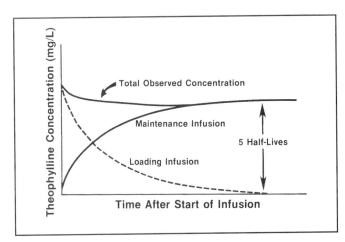

FIGURE 14-1.

Plasma concentrations with a loading dose and continuous infusion of theophylline or aminophylline.

laboratory as 22 mcg/mL. The infusion is stopped. Determine JM's actual clearance, a new infusion rate to achieve a serum concentration of 13 mcg/mL, and how long the nurse must wait before starting the new infusion.

To determine JM's actual theophylline clearance, we can rearrange Equation 14-4 in Problem 1-C and calculate this parameter as follows:

$$D = \frac{\overline{C}p_{ss}\ Cl\ \tau}{SF}$$

Rearrange to solve for Cl:

$$Cl = \frac{DSF}{\overline{C}p_{ss}\ \tau}$$

(See **Equation 14-4**.)
where:
  Cl = clearance (L/hour),
  D = maintenance dose (mg/hour),
  S = salt form,
  F = bioavailability, and
  $\overline{C}p_{ss}$ = average steady state concentration (mcg/mL).

$$Cl = \frac{45\ mg/hr \times 0.8}{22\ mcg/mL}$$
$$= 1.64\ L/hr$$

Notice that we estimated JM's theophylline Cl as 2.8 L/hour, but his actual value is 1.64 L/hour.

Now that we have his actual clearance, we can calculate a new maintenance dose that will give us the desired theophylline serum concentration of 13 mcg/mL:

$$D = \frac{\overline{C}p_{ss}\ Cl\ \tau}{SF}$$

(See **Equation 14-4**.)

$$D = \frac{13\ mcg/mL \times 1.64\ L/hr \times 1\ hr}{0.8}$$
$$= 26.65\ mg/hr$$
$$\sim 25\ mg/hr$$

The resulting serum concentration from this dose will be slightly less than 13 mcg/mL.

To determine how long it will be necessary to wait before starting this new maintenance dose, we need to determine JM's theophylline elimination rate. Use the following formula:

$$K = \frac{Cl}{V}$$

(See **Equation 3-4**.)

where:
  K = elimination rate constant (hr^{-1}),
  Cl = clearance (L/hour), and
  V = volume of distribution (L).

$$K = \frac{1.64\ L/hr}{35\ L}$$
$$= 0.047\ hr^{-1}$$

Next we can determine the time we need to wait by using the following equation:

$$C = C_0 e^{-Kt}\ (\text{See Equation 3-2}.)$$

where:
  t = time to wait (hours),
  C = desired concentration (mcg/mL),
  C_0 = current concentration (mcg/mL), and
  K = elimination rate constant (hr^{-1}).

Therefore:

$$13 = 22e^{-0.047t}$$
$$13/22 = e^{-0.047t}$$
$$0.591 = e^{-0.047t}$$
$$\ln 0.591 = \ln e^{-0.047t}$$
$$-0.526 = -0.047t$$
$$t = 11.19\ hours$$
$$\sim 11\ hours$$

JM would receive the new infusion of 25 mg/hour starting 11 hours after discontinuing the previous infusion of 45 mg/hour.

■ CLINICAL CORRELATE

The most significant side effects from theophylline occur at serum concentrations higher than 20 mcg/mL. These include nausea, vomiting, headache, diarrhea, irritability, and insomnia. At concentrations higher than 35 mcg/mL, major adverse effects include hyperglycemia, hypotension, cardiac arrhythmias, seizures, brain damage, and death.

CASE 2

MT is a 32-year-old, 55-kg, white woman. She is admitted to the hospital for treatment of chronic bronchitis.

She has a history of heavy marijuana and tobacco use but no other medical problems. She is not currently taking any medications.

Problem 2A. Estimate MT's volume of distribution and clearance.

To estimate MT's volume of distribution (see **Equation 14-1**),

$$V \text{ (L)} = \text{weight (kg)} \times 0.5 \text{ L/kg}$$

$$= 55 \text{ kg } (0.5 \text{ L/kg})$$

$$= 27.5 \text{ L}$$

To estimate MT's clearance (see **Equation 14-3**),

$$Cl = (0.04 \text{ L/kg/hr}) \times \text{weight (kg)} \times \text{(adjustment factors)}$$

$$= (0.04 \text{ L/kg/hr}) \times 55 \text{ kg} \times (2.2)$$

$$= 4.84 \text{ L/hr}$$

(The clearance adjustment factor of 2.2 is found in Table 14-1 for cigarette and marijuana smoking.)

Problem 2B. Calculate an aminophylline loading dose for MT that will achieve an initial plasma concentration of 15 mcg/mL. The dose will be given as an infusion over 30 minutes.

To calculate the loading dose,

$$D = \frac{CpdV}{SF}$$

(See **Equation 14-2**.)

$$D = \frac{15 \text{ mg/L} \times (27.5 \text{ L})}{0.8}$$

$$= 515.63 \text{ mg}$$

$$\sim 500 \text{ mg}$$

Problem 2C. Calculate an infusion rate of aminophylline that will maintain MT's serum concentration at 12 mcg/mL.

To determine the infusion rate,

$$D = \frac{\overline{Cp}_{ss} \, Cl \, \tau}{SF}$$

(See **Equation 14-4**.)

$$D = \frac{12 \text{ mcg/mL} \times 4.84 \text{ L/hr} \times 1 \text{ hr}}{0.8}$$

$$= 72.6 \text{ mg/hr}$$

$$\sim 70 \text{ mg/hr}$$

CASE 3

Patient KT, a 65-kg, 17-year-old boy, has been stabilized on 30 mg/hour theophylline for an acute asthmatic attack he experienced 36 hours ago. His plasma theophylline level is now 12 mcg/mL. KT is ready to be discharged on an oral theophylline regimen to be given every 12 hours. Calculate a dose for KT.

Problem 3A. Calculate KT's clearance.

$$Cl = \frac{DSF}{\overline{Cp}_{ss} \, \tau}$$

(See **Equation 14-4**.)

$$Cl = \frac{30 \text{ mg/hr} \times 1 \times 1}{12 \text{ mcg/mL} \times 1}$$

$$= 2.5 \text{ L/hr}$$

Notice that both S and F for theophylline are 1.

Problem 3B. Suggest an oral dosage regimen that will produce a $\overline{C}p_{ss}$ average of approximately 12 mcg/mL, using a sustained released product dosed every 12 hours.

$$D = \frac{\overline{C}p_{ss} \, Cl \, \tau}{SF}$$

(See **Equation 14-3**.)
where:
  D = the maintenance dose (mg);
  $\overline{C}p_{ss}$ = the average steady state concentration (mcg/mL);
  Cl = clearance (L/hour);
  τ = dosing interval (hours);
  S = salt form, which is 1 for theophylline; and
  F = bioavailability, which is 1 for many of the sustained-release oral formulations.

$$D = \frac{(12 \text{ mcg/mL})(2.5 \text{ L/hr})(12 \text{ hr})}{1 \times 1}$$

$$= 360 \text{ mg}$$

$$\sim 350 \text{ mg}$$

KT should receive 350 mg of sustained-release theophylline orally every 12 hours.

REFERENCES

1. *Guidelines for the Diagnosis and Management of Asthma: Expert Panel Report 2.* Bethesda, MD: U.S. Department of Health and Human Services, Public Health Service, National Institutes of

Health, National Heart, Lung, and Blood Institute; 1997. NIH publication no. 97–4051. Also available at http://www.nhlbi.nih.gov/guidelines/asthma/asthgdln.htm.

2. Markham A, Faulds D. Theophylline. A review of its potential steroid sparing effects in asthma. *Drugs* 1998;56:1081–91.

3. Page CP. Recent advances in our understanding of the use of theophylline in the treatment of asthma. *J Clin Pharmacol* 1999;39:237–40.

4. Wagner JG. Theophylline: pooled Michaelis-Menten behavior of theophylline and its parameters (V_{max} and K_m)

among asthmatic children and adults. *Ther Drug Monit* 1987;9:11.

5. Adebayo GI, Coker HA. Cimetidine inhibition of theophylline elimination: influence of adult age and time course. *Biopharm Drug Dispos* 1987;8:149.

6. Ludden TM. Pharmacokinetic interactions of macrolide antibiotics. *Clin Pharmacokinet* 1985;10:63.

7. Edwards DJ, Zarowitz BJ, Slaughter RL. Theophylline. In: Evans WE, Schentag JJ, Jusko WJ, editors. *Applied Pharmacokinetics*. 3rd ed. Vancouver, WA: Applied Therapeutics; 1992. pp. 13-1–13-38.

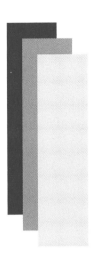

LESSON
15

Phenytoin and Digoxin

PHENYTOIN

Phenytoin is an anticonvulsant medication used for many types of seizure disorders. Phenytoin is usually administered either orally or intravenously and exhibits nonlinear or Michaelis–Menten kinetics (see Lesson 10). Unlike drugs undergoing first-order elimination (Figure 15-1), the plot of the natural logarithm of concentration versus time is nonlinear with phenytoin (Figure 15-2). Phenytoin is 90% protein bound; only the unbound fraction is active. (Note that patients with low serum albumin concentrations will have a higher unbound or active fraction of phenytoin. This should be factored in when dosing these patients.)

Phenytoin is metabolized by hepatic enzymes that can be saturated with the drug at concentrations within the therapeutic range. Consequently, as the phenytoin dose increases, a disproportionately greater increase in plasma concentration is achieved. This enzyme saturation process can be characterized with an enzyme-substrate model first developed by the biochemists Michaelis and Menten in 1913. In this metabolic process, drug clearance is constantly changing (in a nonlinear fashion) as dose changes. Drug clearance decreases as drug concentration increases (Figures 15-3 and 15-4).

To describe the relationship between concentration and dose, a differential equation can be written as shown below:

$$\frac{dX}{dt} = \frac{V_{max} \times C_{ss}}{K_m + C_{ss}}$$

(See **Equation 10-1**.)
where:
  dX = change in amount of drug;
  dt = change in time;
  V_{max} = maximum amount of drug that can be metabolized per unit time, usually expressed as mg/day;
  K_m = Michaelis–Menten constant, representing the concentration of phenytoin at which the rate of this enzyme-saturable hepatic metabolism is one-half of maximum; and
  C_{ss} = average steady-state phenytoin concentration.

Next, this differential equation can be expressed algebraically by assuming that we are at steady state and dX/dt is held constant. Then dX/dt, the change in the amount of drug (X) over time (t), can be expressed as X_0/τ (dose over dosing interval), as shown in the following equation:

$$X_0/\tau \, (S) = \frac{V_{max} \times C_{ss}}{K_m + C_{ss}}$$

(See **Equation 10-1**.)
where:
  X_0/τ = amount of phenytoin free acid divided by dosing interval (which can also be expressed as X_d, meaning daily dose of phenytoin free acid); and
  S = the salt factor or the fraction of phenytoin free acid in the salt form used. S equals 0.92 for phenytoin sodium injection and capsules and 1.0 for phenytoin suspension and chewable tablets (i.e., the free acid form of phenytoin), and 0.66 for fosphenytoin injection. The oral bioavailability of phenytoin is considered to be 100%, so an F factor is not needed in these calculations.

◼ CLINICAL CORRELATE

Although fosphenytoin contains only 66% phenytoin free acid, it is correctly prescribed and labeled in units of "PE," meaning "phenytoin sodium equivalents." The commercial fosphenytoin product is packaged to be very similar to phenytoin sodium injection; it contains 150 mg fosphenytoin per 2-mL ampul, providing 100 mg PE (100 mg phenytoin sodium equivalents).

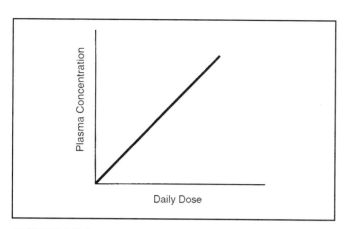

FIGURE 15-1.
First-order elimination model.

This Michaelis–Menten equation (MME) can then be rearranged to solve for C_{ss} as follows:

$$X_0/\tau\,(S) = \frac{V_{max} \times C_{ss}}{K_m + C_{ss}}$$

(See **Equation 10-1**.)

First, cross-multiply by the denominator:

$$[X_0/\tau(S) \times K_m] + [X_0/\tau(S) \times C_{ss}] = V_{max} \times C_{ss}$$

Then transpose "$[X_0/\tau(S) \times C_{ss}]$" to the right side of the equation:

$$[X_0/\tau(S) \times K_m] = [V_{max} \times C_{ss}] - [X_0/\tau(S) \times C_{ss}]$$

Factor out C_{ss}:

$$[X_0/\tau(S) \times K_m] = C_{ss}\,[V_{max} - X_0/\tau(S)]$$

Transpose "$[V_{max} - X_0/\tau(S)]$" to the left side of the equation:

$$C_{ss} = \frac{X_0/\tau(S) \times K_m}{V_{max} - X_0/\tau(S)}$$

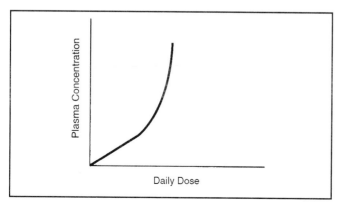

FIGURE 15-2.
Michaelis–Menten elimination model.

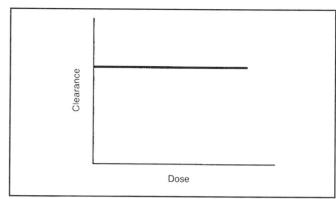

FIGURE 15-3.
First-order elimination model.

The two representations of the MME below can now be used for phenytoin dosing, as illustrated in the following cases:

$$X_0/\tau\,(S) = \frac{V_{max} \times C_{ss}}{K_m + C_{ss}}$$

(See **Equation 10-1**.)

⚠ 15-1 $$C_{ss} = \frac{X_0/\tau(S) \times K_m}{V_{max} - X_0/\tau(S)}$$

CASE 1

JH, a 23-year-old white man, is admitted to the hospital after a generalized seizure that was successfully treated with intravenous (IV) diazepam. His physician has written an order for pharmacy to calculate and order an IV phenytoin loading dose and recommend an initial oral maintenance dose and timing of plasma concentrations. Other pertinent clinical data include: weight, 75 kg;

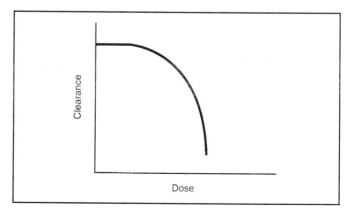

FIGURE 15-4.
Michaelis–Menten elimination model.

height, 5 feet, 11 inches; serum creatinine, 1.0 mg/dL; and serum albumin, 4.8 g/dL.

Problem 1A. What intravenous loading dose and oral maintenance dose would you recommend to achieve and maintain a phenytoin concentration of approximately 20 mg/L?

Calculation of the loading dose is not affected by the nonlinear pharmacokinetics of multiple-dose phenytoin regimens. The loading dose calculation is based on the patient's weight, estimated volume of distribution, serum albumin concentration, and renal function assessment as well as the salt form of phenytoin used. The generally accepted population parameter for phenytoin's volume of distribution is 0.65 L/kg of body weight.[1] The loading dose (X_0) formula is:

$$X_0 = \frac{V \times C_{desired}}{S}$$

(See **Equation 1-1**.)
where:

V = volume of distribution estimate of 0.65 L/kg (V = 0.65 L/kg(75 kg) = 48.8 L for JH),

$C_{desired}$ = concentration desired 1 hour after the end of the infusion (20 mg/L for JH), and

S = salt factor (0.92 for injection).

Therefore:

$$X_0 = \frac{(48.8\ L)(20\ mg/L)}{0.92}$$
$$= 1060\ mg\ of\ phenytoin\ sodium\ injection$$

We could then order a dose of 1000 mg of phenytoin mixed in 100 mL of normal saline given intravenously via controlled infusion. The administration rate should not exceed 50 mg/minute to avoid potential cardiovascular toxicity associated with the propylene glycol diluent of the phenytoin injection. A rate of 25 mg/minute or less is preferred for elderly patients. The accuracy of this loading dose estimate can be checked by obtaining a phenytoin plasma drug concentration at approximately 1 hour after the end of the loading dose infusion.

■ CLINICAL CORRELATE

Phenytoin sodium injection uses a propylene glycol base as its vehicle and will precipitate in most IV fluids. It is most compatible in normal saline but can even precipitate in this fluid and clog an existing inline IV filter if one is being used. Propylene glycol is a cardiotoxic agent and can cause various complications such as bradycardia and hypotension. An alternative is to use the newer fosphenytoin injection, which is compatible with many IV fluids and can also be administered safely at a faster rate (up to 150 mg/minute). Fosphenytoin is, however, much more expensive than phenytoin sodium injection.

There are two methods to calculate an initial daily maintenance dose (X_d): an empiric method and a method based on estimating the patient's V_{max} and K_m.

Method 1 (Empiric)

Multiply JH's weight of 75 kg by 5 mg/kg/day to get an estimated dose of 375 mg of free acid phenytoin or 408 mg of phenytoin sodium, which would be rounded to 400 mg. This dose of 400 mg/day may be divided into 200 mg twice daily if necessary to decrease the likelihood of enzyme saturation and reduce concentration-dependent side effects. This assumes that the patient has an average K_m and V_{max}.

Method 2

Substitute population estimates for V_{max} and K_m into the MME and solve for the dose as follows:

$$X_d \times S = \frac{V_{max} \times C_{ss}}{K_m + C_{ss}}$$

(See **Equation 10-1**.)
where:

V_{max} = population estimate of maximum rate of drug metabolism (7 mg/kg/day[1] × 75 kg = 525 mg/day),

K_m = population estimate of Michaelis–Menten constant (4 mg/L[1]),

C_{ss} = desired average steady-state plasma concentration of 15 mg/L, and

S = salt factor (0.92 for phenytoin sodium capsules).

Therefore:

$$X_d(0.92) = \frac{525\ mg/day\ \times\ 15\ mg/L}{4\ mg/L + 15\ mg/L}$$
$$= \frac{7875\ mg^2\ L/day}{19\ mg/L}$$
$$= \sim 415\ mg/day\ of\ phenytoin\ free\ acid$$
$$X_d = \frac{415\ mg/day}{0.92}$$
$$= 451\ mg/day\ of\ the\ sodium\ salt\ of$$
$$phenytoin,\ round\ to\ 450\ mg/day$$

Note how the units in the equation cancel out, yielding "mg/day" as the final units.

This calculation of 415 mg of phenytoin free acid is larger than our empiric estimate of 375 mg/day, showing that the empiric method of 5 mg/kg/day results in a lower value for JH's initial phenytoin maintenance dose. In JH's case, although this would equal a daily dose of four 100-mg phenytoin sodium capsules plus one 50-mg phenytoin tablet (which is phenytoin free acid), a patient would usually be begun on 400 mg/day (200 mg BID) and titrated up to 450 mg if needed based on plasma phenytoin drug concentrations.

Problem 1B. When would you recommend that steady-state plasma concentrations be drawn?

It is difficult to calculate when multiple dosing with phenytoin will reach steady state because the time to steady state is concentration dependent. With drugs that undergo first-order elimination, steady state can be reached in three to five drug half-lives because this model assumes that clearance and volume of distribution are constant. However, because of its capacity-limited metabolism, phenytoin clearance decreases with increasing concentration. Therefore, the calculation of time to reach steady state is quite complicated and cannot be based on half-life. In fact, phenytoin does not have a true half-life; its half-life is dependent on drug concentration.

The major factor in determining how long it will take to attain steady state is the difference between V_{max} and the daily dose. The closer V_{max} is to the dose, the longer it will take to achieve steady state. This relationship between V_{max} and concentration can be derived mathematically by examining the equations used to calculate dose for first- and zero-order models. We will start by rearranging two definitions in the first-order model:

$$C_{ss} = \frac{X_0}{V} \qquad \text{rearranges to} \qquad X_0 = C_{ss} \times V$$

(See **Equation 1-1**.)
and

$$Cl_t = VK \qquad \text{rearranges to} \qquad V = \frac{Cl_t}{K}$$

so, by substituting for V:

$$X_0 = \frac{C_{ss} \times Cl_t}{K} \qquad \text{or} \qquad X_0 \times K = C_{ss} \times Cl_t$$

$C_{ss} \times Cl_t$ from our first-order equation can be substituted for X_0/τ in the zero-order equation derived in the introduction:

$$X_0/\tau = \frac{V_{max} \times C_{ss}}{K_m + C_{ss}}$$

(See **Equation 10-1**.)
Substituting $C_{ss} \times Cl_t$ for X_0/τ yields:

$$Cl_t \times C_{ss} = \frac{V_{max} \times C_{ss}}{K_m + C_{ss}}$$

Solving for Cl_t:

$$(C_{ss} \times Cl_t \times K_m) + (Cl_t \times C_{ss}^2) = V_{max} \times C_{ss}$$

$$\frac{C_{ss} \times Cl_t \times K_m}{C_{ss}} + \frac{Cl_t \times C_{ss}^2}{C_{ss}} = V_{max}$$

$$(Cl_t \times K_m) + (Cl_t \times C_{ss}) = V_{max}$$

$$Cl_t(K_m + C_{ss}) = V_{max}$$

This equation can now be rearranged to represent clearance in terms of V_{max} and C_{ss} as shown:

$$Cl_t = \frac{V_{max}}{K_m + C_{ss}}$$

where:
  Cl_t = clearance of phenytoin;
  V_{max} = maximum rate of drug metabolism, usually expressed as mg/day;
  K_m = Michaelis–Menten constant, representing the concentration of phenytoin at which the rate of this enzyme-saturable hepatic metabolism is half of maximum; and
  C_{ss} = average steady-state phenytoin concentration.

Examination of this equation shows that when C_{ss} is very small compared to K_m, Cl_t will approximate V_{max}/K_m, a relatively constant value. Therefore, at low concentrations, the metabolism of phenytoin follows a first-order process. However, as C_{ss} increases to exceed K_m, as is usually seen with therapeutic concentrations of phenytoin, Cl_t will decrease and metabolism will convert to zero order. We can calculate an estimate of the time it takes to get to 90% of steady state using the following equation:

$$t_{90\%} = \frac{K_m \times V}{(V_{max} - X_d)^2}[(2.3 \times V_{max}) - (0.9 \times X_d)]$$

(See **Equation 10-4**.)
where:
  $t_{90\%}$ = estimated number of days to get to 90% of steady state,
  X_d = daily dose of phenytoin (in mg/day),
  V = volume of distribution,
  V_{max} = maximum rate of drug metabolism (in mg/day), and
  K_m = Michaelis–Menten constant.

This equation is derived from a complex integration of the differential equation describing the difference between the rate of drug coming in (i.e., the daily dose) and the rate of drug going out of the body. This equation gives us an estimate of when to draw steady-state plasma concentrations and is based on the assumption that the beginning phenytoin concentration is zero. In patients such as JH, who have previously received a loading dose, $t_{90\%}$ may be different, usually shorter, unless the loading dose yielded an initial concentration greater than that desired, in which case $t_{90\%}$ would be even longer.

CLINICAL CORRELATE

The $t_{90\%}$ equation is a very rough estimate of time to 90% of steady state and should be used only as a general guide. The clinician should check nonsteady-state phenytoin concentrations before this time to avoid serious subtherapeutic or supratherapeutic concentrations.

In patient JH's case, $t_{90\%}$ is calculated as follows:

$$t_{90\%} = \frac{K_m \times V}{(V_{max} - X_d)^2}[(2.3 \times V_{max}) - (0.9 \times X_d)]$$

(See **Equation 10-4**.)
where:
  K_m = 4 mg/L,
  V_{max} = 7 mg/kg/day × 75 kg (525 mg/day),
  X_d = 418 mg/day of phenytoin (free acid), and
  V = 0.65 L/kg × 75 kg (48.8 L).

Therefore:

$$t_{90\%} = \frac{4 \text{ mg/L} \times 48.8 \text{ L}}{(525 \text{ mg/day} - 418 \text{ mg/day})^2}[(2.3 \times 525 \text{ mg/day}) - (0.9 \times 418 \text{ mg/day})]$$

$$= 14.13 \text{ days}$$

Note how the units cancel out in this equation, leaving the answer expressed in days, not hours. This equation estimates that it will take JH approximately 14 days for his phenytoin concentration to reach steady state with a desired C_{ss} concentration of 15 mg/L.

Close inspection of this calculation illustrates the impact that the denominator—the difference of V_{max} and daily dose—has on the time it takes to reach steady state. For example, if we assume that JH's daily dose was 500 mg/day, we can re-solve the $t_{90\%}$ equation as shown below, where strikeouts show the changes:

$$t_{90\%} = \frac{4 \text{ mg/L} \times 48.8 \text{ L}}{(525 \text{ mg/day} - 500 \; \cancel{418} \text{ mg/day})^2}[(2.3 \times 500 \; \cancel{525} \text{ mg/day}) - (0.9 \times 500 \; \cancel{418} \text{ mg/day})]$$

$$= 236.6 \text{ days}$$

This means that, theoretically, it would now take approximately 237 days for patient JH to reach steady state on a dose of 500 mg/day. Of course, JH would actually show signs of toxicity long before he reached steady state, but this illustrates the effect the difference of dose and V_{max} has on the calculation of time to steady state. In fact, if the daily dose exceeds V_{max}, steady state is never achieved.

CASE 2

For this case, we use the data presented in Case 1 and continue treating patient JH. A phenytoin plasma concentration of 6 mg/L is drawn 18 days after the beginning of therapy. Although JH's seizure frequency has decreased, he is still having occasional seizures, and his physician has decided to adjust his dosing regimen to attain a plasma concentration of 15 mg/L.

Problem 2A. Calculate an appropriate dosing regimen to attain our desired concentration of 15 mg/L.

Now that we have one steady-state concentration, we can calculate a new maintenance dose for JH. This is done using the basic MME with two unknowns, V_{max} and K_m. We can use a population estimate for one of the unknowns (usually K_m), solve for the other unknown, and then recalculate the new dose once again using the MME. This method is preferred over using population estimates for both unknowns. For JH, this calculation is as follows:

$$X_d \times S = \frac{V_{max} \times C_{ss}}{K_m + C_{ss}}$$

(See **Equation 10-1**.)
First, rearrange the MME to isolate V_{max}:

$$V_{max} = \frac{(X_d \times S)(K_m + C_{ss})}{C_{ss}}$$

(See **Equation 10-1**.)
where:
  V_{max} = calculated estimate of patient's V_{max},
  K_m = population estimate of 4 mg/L,
  $X_d \times S$ = patient's daily dose of phenytoin (418 mg/day of free acid), and
  C_{ss} = reported steady-state concentration (6 mg/L).

$$V_{max} = \frac{(418 \text{ mg/day})(4 \text{ mg/L} + 6 \text{ mg/L})}{(6 \text{ mg/L})}$$

$$= \frac{(418 \text{ mg/day})(10 \text{ mg/L})}{(6 \text{ mg/L})}$$

$$= \frac{(4180 \text{ mg}^2/\text{day} \times \text{L})}{(6 \text{ mg/L})}$$

$$= 696.67 \text{ mg/day, rounded to 697 mg/day}$$

So JH's new estimated V_{max} is 697 mg/day, which is larger than the population estimate of 525 mg/day, meaning that he has a greater phenytoin clearance than first estimated.

We now take the new V_{max} and the MME for our new dose and use it in the MME to solve for X_d as follows:

$$X_d \times S = \frac{V_{max} \times C_{ss}}{K_m + C_{ss}}$$

(See **Equation 10-1**.)

where:

$X_d \times S$ = new dose of phenytoin sodium ($S = 0.92$),
C_{ss} = desired steady-state concentration of 15 mg/L,
K_m = population estimate of 4 mg/L, and
V_{max} = calculated estimate (697 mg/day).

$$X_d \times S = \frac{697 \text{ mg/day} \times 15 \text{ mg/L}}{4 \text{ mg/L} + 15 \text{ mg/L}}$$

$$= \frac{10{,}455 \text{ mg}^2/\text{day} \times L}{19 \text{ mg/L}}$$

$X_d (0.92)$ = 550 mg/day of phenytoin free acid
X_d = 598 mg/day of phenytoin sodium, rounded to 600 mg/day

Therefore, JH's new dose would be 600 mg/day as phenytoin sodium capsules in divided doses, which is equivalent to 552 mg of phenytoin free acid. Because this is a large increase in dose, it may saturate the patient's hepatic enzymes, causing the plasma concentration to increase disproportionately. The practitioner may decide to give a lower dose initially.

▪ CLINICAL CORRELATE

Phenytoin doses are usually increased by 25–100 mg/day. Phenytoin pharmacokinetic dosing calculations are not as accurate and predictive as those for the aminoglycosides and theophylline; therefore, good clinical judgment is required when recommending a dose.

Problem 2B. When should a plasma phenytoin concentration be drawn?

We can recalculate when JH's phenytoin concentration will reach steady state on this new dose. Remember, time to 90% of steady state ($t_{90\%}$) is dependent on plasma drug concentration. JH's new estimate of $t_{90\%}$ is calculated as follows:

$$t_{90\%} = \frac{K_m \times V}{(V_{max} - X_d)^2}[(2.3 \times V_{max}) - (0.9 \times X_d)]$$

(See **Equation 10-4**.)

where:

K_m = population estimate (4 mg/L),
V_{max} = calculated estimate based on one steady-state concentration (697 mg/day),
X_d = daily dose of 552 mg/day of phenytoin free acid, and
V = population estimate of volume of distribution (48.8 L).

Therefore:

$$t_{90\%} = \frac{4 \text{ mg/L} \times 48.8 \text{ L}}{(697 \text{ mg/day} - 552 \text{ mg/day})^2}[(2.3 \times 697 \text{ mg/day}) - (0.9 \times 552 \text{ mg/day})]$$

$$= 10.3 \text{ days for new } t_{90\%} \text{ to be reached}$$

Note that our new $t_{90\%}$ is slightly smaller than the previous estimate because the difference between V_{max} and dose is now greater.

Problem 2C. Three weeks later, JH's plasma phenytoin concentration is 20 mg/L. He is now seizure free, and his physician would like to adjust his dose to get his plasma concentration back to 15 mg/L. Note that JH states that he has been taking his phenytoin exactly as prescribed. What dose would you now recommend to achieve a plasma phenytoin concentration of 15 mg/L?

Now that we have measured two different steady-state concentrations at two different doses, we can make an even more accurate dosing change.

As shown in Lesson 14, clearance can be expressed as X_d/C_{ss}, resulting in the plot in Figure 15-5.

We can now plot both steady-state doses (X_1 of 418 mg/day and X_2 of 552 mg/day) on the y-axis and both steady-state X_d/C_{ss} values ($X_1/C_1 = 418/6$ L/day and $X_2/C_2 = 552/20$ L/day) on the x-axis, thus linearizing these relationships. This allows us to express the relationship in the algebraic form for a straight line, $Y = mX + b$, where m, the slope of the line, equals the negative value of the patient's K_m (i.e., $m = -K_m$) and the y-inter-

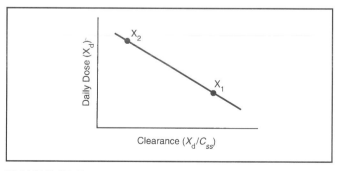

FIGURE 15-5.

Relationship of daily dose to clearance.

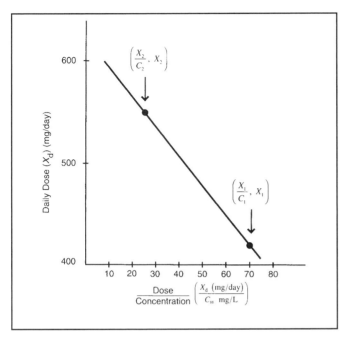

FIGURE 15-6.
Relationship of daily dose to the dose divided by steady-state concentration achieved.

cept is the patient's V_{max}. For JH, this graph is drawn as in Figure 15-6.

The slope of the line, which represents $-K_m$, can now be calculated as follows:

$$-K_m = \frac{X_1 - X_2}{\dfrac{X_1}{C_1} - \dfrac{X_2}{C_2}}$$

$$= \frac{418 \text{ mg/day} - 552 \text{ mg/day}}{\dfrac{418 \text{ mg/day}}{6 \text{ mg/day}} - \dfrac{552 \text{ mg/day}}{20 \text{ mg/day}}}$$

$$K_m = 3.18 \text{ mg/L}$$

(See **Equation 10-2**.)

Next, we substitute this new value for K_m into the MME and solve for a V_{max} as follows:

$$V_{max} = \frac{(X_d \times S)(K_m + C_{ss})}{C_{ss}}$$

(See **Equation 10-1**.)
where:
$X_d \times S$ = either of the doses JH received (418 or 552 mg/day of free acid),
C_{ss} = steady-state concentration at the dose selected, and
K_m = calculated value of 3.19 mg/L.

Using the 418-mg/day dose, C_{ss} = 6 mg/L.

$$V_{max} = \frac{(418 \text{ mg/day})(3.18 \text{ mg/L} + 6 \text{ mg/L})}{6 \text{ mg/L}}$$

$$= 639.5 \text{ mg/day}$$

Using the 552 mg/day dose, C_{ss} = 20 mg/L.

$$V_{max} = \frac{(552 \text{ mg/day})(3.18 \text{ mg/L} + 20 \text{ mg/L})}{(20 \text{ mg/L})}$$

$$= 639.5 \text{ mg/day}$$

which we will round to 640 mg/day. Note that either set of doses and concentrations will give the same V_{max}.

Finally, we substitute our new V_{max} of 640 mg/day and our calculated K_m of 3.18 mg/mL into the MME and solve for X_d as follows:

$$X_d \times S = \frac{V_{max} \times C_{ss}}{K_m + C_{ss}}$$

(See **Equation 10-1**.)
where:
V_{max} = 640 mg/day of phenytoin free acid,
K_m = 3.18 mg/L,
C_{ss} = desired average steady-state plasma concentration of 15 mg/L, and
S = salt factor (0.92 for phenytoin sodium capsules).

$$X_d(0.92) = \frac{(640 \text{ mg/day})(15 \text{ mg/L})}{3.18 \text{ mg/L} + 15 \text{ mg/L}}$$

X_d (0.92) = 528 mg/day of phenytoin free acid
X_d = 574 mg/day of phenytoin sodium

Therefore, we could give JH 560 mg (five 100-mg phenytoin capsules plus two 30-mg phenytoin capsules) daily in divided doses. This would give slightly less than the calculated amount of 574 mg/day.

▮ CLINICAL CORRELATE

It is important to dose phenytoin correctly so side effects do not occur. Dose-related side effects at serum concentrations greater than 20 mcg/mL include nystagmus, whereas concentrations greater than 30 mcg/mL and more may result in nystagmus and ataxia. Concentrations greater than 40 mcg/mL may produce ataxia, lethargy, and diminished cognitive function. Adverse effects that may occur at therapeutic concentrations include gingival hyperplasia, folate deficiency, peripheral neuropathy, hypertrichosis, and thickening of facial features.

DIGOXIN

Digoxin is an inotropic medication used primarily for the treatment of heart failure. It may also be used in the management of atrial fibrillation. Doses of digoxin are usually administered orally or intravenously. The accepted therapeutic range for digoxin is 0.5–1.2 ng/mL (average, 0.75 ng/mL) in heart failure with some patients experiencing additional benefits with levels up to 1.5 ng/mL. For atrial fibrillation, the acceptable range is between 0.8 and 1.5 ng/mL, with certain patients experiencing additional benefits with levels up to 2.0 ng/mL (although concentrations greater than 2.0 ng/mL may be required for atrial fibrillation in some cases). Note that the units of plasma concentrations for digoxin are different (nanograms per milliliter) from those of other commonly monitored drugs (usually milligrams per liter).

The steady-state volume of distribution (V_{ss}) of digoxin is large and extremely variable. Differences in renal function account for some of the interpatient variation. The V_{ss} ranges from:

⚠️ 4 to 9 L/kg ideal body weight (IBW)
15-2 (average, 6.7 L/kg IBW)

in subjects with normal renal function, whereas in patients with renal failure the average V_{ss} is 4.7 L/kg IBW. Digoxin is approximately 25% bound to serum protein in patients with normal creatinine clearance.[1] In patients with severe renal dysfunction, digoxin is only 18% protein bound.[2] This reduction in protein binding of digoxin is thought to be due to displacement of digoxin by endogenous substances that are not cleared efficiently in patients with renal dysfunction.

When calculating digoxin dosage, the bioavailability (F) of oral dosage forms is an important consideration. For patients with normal oral absorption, digoxin tablets are 50–90% (average, 75%) absorbed ($F = 0.75$), digoxin elixir is 80% absorbed ($F = 0.80$), and digoxin liquid-filled capsules are nearly 100% absorbed ($F = 1.0$).

Systemic clearance (Cl_t) of digoxin is determined by both renal (Cl_r) and nonrenal, or metabolic, clearance (Cl_m). Cl_t, expressed in units of mL/minute/1.73 m² body surface area, can be calculated as follows[1]:

⚠️ $Cl_t = (1.101 \times Cl_r) + Cl_m$
15-3
(See **Equation 2-1**.)
where:

⚠️ Cl_r (expressed as mL/minute/1.73 m²) = 0.927 ×
15-4 creatinine clearance (mL/minute/1.73 m²),[3]

and:

Cl_m = 36 mL/minute/1.73 m² in patients with resolved or no history of heart failure and 20 mL/minute/1.73 m² in patients with severe heart failure.[1]

CLINICAL CORRELATE

Although the equations for estimating total body, renal, and metabolic clearances for digoxin state that adjustments to these calculations must be made based on the patient's body surface area, this is rarely necessary in clinical practice except in extreme situations.

CASE 3

A 68-year-old woman, patient JS, is being treated for rapid ventricular rate (140 beats per minute) associated with atrial fibrillation. Her medical history includes two myocardial infarctions, hypertension, and gout. She is 65 inches tall and weighs 57 kg, her blood pressure is 130 mm Hg/84 mm Hg, and her serum creatinine concentration is 1.2 mg/dL.

Over the past 24 hours, the physician has given her a 1-mg IV loading dose (given as 0.5 mg, 0.25 mg, and 0.25 mg given at 6-hour intervals) and a 0.25-mg IV dose of digoxin for an acute increase in her heart rate to 160 beats per minute. Her physician would like to begin a daily oral maintenance dose to achieve a steady-state plasma concentration of 1.8 ng/mL.

Problem 3A. Recommend an oral maintenance dose of digoxin in this patient to achieve a steady-state plasma concentration of 1.8 ng/mL.

The relationship between the steady-state plasma concentration, maintenance dose, and total systemic clearance is shown below:

⚠️ $$C_{ss} = \frac{X_d \times 10^6 \times F}{Cl_t \times \tau}$$
15-5
(See **Equation 4-3**.)

The above equation can be rearranged and written as follows:

$$X_d = \frac{C_{ss} \times Cl_t \times \tau}{10^6 \times F}$$

where:
X_d = maintenance dose of digoxin, in mg/day;
C_{ss} = steady-state plasma concentration, in ng/mL;
Cl_t = total body clearance;
τ = dosing interval, in minutes (1440 minutes = 1 day);
10^6 = conversion from nanograms to milligrams (i.e., 10^6 ng = 1 mg); and
$F = 0.75$ for tablets.

To determine systemic clearance, we must estimate JS's creatinine clearance. We use the Cockcroft–Gault equation:

$$CrCl_{(female)} = (0.85)\frac{(140 - age)(IBW)}{72 \times SCr}$$

(See **Equation 9-1**.)
where:
CrCl = creatinine clearance, in mL/minute;
IBW = ideal body weight, in kg; and
SCr = serum creatinine, in mg/dL.

Therefore:

$$CrCl_{(female)} = (0.85)\frac{(140 - 68)(57)}{72 \times 1.2}$$

$$= 40 \text{ mL/minute}$$

Renal clearance is calculated as follows:

$$Cl_r = 0.927 \times CrCl \text{ (See Equation 15-4.)}$$

$$= 0.927 \times 40 \text{ mL/minute/1.73 m}^2$$

$$= 37 \text{ mL/minute/1.73 m}^2$$

Nonrenal clearance (Cl_m) for this patient would be the population estimate of 36 mL/minute/1.73 m² (JS has no history of heart failure).

Therefore, total body clearance of digoxin would be:

$$Cl_t = (1.101 \times Cl_r) + Cl_m \text{ (See Equation 15-3.)}$$

$$= (1.101 \times 37 \text{ mL/minute/1.73 m}^2) + 36 \text{ mL/minute/} 1.73 \text{ m}^2$$

$$= 77 \text{ mL/minute/1.73 m}^2$$

The daily maintenance dose required to achieve a steady-state concentration of 1.8 ng/mL would be:

$$X_d = \frac{C_{ss} \times Cl_t \times \tau}{10^6 \times F}$$

$$= \frac{1.8 \text{ ng/mL} \times 77 \text{ mL/min} \times 1440 \text{ min}}{10^6 \text{ ng/mg} \times 0.75}$$

$$= 0.266 \text{ mg}$$

(See **Equation 15-5**.)
This patient would probably take 0.25 mg of oral digoxin daily to achieve a steady-state digoxin concentration of slightly less than 1.8 ng/mL.

Problem 3B. After receiving 0.25 mg of digoxin daily for 1 month, patient JS comes to the emergency room with severe nausea and vomiting. Her steady-state plasma digoxin concentration is 3.2 ng/mL. The physician holds digoxin therapy for 2 days and asks you to recommend a new dose to achieve a target concentration of 1.8 ng/mL.

In this problem, the patient may have deteriorating renal function, or, she may have consumed more digoxin than was prescribed. To determine a new dose, we will assume the former. First, the patient's actual Cl_t must be calculated based on the steady-state plasma digoxin concentration. To solve for Cl_t, we must rearrange the following equation:

$$C_{ss} = \frac{X_d \times 10^6 \times F}{Cl_t \times \tau}$$

(See **Equation 15-5**.)
to:

$$Cl_t = \frac{X_d \times 10^6 \times F}{C_{ss} \times \tau}$$

where:
Cl_t = total body clearance,
X_d = maintenance dose of digoxin, in mg/day;
C_{ss} = steady-state plasma concentration, in ng/mL;
τ = 1440 minutes (1 day);
10^6 = conversion from nanograms to milligrams (i.e., 10^6 ng = 1 mg); and
F = bioavailability (0.75 for digoxin tablets).

Plugging in our values for patient JS:

$$Cl_t = \frac{0.25 \text{ mg/day} \times 10^6 \text{ ng/mg} \times 0.75}{3.2 \text{ ng/mL} \times 1440 \text{ min/day}}$$

$$= 41 \text{ mL/min}$$

Then we use patient JS's actual Cl_t to calculate the appropriate dose to achieve our desired C_{ss} of 1.8 ng/mL.

$$= \frac{1.8 \text{ ng/mL} \times 41 \text{ mL/min} \times 1440 \text{ min}}{10^6 \text{ ng/mg} \times 0.75}$$

$$= 0.142 \text{ mg}$$

This dose could be rounded to 0.125 mg/day to achieve a C_{ss} of slightly less than 1.8 ng/mL.

CASE 4

A 48-year-old man, patient MS, presents to the emergency room with shortness of breath and significant peripheral edema of his lower extremities. He has chronic renal insufficiency and is diagnosed as having heart failure, for which his physician recommends beginning digoxin. Patient MS is 68 inches tall and weighs 88 kg, and his serum creatinine concentration is 2.4 mg/dL.

Therefore, for this patient,

IBW = 50 kg + 2.3 kg for each inch over 5 feet in height

= 50 kg + 2.3 kg (8 inches)

= 50 kg + 18.4 kg

= 68.4 kg

And

$$CrCl_{(male)} = \frac{(140 - age)(IBW)}{72 \times SCr}$$
$$= \frac{(140 - 48)(68.4)}{72 \times 2.4}$$
$$= 36 \text{ mL/min}$$

■ CLINICAL CORRELATE

Patients with heart failure usually do not require a loading dose of digoxin before initiating maintenance dose therapy.

Problem 4A. Calculate a maintenance dose of digoxin to achieve a steady-state digoxin concentration of 0.9 ng/mL.

Recall that the total systemic clearance and renal clearance of digoxin must be calculated:

Cl_r (mL/minute) = 0.927 × CrCl (See **Equation 15-4.**)

= 0.927 × 36

= 33 mL/minute

and:

Cl_t (mL/minute) = (1.101 × Cl_r) + Cl_m
(See **Equation 15-3.**)

= (1.101 × 33) + 20

= 36 + 20

= 56 mL/minute

Note that because this patient has severe heart failure, Cl_m is approximately 20 mL/minute.

Now we can calculate a daily digoxin maintenance dose for this patient:

$$X_d = \frac{C_{ss} \times Cl_t \times \tau}{10^6 \times F}$$

(See **Equation 15-5.**)
where:
  X_d = maintenance dose of digoxin, in mg/day;
  C_{ss} = steady-state plasma concentration (0.9 ng/mL);
  CL_t = systemic clearance (56 mL/minute);
  τ = 1440 minutes (1 day);
  10^6 = conversion from nanograms to milligrams (i.e., 10^6 ng = 1 mg); and
  F = bioavailability (0.75 for tablets).

The maintenance dose (X_d) to achieve a steady-state concentration of 0.9 ng/mL would be:

$$X_d = \frac{0.9 \text{ ng/mL} \times 56 \text{ mL/min} \times 1440 \text{ min}}{10^6 \text{ ng/mg} \times 0.75}$$
$$= \frac{72{,}576 \text{ ng}}{750{,}000 \text{ ng/mg}}$$
$$= 0.097 \text{ mg}$$

Therefore, this patient with severe heart failure and chronic renal insufficiency would require an oral digoxin dose of 0.125 mg alternating with 0.0625 mg every other day, which will achieve a plasma digoxin concentration slightly less than 0.9 ng/mL.

■ CLINICAL CORRELATE

IV administration of digoxin should be given by slow IV push. This method of administration prevents the propylene glycol contained in this formulation from causing cardiovascular collapse.

REFERENCES

1. Koup JR, Jusko WJ, Elwood CM, et al. Digoxin pharmacokinetics: role of renal failure in dosage regimen design. *Clin Pharmacol Ther* 1975;18:9–21.
2. Reuning RH, Sams RA, Notari RE. Role of pharmacokinetics in drug dosage adjustment. I. Pharmacologic effect kinetics and apparent volume of distribution of digoxin. *J Clin Pharmacol* 1973;13:127–41.
3. Keys PW. Digoxin. In: Evans WE, Schentag JJ, Jusko WJ, editors. *Applied Pharmacokinetics: Principles of Therapeutic Drug Monitoring.* 3rd ed. Spokane, WA: Applied Therapeutics; 1992.

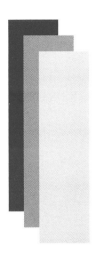

APPENDIX
A

Basic and Drug-Specific Pharmacokinetic Equations

BASIC PHARMACOKINETIC EQUATIONS

Equation Showing the Relationship of Drug Concentration (mg/L), Drug Dose (mg), and Volume of Distribution (Liters)

⚠ 1-1

$$\text{concentration} = \frac{\text{amount of drug in body}}{\text{volume in which drug is distributed}}$$

$$C = \frac{X}{V}$$

(See p. 10.)

Equation for Calculating Total Body Clearance

⚠ 2-1

$$Cl_t = Cl_r + Cl_m + Cl_b + Cl_{other}$$

(See p. 21.)

Equation for Calculating Organ Clearance of a Drug

⚠ 2-2

$$Cl_{organ} = Q \times \frac{C_{in} - C_{out}}{C_{in}} \text{ or } Cl_{organ} = QE$$

(See p. 21.)

Elimination Rate Constant (K) for First-Order, One-Compartment Model

⚠ 3-1

$$\text{slope} = -K = \frac{\ln C_1 - \ln C_0}{t_1 - t_0}$$

(See p. 31.)

or:

$$-K = \frac{\ln \dfrac{C_1}{C_0}}{t_1 - t_0}$$

Concentration at Any Given Time, Based on a Previous Concentration (C_0) and K for First-Order, One-Compartment Model

⚠ 3-2

$$C = C_0 e^{-Kt}$$

(See p. 32.)

where:

C = plasma drug concentration at time = t,

C_0 = plasma drug concentration at time = 0,

K = elimination rate constant,

t = time after dose, and

e^{-Kt} = percent or fraction remaining after time (t).

Note: used often to calculate Cp_{min} from Cp_{max}.

Calculation of $T^{1/2}$ from K, or K from $T^{1/2}$ for First-Order, One-Compartment Model

⚠ 3-3
$$T^{1/2} = \frac{0.693}{K}$$

(See p. 33.)

or:

$$K = \frac{0.693}{T^{1/2}}$$

Mathematical Relationship Between Systemic Clearance (Cl_t) to Both V and K for First-Order, One-Compartment Model

⚠ 3-4
$$Cl_t/V = K$$

(See p. 34.)

or:

$$Cl_t = V \times K \text{ or } V = Cl_t/K$$

Calculation of Area Under the Plasma Drug Concentration Curve (AUC) and Its Relationship to Both Drug Clearance ($K \times V$) and Dose Administered

⚠ 3-5
$$AUC = \frac{\text{dose administered}}{\text{drug clearance}}$$

(See p. 35.)

or:

$$\text{drug clearance} = \frac{\text{dose administered}}{AUC}$$

or:

$$AUC = \frac{\text{initial concentration } (C_0)}{\text{elimination rate constant } (K)}$$

"Accumulation Factor" When Not at Steady State for a One-Compartment, First-Order Model

⚠ 4-1
$$\text{accumulation factor} = \frac{(1 - e^{-nK\tau})}{(1 - e^{-K\tau})}$$

(See p. 47.)

"Accumulation Factor" When at Steady State for a One-Compartment, First-Order Model

⚠ 4-2
$$\frac{1}{(1 - e^{-K\tau})}$$

(See p. 51.)

Calculation of Average Drug Concentration from AUC and Dosing Interval or from Dose/Cl

$$\bar{C} = \frac{AUC}{\tau}$$

and because:

$$AUC = \frac{\text{dose}}{\text{drug clearance}}$$

$$\bar{C} = \frac{\text{dose}}{\text{drug clearance} \times \tau}$$

or:

⚠ 4-3
$$\bar{C} = \frac{\text{dose}}{Cl_t \times \tau}$$

(See p. 52.)

Cockcroft–Gault Equations for Calculating Creatinine Clearance (CrCl) in Men and Women

⚠ 9-1
$$CrCl_{male} = \frac{(140 - age)IBW}{72 \times SCr}$$

(See p. 122.)

or:

$$CrCl_{female} = \frac{(0.85)(140 - age)IBW}{72 \times SCr}$$

Note: IBW = ideal body weight.

Equations for Estimating IBW in Men and Women

⚠ 9-2
$$IBW_{males} = 50 \text{ kg} + 2.3 \text{ kg for each inch over 5 feet in height}$$

(See p. 123.)

$$IBW_{females} = 45.5 \text{ kg} + 2.3 \text{ kg for each inch}$$
$$\text{over 5 feet in height}$$

Adjusted Body Weight (AdjBW) Equation for Patients Whose Total Body Weight (TBW) is More Than 20% Over Their IBW

$$AdjBW = IBW + 0.4(TBW - IBW)$$

9-3
(See p. 123.)

Michaelis–Menten Equation (MME)

$$\text{daily dose} = \frac{V_{max}C}{K_m + C}$$

10-1
(See p. 132.)
or:

$$\text{daily dose}(K_m + C) = V_{max}C$$
$$\text{daily dose}(K_m) + \text{daily dose}(C) = V_{max}C$$
$$\text{daily dose}(C) = V_{max}C - \text{daily dose}(K_m)$$

Note: relates V_{max}, K_m, plasma drug concentration, and daily dose (at steady state) for zero-order (i.e., non-linear) model.

Calculation of K_m, the "Michaelis Constant" (mg/L), Representing the Drug Concentration at Which the Rate of Elimination is Half the Maximum Rate (V_{max}) for Zero-Order (i.e., Non-Linear) Model

$$\text{slope} = -K_m = \frac{\text{dose}_{initial} - \text{dose}_{increased}}{\text{dose}/C_{initial} - \text{dose}/C_{increased}}$$

10-2
(See p. 132.)

Calculating Steady-State Concentration from Estimates of K_m, V_{max}, and Dose (Rearrangement of the MME) for Zero-Order (i.e., Non-Linear) Model

$$C = \frac{K_m(\text{daily dose})}{V_{max} - \text{daily dose}}$$

10-3
(See p. 133.)

AMINOGLYCOSIDE DOSING EQUATIONS

Calculation of Population Estimates for K Based on CrCl

$$K = 0.00293(CrCl) + 0.014$$

12-1
(See p. 159.)

Calculation of Population Estimates for Volume of Distribution (V) Based on Body Weight or AdjBW$_{AG}$

$$V = 0.24 \text{ L/kg (IBW)}$$

12-2
(See p. 159.)
or:

$$V = 0.24 \text{ L/kg AdjBW}_{AG}$$

where:

$$AdjBW_{AG} = IBW + 0.1(TBW - IBW)$$

12-3
(See p. 159.)

Calculation of Best Dosing Interval (τ) Based on Desired Peak and Trough Concentrations

$$\tau = \frac{1}{-K}(\ln C_{trough(desired)} - \ln C_{peak(desired)}) + t$$

12-4
(See pp. 161 and 168.)
where t is the duration of the infusion in hours.

Note: should be rounded off to a practical dosing interval such as Q 8 hours, Q 12 hours, etc.

Calculation of Initial Maintenance Dose (K_0) Based on Estimates of K, V, Desired C_{peak}, and τ

$$C_{peak(steady state)} = \frac{K_0(1 - e^{-Kt})}{VK(1 - e^{-K\tau})}$$

5-1
(See p. 66.)
where:

$C_{peak(steady state)}$ = desired peak drug concentration at steady state (milligrams per liter),

K_0 = drug infusion rate (also maintenance dose you are trying to calculate, in milligrams per hour),

V = volume of distribution (population estimate for aminoglycosides, in liters),

K = elimination rate constant (population estimate for aminoglycosides, in reciprocal hours),

t = duration of infusion (hours), and

τ = desired or most appropriate dosing interval (hours).

Calculation of C_{trough} Concentration Expected from Dose (K_0) and Dosing Interval Used (τ)

⚠ $C = C_0 e^{-Kt}$
3-2

(See p. 32.)

or:

⚠ $C_{trough(steady\ state)} = C_{peak(steady\ state)} e^{-Kt'}$
3-2

(See p. 32.)

where $t' = \tau$ – time of infusion (t), or the change in time from the first concentration to the second.

Calculation of Loading Dose Based on Initial Calculated Maintenance Dose and Accumulation Factor

⚠ $\text{loading dose} = \dfrac{K_0}{(1 - e^{-K\tau})}$
12-5

(See p. 164.)

where:

K_0 = estimated maintenance dose,

$1/(1 - e^{-K\tau})$ = accumulation factor at steady state, and

τ = dosing interval at which estimated maintenance dose is given.

Calculation of Patient-Specific (i.e., Actual) K Based on Two Drug Concentrations and Dosing Interval

⚠ $K = -\dfrac{\ln C_{trough} - \ln C_{peak}}{\tau - t}$
3-1

(See p. 31.)

or:

$-K = \dfrac{\ln C_{peak} - \ln C_{trough}}{\tau - t}$

Remembering a rule of logarithms: $\ln a - \ln b = \ln (a/b)$, we can simplify this equation for hand-held calculators:

$$K = -\dfrac{\ln\left(\dfrac{C_{trough}}{C_{peak}}\right)}{\tau - t}$$

or:

$$-K = \dfrac{\ln\left(\dfrac{C_{peak}}{C_{trough}}\right)}{\tau - t}$$

Either equation may be used to calculate K.

Calculation of Patient-Specific (i.e., Actual) V Based on Actual K, and Dose (K_0), τ, and Two Drug Concentrations

⚠ $C_{peak(steady\ state)} = \dfrac{K_0(1 - e^{-Kt})}{VK(1 - e^{-K\tau})}$
5-1

(See p. 66.)

where:

$C_{peak(steady\ state)}$ = C_{peak} measured at steady state,

K_0 = maintenance dose infused at time C_{peak} and C_{trough} were measured,

V = patient's actual volume of distribution that you are trying to determine based on C_{peak} and C_{trough} values,

K = elimination rate constant calculated from patient's C_{peak} and C_{trough} values,

t = duration of infusion (hours), and

τ = patient's dosing interval at time C_{peak} and C_{trough} were measured.

Calculation of Actual (i.e., New) Dosing Interval Based on Patient-Specific Value for K

⚠ $\tau = \dfrac{1}{-K}(\ln C_{trough\ (desired)} - \ln C_{peak\ (desired)}) + t$
12-4

(See pp. 161 and 168.)

where t is the duration of infusion in hours and K is the actual elimination rate calculated from patient's peak and trough values.

Calculation of Patient-Specific or Adjusted Maintenance Dose (K_0) Based on Actual Values for K and V

⚠ $C_{peak(steady\ state)} = \dfrac{K_0(1 - e^{-Kt})}{VK(1 - e^{-K\tau})}$
5-1

(See p. 66.)

where:

$C_{peak(steady\ state)}$ = desired steady-state C_{peak};

K_0 = drug infusion rate (also adjusted maintenance dose you are trying to calculate, in milligrams per hour);

V = actual volume of distribution determined from patient's measured C_{peak} and C_{trough} values, in liters;

K = actual elimination rate constant calculated from patient's measured C_{peak} and C_{trough} values, in reciprocal hours;

t = infusion time, in hours; and

τ = adjusted dosing interval rounded to a practical number.

Calculation of New Expected $C_{trough(steady\ state)}$ That Would Result from New Maintenance Dose and Interval Used

⚠
3-2

$$C_{trough(steady\ state)} = C_{peak(steady\ state)}e^{-Kt'}$$

(See p. 32.)

where K is actual patient-specific K.

Calculation of "Time to Hold" Dose When Actual C_{trough} from Laboratory Is Too High

$$C_{trough(steady\ state)(desired)} = C_{trough(steady\ state)}e^{-Kt'}$$

where t' is the amount of time to hold the dose after the end of the dosing interval.

Next, take the natural log of both sides: number = number (t') and then simply solve for t', which is now not an exponent

Average Dose for Gentamicin or Tobramycin When Given as an Extended (i.e., Once Daily) Interval Dose Based on Actual Body Weight

⚠
12-6

$$X_0 = 4\text{–}7\ mg/kg\ actual\ body\ weight$$

(See p. 170.)

VANCOMYCIN DOSING EQUATIONS

Calculation of Population Estimate for K Based on CrCl

⚠
13-2

$$K = 0.00083\ hr^{-1}\ [CrCl\ (in\ mL/minute)] + 0.0044$$

(See p. 173.)

Calculation of Population Estimate for Volume of Distribution (V) Based on TBW

⚠
13-1

$$V = 0.9\ L/kg\ TBW$$

(See p. 173.)

Note that, unlike the aminoglycosides, it is recommended that TBW be used to calculate the volume of distribution.

Calculation of Best Dosing Interval (τ) Based on Desired Peak and Trough Concentrations

⚠
13-4

$$\tau = \frac{1}{-K}\left[\ln C_{trough\ (desired)} - \ln C_{peak\ (desired)}\right] + t + t'$$

(See p. 175 and **Equation 12-4**.)

where:

t = duration of infusion (usually 1 or 2 hours for vancomycin), and

t' = time between end of infusion and collection of blood sample (usually 2 hours).

Calculation of Initial Maintenance Dose (K_0) Based on Estimates of K, V, Desired C_{peak}, τ, and t

⚠
13-3

$$C_{peak(steady\ state)} = \frac{K_0(1-e^{-Kt})}{VK(1-e^{-K\tau})}e^{-Kt'}$$

(See p. 175 and **Equation 5-1**.)

where:

$C_{peak(steady\ state)}$ = desired peak concentration (usually 2 hours after end of infusion;

K_0 = drug infusion rate (dose/infusion time);

t = duration of infusion (usually 1 or 2 hours for vancomycin);

K = estimated elimination rate constant;

V = estimated volume of distribution;

t' = time between end of infusion and collection of blood sample (usually 2 hours) (inclusion of t' is different from the calculation for aminoglycosides because sampling time for vancomycin is often at least 4 hours after the beginning of the infusion); and

τ = desired dosing interval, as determined above.

Calculation of C_{trough} Concentration Expected from Dose (K_0) and Dosing Interval Used (τ)

⚠
13-5 $C_{trough} = C_{peak(steady\ state)} e^{-Kt''}$

(See p. 175 and **Equation 3-2**.)
where t'' is the difference in time between the two plasma concentrations.

Calculation of Patient-Specific (i.e., Actual) K Based on Two Drug Concentrations and Dosing Interval

$$K = -\frac{\ln C_{trough} - \ln C_{peak}}{\tau - t - t'}$$

(See **Equation 3-1**.)

Calculation of Patient-Specific (i.e., Actual) V Based on Actual K, and Dose (K_0), τ, and Two Drug Concentrations

⚠
13-3 $C_{peak(steady\ state)} = \dfrac{K_0(1 - e^{-Kt})}{VK(1 - e^{-K\tau})} e^{-Kt'}$

(See p. 175.)
where:

$C_{peak(steady\ state)}$ = measured steady-state peak plasma concentration drawn 2 hours after end of infusion.

Calculation of Actual (i.e., New) Dosing Interval Based on Patient-Specific Value for K

⚠
13-4 $\tau = \dfrac{1}{-K}[\ln C_{trough\ (desired)} - \ln C_{peak\ (desired)}] + t + t'$

(See p. 175.)

Calculation of Patient-Specific Maintenance Dose (K_0) Based on Actual Values for K and V

⚠
13-3 $C_{peak(steady\ state)} = \dfrac{K_0(1 - e^{-Kt})}{VK(1 - e^{-K\tau})} e^{-Kt'}$

(See p. 175.)

where:

$C_{peak(steady\ state)}$ = desired peak concentration at steady state;

K_0 = drug infusion rate (also maintenance dose you are trying to calculate, in milligrams per hour),

V = volume of distribution,

K = elimination rate constant calculated from C_{peak} and C_{trough},

t = infusion time (usually 1 or 2 hours),

t' = time from end of infusion until concentration is determined (usually 2 hours for peak), and

τ = desired or most appropriate dosing interval.

Calculation of New Expected $C_{trough(steady\ state)}$ That Would Result from New Maintenance Dose and Interval Used

⚠
13-5 $C_{trough\ (steady\ state)} = C_{peak(steady\ state)} e^{-Kt''}$

(See p. 175.)
where t'' is now the number of hours between the peak and trough ($t'' = \tau - t - t'$).

Calculation of "Time to Hold" Dose When Actual C_{trough} from Laboratory Is Too High

⚠
3-2 $C_{trough(desired)} = C_{trough(actual)} e^{-Kt}$

(See p. 32.)
where:

t is the amount of time to hold the dose.

Next, take the natural log of both sides:
'number' = 'number' (t') and then simply solve for t' which is now not an exponent

THEOPHYLLINE DOSING EQUATIONS

Equation for Calculating the Volume of Distribution for Theophylline and Aminophylline

⚠
14-1 $V(L) = weight(kg) \times 0.5\ L/kg$

(See p. 188.)

Equation for Calculating a Loading Dose of Theophylline or Aminophylline

$$D = \frac{CpdV}{SF}$$

14-2

(See p. 188.)

Equation for Calculating Clearance for Theophylline or Aminophylline

$$Cl = (0.04 \text{L/kg/hr}) \times \text{weight (kg)}$$

14-3

(See p. 189.)

Equation for Calculating a Theophylline or Aminophylline Maintenance Dose

$$D = \frac{\overline{C}p_{ss}\, Cl\, \tau}{SF}$$

14-4

(See p. 189.)

PHENYTOIN DOSING EQUATIONS

Calculation of Population Estimate for Volume of Distribution (V)

$$V = 0.65 \text{ L/kg}$$

Michaelis–Menten Constant, Representing the Concentration of Phenytoin at Which the Rate of Enzyme-Saturable Hepatic Metabolism Is One-Half of Maximum ($^{1}/_{2}V_{max}$)

$$K_m = 4 \text{ mg/L}$$

Maximum Amount of Drug That Can Be Metabolized Per Unit Time

$$V_{max} = 7 \text{ mg/kg/day}$$

Note: usually expressed as mg/day.

Calculation of Phenytoin Loading Dose

$$X_0 = \frac{V \times C_{desired}}{S}$$

1-1

(See p. 10.)

where:
  V = volume of distribution estimate of 0.65 L/kg,
  $C_{desired}$ = concentration desired 1 hour after the end of the infusion, and
  S = salt factor.

Two Representations of Michaelis–Menten Equation Used To Calculate Daily Dose [X_0/τ (S)] or Expected Serum Concentration C_{ss}

$$X_0/\tau\ (S) = \frac{V_{max} \times C_{ss}}{K_m + C_{ss}}$$

10-1

(See p. 132.)

$$C_{ss} = \frac{X_0/\tau\ (S) \times K_m}{V_{max} - X_0/\tau\ (S)}$$

15-1

(See p. x.)

Calculation of Time (in Days) for Phenytoin Dosing Regimen to Reach Approximately 90% of Its Steady-State Concentration

$$t_{90\%} = \frac{K_m \times V}{(V_{max} - X_d)^2}[(2.3 \times V_{max}) - (0.9 \times X_d)]$$

10-4

(See p. 133.)

where:
  X_d = daily dose of phenytoin (in mg/day),
  V = volume of distribution,
  V_{max} = maximum rate of drug metabolism (in mg/day), and
  K_m = Michaelis–Menten constant.

Phenytoin Dosing Methods

Empiric Dosing Method 1A

Use 5 mg/kg/day

Empiric Dosing Method 1B

Use population estimates for the Michaelis–Menten values for K_m of 4 mg/L and V_{max} of 7 mg/kg/day and solve the general MME formula as shown below:

$$X_0/\tau\ (S) = \frac{V_{max} \times C_{ss-desired}}{K_m + C_{ss-desired}}$$

Dosing Method 2

Use this method after you have one steady-state phenytoin serum drug concentration to solve for V_{max} while still using the population parameter for K_m.

First, to solve for V_{max}:

⚠ 10-1
$$V_{max} = \frac{(X_d \times S)(K_m + C_{ss-lab})}{C_{ss-lab}}$$

(See p. 132.)
where:
  V_{max} = calculated estimate of patient's V_{max},
  K_m = population estimate of 4 mg/L,
  $X_d \times S$ = patient's daily dose of phenytoin free acid), and
  C_{ss} = reported steady-state concentration.

Second, after solving for this "better" value for V_{max}, use it plus the old K_m value in the MME to re-solve for dose, as shown below:

⚠ 10-1
$$X_d \times S = \frac{V_{max} \times C_{ss}}{K_m + C_{ss}}$$

(See p. 132.)
where:
  $X_d \times S$ = new dose of phenytoin (either free acid or salt),
  C_{ss} = desired steady-state concentration (usually 15 mg/L),
  K_m = population estimate of 4 mg/L, and
  V_{max} = calculated estimate from above.

Dosing Method 3

Use after you have two steady-state phenytoin concentrations from two different phenytoin doses. You can now work another equation to solve for a better value for K_m (shown below). Then use this better K_m value to once again re-solve for an even better V_{max} value than used in Method 2. Once you get new (i.e., real) K_m and V_{max}, re-solve the MME equation for dose.

First, solve for "real" K_m. The slope of the line, which represents $-K_m$, can now be calculated as follows:

⚠ 10-2
$$-K_m = \frac{X_1 - X_2}{\dfrac{X_1}{C_1} - \dfrac{X_2}{C_2}}$$

(See p. 132.)
where:
  X = dose, and
  C = concentration.

Next, we substitute this new value for K_m into the MME and solve for a V_{max} as follows:

⚠ 10-1
$$V_{max} = \frac{(X_d \times S)(K_m + C_{ss})}{C_{ss}}$$

(See p. 132.)
where:
  $X_d \times S$ = either of the doses the patient received, expressed as free acid,

  C_{ss} = steady-state concentration at the dose selected, and
  K_m = calculated value.

Finally, we substitute our new V_{max} value (mg/day) and our calculated K_m value (mg/mL) into the MME and solve for X_d as follows:

⚠ 10-1
$$X_d \times S = \frac{V_{max} \times C_{ss}}{K_m + C_{ss}}$$

(See p. 132.)

DIGOXIN DOSING EQUATIONS

Volume of Distribution of Digoxin in Patients with Normal Renal Function

⚠ 15-2
$$V_{ss} = 4 \text{ to } 9 \text{ L/kg IBW (average, 6.7 L/kg IBW)}$$

(See p. 200.)

Equation for Estimating Total Systemic Clearance for Digoxin

⚠ 15-3
$$Cl_t = (1.101 \times Cl_r) + Cl_m$$

(See p. 200.)
where:
  Cl_r is expressed as mL/minute/1.73 m^2,
  Cl_m = 36 mL/minute/1.73 m^2 in patients without active heart failure, and
    = 20 mL/minute/1.73 m^2 in patients with severe heart failure.

Equation for Estimating Renal Clearance of Digoxin

⚠ 15-4
$$Cl_r = 0.927 \times \text{creatinine clearance (mL/minute/1.73 m}^2)$$

(See p. 200.)

Equation Showing Relationship between Steady-State Plasma Concentration, Maintenance Dose, and Total Systemic Clearance

⚠ 15-5
$$C_{ss} = \frac{X_d \times 10^6 \times F}{Cl_t \times \tau}$$

(See p. 200.)

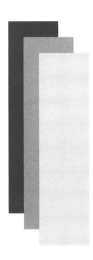

APPENDIX
B

Supplemental Problems*

QUESTIONS

SP1. Antipyrine (a drug used for pharmacologic and pharmacokinetic studies in the evaluation of hepatic mixed-function oxidase activity) was administered as a single intravenous (IV) bolus dose (1200 mg). The following plasma drug concentration and time data were collected:

Time after Dose (hours)	Plasma Drug Concentration (mg/L)
2	26.1
4	24.3
8	20.7
18	14.2
32	8.6
48	4.5

Using semilog graph paper, determine the approximate time after the dose when the plasma drug concentration falls to 3.0 mg/L.

A. 50 hours

B. 40 hours

C. 70 hours

D. 60 hours

SP2. Using the same data for antipyrine dosing above, estimate the volume of distribution.

A. 50.2 L

B. 42.9 L

C. 45.3 L

D. 24.9 L

SP3. Just after an IV dose of antibiotic X, the plasma drug concentration was 7.3 mg/L. Six hours later, the concentration was 2.9 mg/L. Predict the plasma drug concentration at 10 hours after the dose.

A. 2.9 mg/L

B. 2.1 mg/L

C. 1.63 mg/L

D. 3.1 mg/L

SP4. The following plasma drug concentration and time data were obtained after an IV bolus dose of procainamide (420 mg):

Time after Dose (hours)	Plasma Drug Concentration (mg/L)
0	3.86
0.5	3.36
1.0	3.00
2.0	2.29
3.0	1.77
5.0	1.06
7.0	0.63
10.0	0.29

Calculate clearance by the area method.

A. 27.83 L/hour

B. 19.4 L/hour

C. 33.6 L/hour

D. 11.8 L/hour

*These problems supplement material presented in Lessons 1–11.

SP5. What will be the minimum concentration after the thirteenth IV dose of drug X if C_{max} equals 100 mg/L after the first dose, K equals 0.4 hr^{-1}, and τ equals 6 hours? (Assume an IV bolus dose model.)

A. 8.98 mg/L

B. 9.98 mg/L

C. 13.9 mg/L

D. 7.36 mg/L

SP6. An IV bolus dose of antibiotic Q (500 mg) was administered to a patient on an every-6-hour schedule. Predict the plasma drug concentrations at 3 and 6 hours after dosing. Assume: (1) a one-compartment model, (2) $T^{1/2}$ = 4.95 hours, (3) Cl_t = 14.2 L/hour, and (4) the attainment of steady state.

A. 5.7 and 3.7 mg/L, respectively

B. 7.1 and 9.8 mg/L, respectively

C. 3.7 and 2.9 mg/L, respectively

D. 6.9 and 5.7 mg/L, respectively

SP7. For the same patient, predict the plasma concentrations at 3 and 6 hours after the second dose.

A. 6.46 and 5.02 mg/L, respectively

B. 3.32 and 2.19 mg/L, respectively

C. 8.12 and 5.78 mg/L, respectively

D. 4.64 and 3.05 mg/L, respectively

SP8. An 80-kg patient receives 500 mg of drug Y intravenously by bolus injection every 6 hours. Assume that V = 0.5 L/kg, and $T^{1/2}$ = 6.4 hours. Predict the steady-state peak and trough concentrations.

A. 28.6 and 14.7 mg/L, respectively

B. 26.2 and 13.7 mg/L, respectively

C. 24.3 and 12.9 mg/L, respectively

D. 19.8 and 9.6 mg/L, respectively

SP9. Calculate the theophylline clearance (Cl_t) for a 52-kg patient receiving a continuous IV infusion of aminophylline at 75 mg/hour. The patient's steady-state plasma theophylline concentration with this dose rate is 20.2 mg/L. Assume that the patient's V = 0.45 L/kg. Remember, aminophylline = 80% theophylline.

A. 2.97 L/hour

B. 3.75 L/hour

C. 3.71 L/hour

D. 2.37 L/hour

SP10. The following plasma concentration and time data were collected after a single 500-mg IV dose of amikacin:

Time after Dose (hours)	Amikacin Concentration (mg/L)
2	22.5
4	18.4
8	12.3
16	5.6
24	2.5
36	0.75
48	0.23

Calculate K, V_{area}, and Cl_t for this patient.

A. 0.20 hr^{-1}, 28.2 L, and 2.82 L/hour, respectively

B. 0.01 hr^{-1}, 1.82 L, and 0.182 L/hour, respectively

C. 0.10 hr^{-1}, 18.2 L, and 1.82 L/hour, respectively

D. 0.10 hr^{-1}, 182 L, and 18.2 L/hour, respectively

SP11. Seven healthy female subjects were each given 1250 mg of an experimental drug (BB-K8) by IV bolus administration. The drug follows first-order kinetics. The following mean plasma concentration and time data were obtained:

Time after Dose (hours)	Mean Plasma Drug Concentration (mg/L)
0	116.0
0.08	108.3
0.17	92.8
0.25	83.3
0.50	59.2
0.75	38.2
1.0	30.6
1.5	22.9
2.0	19.7
3.0	13.2
4.0	9.3
5.0	7.3
6.0	5.1
7.0	4.1
8.0	2.8

Plot the plasma concentration versus time profile on semilog paper. From your graph, determine A, B, α, β, V_{area}, and Cl_t (in milliliters per minute).

A. 3.60 hr^{-1}, 0.41 hr^{-1}, 39.1 L, and 11 L/hour, respectively

B. 2.60 hr^{-1}, 0.31 hr^{-1}, 29.1 L, and 9 L/hour, respectively

C. 1.60 hr^{-1}, 0.21 hr^{-1}, 19.1 L, and 7 L/hour, respectively

D. 4.60 hr^{-1}, 0.35 hr^{-1}, 49.1 L, and 12 L/hour, respectively

SP12. Calculate V_{area} given the data in Supplemental Problem 1. Compare it with the V calculated (using the back-extrapolation method) in Supplemental Problem 2.

A. 54.6 L

B. 43.6 L

C. 10.3 L

D. 42.96 L

SP13. An outpatient had been taking 400 mg of phenytoin per day for 1 month and had a plasma concentration of 6.0 mg/L when sampled 6 hours after the dose. Because of continued seizures, the dose was increased to 500 mg/day. Four weeks later, the patient was seen in a clinic, and the plasma drug concentration 6 hours after the dose was 9.0 mg/L (assume steady state). The physicians asked that the dose be increased to provide a plasma concentration of 12 mg/L 6 hours after the dose. What dose would you recommend?

A. 552 mg phenytoin free acid/day

B. 600 mg phenytoin free acid/day

C. 652 mg phenytoin free acid/day

D. 900 mg phenytoin free acid/day

ANSWERS

SP1. A, B, C. Incorrect answers

D. CORRECT ANSWER

SP2. A, C, D. Incorrect answers

B. CORRECT ANSWER.

$$C_0 = 28 \text{ mg/L}$$

$$V = \frac{\text{dose}}{C_0} = \frac{1200 \text{ mg}}{28 \text{ mg/L}} = 42.9 \text{ L}$$

SP3. A, B, D. Incorrect answers

C. CORRECT ANSWER. First, calculate the elimination rate constant (K):

$$K = -\frac{(\ln 7.3 - \ln 2.9)}{(0 - 6 \text{ hr})} = 0.15 \text{ hr}^{-1}$$

Then use these equations:

$$C = C_0 e^{-Kt}$$

$$C_{at\ 10\ hr} = (7.3 \text{ mg/L})e^{-0.15\ hr^{-1}(10\ hr)}$$

$$= 1.63 \text{ mg/L}$$

SP4. A. CORRECT ANSWER. To calculate clearance by the area method, we need to know the area under the plasma concentration curve (AUC) and the dose (X_0). Therefore, it is first necessary to calculate AUC using the trapezoidal method as shown below. Note that one way to indicate an AUC from one time point to another is as $AUC_{0\rightarrow0.5}$, which means AUC from 0 to 0.5 hour.

$$AUC_{0\rightarrow0.5} = \frac{(3.84 \text{ mg/L} + 3.36 \text{ mg/L})}{2} \times (0.5 - 0 \text{ hr}) = 1.80 (\text{mg/L}) \times \text{hr}$$

$$AUC_{0.5\rightarrow1} = \frac{(3.36 + 3.00)}{2} \times (1 - 0.5) = 1.59 (\text{mg/L}) \times \text{hr}$$

$$AUC_{1\rightarrow2} = \frac{(3.00 + 2.29)}{2} \times (2 - 1) = 2.65 (\text{mg/L}) \times \text{hr}$$

$$AUC_{2\rightarrow3} = \frac{(2.29 + 1.77)}{2} \times (3 - 2) = 2.03 (\text{mg/L}) \times \text{hr}$$

$$AUC_{3\rightarrow5} = \frac{(1.77 + 1.06)}{2} \times (5 - 3) = 2.83 (\text{mg/L}) \times \text{hr}$$

$$AUC_{5\rightarrow7} = \frac{(1.06 + 0.63)}{2} \times (7 - 5) = 1.69 (\text{mg/L}) \times \text{hr}$$

$$AUC_{7\rightarrow10} = \frac{(0.63 + 0.29)}{2} \times (10 - 7) = 1.38 (\text{mg/L}) \times \text{hr}$$

$$AUC_{10\rightarrow\infty} = \frac{C_{10\ hr}}{K} = \frac{0.29 \text{ mg/L}}{0.26 \text{ hr}^{-1}} = 1.12 (\text{mg/L}) \times \text{hr}$$

$$AUC = 1.80 + 1.59 + 2.65 + 2.03 + 2.83 + 1.69 + 1.38 + 1.12 = 15.09 \text{ (mg/L)} \times \text{hr}$$

$$Cl_t = \frac{X_0}{AUC} = \frac{420 \text{ mg}}{15.09 \text{ (mg/L)} \times \text{hr}} = 27.83 \text{ L/hr}$$

B, C, D. Incorrect answers

SP5. A, C, D. Incorrect answers

B. CORRECT ANSWER. To determine C_{min} after the thirteenth dose, first calculate C_{max} after the thirteenth dose using the multiple-dose equation:

$$C_{max(nth\ dose)} = C_{max(nth\ dose)} \frac{(1 - e^{-nK\tau})}{(1 - e^{-K\tau})}$$

$$C_{max13} = C_{max1} \frac{(1 - e^{-13K\tau})}{(1 - e^{-K\tau})}$$

$$C_{max13} = (100 \text{ mg/L})\frac{(1-e^{(-13)(0.4 \text{ hr}^{-1})(6 \text{ hr})})}{(1-e^{(-0.4 \text{ hr}^{-1})(6 \text{ hr})})}$$

$$= 110 \text{ mg/L}$$

Then:

$$C_{min13} = C_{max13}e^{-K\tau} = (110 \text{ mg/L})e^{(-0.4 \text{ hr}^{-1})(6 \text{ hr})}$$

$$= 9.98 \text{ mg/L}$$

SP6. A. CORRECT ANSWER. To predict plasma concentrations 3 and 6 hours after a dose at steady state, we should first estimate the C_{max} (at 0 hour after the dose) using the steady-state IV equation:

$$C_{max} = \frac{X_0}{V(1-e^{-K\tau})}$$

So we first need to estimate V and K. V can be estimated from:

$$Cl_t = VK$$

Then:

$$V = \frac{Cl_t}{K} = \frac{14.2 \text{ L/hr}}{\left(\dfrac{0.693}{4.95 \text{ hr}}\right)}$$

$$V = 101.43 \text{ L}$$

Note that:

$$K = \frac{0.693}{T\frac{1}{2}} = 0.14 \text{ hr}^{-1}$$

Then:

$$C_{max} = \frac{500 \text{ mg}}{(101.43 \text{ L})(1-e^{-0.14 \text{ hr}^{-1}(6 \text{ hr})})}$$

$$= 8.67 \text{ mg/L}$$

From C_{max}, the concentration at anytime after a dose can be calculated by:

$$C_t = C_{max}e^{-Kt}$$

So:

$$C_{3 \text{ hr}} = (8.67 \text{ mg/L})(e^{-0.14 \text{ hr}^{-1})(6 \text{ hr})})$$

$$= 5.7 \text{ mg/L}$$

and:

$$C_{6 \text{ hr}} = (8.67 \text{ mg/L})(e^{-0.14 \text{ hr}^{-1})(6 \text{ hr})})$$

$$= 3.74 \text{ mg/L}$$

B, C, D. Incorrect answers

SP7. A, B, C. Incorrect answers

D. CORRECT ANSWER. The equations used to solve Special Problem 5 can be used here, with the number of doses (n) equal to 2 rather than 13:

$$C_{max(2nd \text{ dose})} = \frac{X_0(1-e^{-nK\tau})}{V(1-e^{-K\tau})}$$

$$= \frac{(500 \text{ mg})(1-e^{(-2)(-0.14 \text{ hr}^{-1})(6 \text{ hr})})}{(101.43 \text{ L})(1-e^{(-0.14 \text{ hr}^{-1})(6 \text{ hr})})}$$

$$= 7.06 \text{ mg/L}$$

Then:

$$C_t = C_{max}e^{-Kt}$$

$$C_{3 \text{ hr}} = (7.06 \text{ mg/L})(e^{(-0.14 \text{ hr}^{-1})(6 \text{ hr})})$$

$$= 4.64 \text{ mg/L}$$

and:

$$C_{6 \text{ hr}} = (7.06 \text{ mg/L})(e^{(-0.14 \text{ hr}^{-1})(6 \text{ hr})})$$

$$= 3.05 \text{ mg/L}$$

SP8. A, C, D. Incorrect answers

B. CORRECT ANSWER. First, determine K and total V:

$$V = 0.5 \text{ L/kg} \times 80 \text{ kg} = 40 \text{ L}$$

$$K = \frac{0.693}{T\frac{1}{2}} = \frac{0.693}{6.4 \text{ hr}} = 0.108 \text{ hr}^{-1}$$

Then use the steady-state multiple-dose equation (for IV bolus doses):

$$C_{peak} = \frac{X_0}{V}\left(\frac{1}{1-e^{-K\tau}}\right)$$

$$= \frac{500 \text{ mg}}{(40 \text{ L})(1-e^{-0.108 \text{ hr}^{-1}(6 \text{ hr})})}$$

$$= 26.2 \text{ mg/L}$$

$$C_{trough} = C_{peak}e^{-K\tau}$$

$$= (26.2 \text{ mg/L})e^{-0.108 \text{ hr}^{-1}(6 \text{ hr})}$$

$$= 13.7 \text{ mg/L}$$

SP9. A. CORRECT ANSWER. To calculate clearance, use the relationship:

$$Cl_t = \frac{K_0}{C_{ss}} = \frac{75 \text{ mg/hr } (0.80)}{20.2 \text{ mg/L}} = 2.97 \text{L/hr}$$

B, C, D. Incorrect answers

SP10. A, B, D. Incorrect answers

C. CORRECT ANSWER. First, the data should be plotted on semilog graph paper to determine if they are linear or nonlinear. When the points are determined to make a straight line, any two may be chosen to calculate K. (It is best, however, to choose two that are not close to each other, such as 2 and 4 hours.) So:

$$K = -\frac{\Delta Y}{\Delta X} = -\left(\frac{\ln 0.75 - \ln 22.5}{36 \text{ hr} - 2 \text{ hr}}\right) = 0.10 \text{ hr}^{-1}$$

Then:

$$T\frac{1}{2} = \frac{0.693}{K} = 6.93 \text{ hr}$$

To calculate V_{area} and Cl_t, we should first estimate the AUC. With a one-compartment, first-order model after IV administration, the calculation of AUC is simplified. In this case:

$$AUC = \frac{C_0}{K}$$

where C_0 is determined by $C_t = C_0 e^{-Kt}$. For $t = 2$ hours:

$$22.5 \text{ mg/L} = C_0 e^{-0.10 \text{ hr}^{-1}(2 \text{ hr})}$$

Then:

$$C_0 = 27.5 \text{ mg/L}$$

and:

$$AUC = \frac{27.5 \text{ mg/L}}{0.1 \text{ hr}^{-1}} = 275 \text{ mg/L} \times \text{hr}$$

Then:

$$V_{area} = \frac{X_0}{AUC \times K}$$
$$= \frac{500 \text{ mg}}{(275 \text{mg/L} \times \text{hr})(0.10 \text{ hr}^{-1})}$$
$$= 18.2 \text{ L}$$

$$Cl_t = \frac{X_0}{AUC}$$
$$= \frac{500 \text{ mg}}{275 \text{ mg/L} \times \text{hr}} = 1.82 \text{ L/hr}$$

Note that the use of AUC for calculation of clearance generally produces a more accurate estimate than the use of $Cl_t = K \times V$.

SP11. A, C, D. Incorrect answers

B. CORRECT ANSWER. A, B, α, and β will be calculated using residuals. First, back-extrapolate the terminal (straight-line) portion of the plot and estimate the back-extrapolated points. Determine the residual points by subtracting the back-extrapolated concentrations from the actual concentrations.

Actual Points		Back-Extrapolated Points		Residual Points
108.3	–	32.0	=	76.3 mg/L
92.8	–	31.0	=	61.8 mg/L
83.3	–	30.0	=	53.3 mg/L
59.2	–	28.0	=	31.2 mg/L
38.2	–	26.0	=	12.2 mg/L
30.6	–	24.0	=	6.6 mg/L
22.9	–	21.0	=	1.9 mg/L

Then plot the residual points on the same graph. From the back-extrapolated line, the intercept = B (equals 33 mg/L) and the terminal slope gives β:

$$\beta = \frac{\ln 2.8 - \ln 13.2}{8 \text{ hr} - 3 \text{ hr}} = -0.31$$
$$= 0.31 \text{ hr}^{-1}$$

Then from the residual line, the intercept = A (equals 84 mg/L) and the slope gives α:

$$\alpha = \frac{\ln 1.9 - \ln 76.3}{1.5 \text{ hr} - 0.08 \text{ hr}} = -2.60$$
$$= 2.60 \text{ hr}^{-1}$$

To calculate V_{area} and Cl_t, the AUC must first be determined. The AUC can be estimated using the trapezoidal rule or by adding the area of each exponential equation:

$$AUC = \frac{A}{\alpha} + \frac{B}{\beta} = 32.3 + 106.5$$
$$= 138.8 \text{ (mg/L)} \times \text{hr}$$

Then:

$$V_{area} = \frac{dose}{AUC \times \beta}$$

$$= \frac{1250 \text{ mg}}{[138.8 \,(\text{mg/L}) \times \text{hr}](0.31 \text{ hr}^{-1})} = 29.1 \text{ L}$$

$$Cl_t = \frac{dose}{AUC}$$

$$= \frac{1250 \text{ mg}}{138.8 \text{ mg/L}} = 9.0 \text{ L/hr}$$

SP12. A, B, C. Incorrect answers

D. CORRECT ANSWER.

$$V_{area} = \frac{dose}{AUC \times K}$$

$$K = 0.037 \text{ hr}^{-1}$$

To calculate the AUC, the C_0 must first be estimated from the plot (C_0 = 28 mg/L):

$$AUC_{0 \to 2} = \frac{(28 + 26.1)(2 - 0)}{2} = 54.1 (\text{mg/L}) \times \text{hr}$$

$$AUC_{2 \to 4} = \frac{(26.1 + 24.3)(4 - 2)}{2} = 50.4 (\text{mg/L}) \times \text{hr}$$

$$AUC_{4 \to 8} = \frac{(24.3 + 20.7)(8 - 4)}{2} = 90.0 (\text{mg/L}) \times \text{hr}$$

$$AUC_{8 \to 18} = \frac{(20.7 + 14.2)(18 - 8)}{2} = 174.5 (\text{mg/L}) \times \text{hr}$$

$$AUC_{18 \to 32} = \frac{(14.2 + 8.6)(32 - 18)}{2} = 159.6 (\text{mg/L}) \times \text{hr}$$

$$AUC_{32 \to 48} = \frac{(8.6 + 4.5)(48 - 32)}{2} = 104.8 (\text{mg/L}) \times \text{hr}$$

$$AUC_{48 \to \infty} = \frac{C_{48}}{K} = \frac{4.5 \text{ mg/L}}{0.037 \text{ hr}^{-1}} = 121.6 (\text{mg/L}) \times \text{hr}$$

Then:

$$AUC = 54.1 + 50.4 + 90.0 + 174.5 + 159.6 + 104.8 + 121.6$$

$$= 755 \,(\text{mg/L}) \times \text{hr}$$

$$V_{area} = \frac{X_0}{AUC \times K}$$

$$= \frac{1200 \text{ mg}}{[755 \,(\text{mg/L}) \times \text{hr}](0.037 \text{ hr}^{-1})} = 42.96 \text{ L}$$

So, in this case, the two estimates for V are similar.

SP13. A, C, D. Incorrect answers

B. CORRECT ANSWER. Phenytoin follows Michaelis–Menten (saturable) pharmacokinetics. To determine V_m and K_m, the daily dose must be plotted (y-axis) versus the daily dose divided by the resulting steady-state concentrations (x-axis). From a plot of the dose (y-axis) versus dose/concentration (x-axis), the following are observed:

V_m = 1000 mg daily (which is equal to the y-intercept)

K_m = 9.0 mg/L (which equals –slope)

Then:

$$\text{dose} = \frac{V_m C_{ss}}{K_m + C_{ss}}$$

where:

C_{ss} = 12 mg/L, the desired concentration:

$$= \frac{(1000 \text{ mg})(12 \text{ mg/L})}{9.0 \text{ mg/L} + 12 \text{ mg/L}} = 571 \text{ mg/day}$$

Therefore, the likely daily dose would be 600 mg/day.

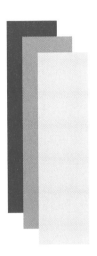

APPENDIX C

Glossary

Area under the moment curve (AUMC)—the area under the (drug concentration × time) versus time (moment) curve, an important model-independent pharmacokinetic parameter.

Area under the plasma concentration versus time curve (AUC)—the area formed under the curve when plasma drug concentration is plotted versus time. Drug clearance is equal to the dose administered divided by AUC.

Bioavailability (F)—the fraction of a given drug dose that reaches the systemic circulation.

Biopharmaceutics—the study of the relationship between the nature and intensity of a drug's biologic effects and various drug formulation or administration factors, such as the drug's chemical nature, inert formulation substances, pharmaceutical processes used to manufacture the dosage form, and routes of administration.

Clearance—the process of removing a drug from plasma (expressed as volume of plasma per a given unit of time).

Clinical pharmacokinetics—the application of pharmacokinetic principles to the safe and effective therapeutic management of drugs in an individual patient.

Compartmental model—a basic type of model used in pharmacokinetics. Compartmental models are categorized by the number of compartments needed to describe the drug's behavior in the body. There are one-compartment, two-compartment, and multi-compartment models. The compartments do not represent a specific tissue or fluid but may represent a group of similar tissues or fluids.

Drug distribution—transport processes that deliver drug to body tissues and fluids after absorption.

50% effective concentration (EC_{50})—the concentration at which 50% of the maximum drug effect is achieved.

Elimination rate constant (K)—a constant representing the fraction of drug removed per unit of time (in units of reciprocal time, usually hr^{-1}).

Extraction ratio (E)—the fraction of drug removed from plasma by one pass through an organ. This ratio is a number between 1 and 0. Organs that are very efficient at eliminating a drug will have an extraction ratio approaching 1 (i.e., 100% extraction).

First-order elimination—occurs when the amount of drug eliminated from the body in a specific time is dependent on the amount of drug in the body at that time. A straight line is obtained from the natural log of plasma drug concentration versus time plot only for drugs that follow first-order elimination.

First-pass effect—drug metabolism by the liver that occurs after absorption but before the drug reaches the systemic circulation.

Formation clearance ($CL_{P \to mX}$)—a model-independent parameter that provides a meaningful estimate of a drug's fractional metabolic clearance.

Half-life ($T\frac{1}{2}$)—the amount of time necessary for a plasma drug concentration to decrease by half.

Kinetic homogeneity—describes the predictable relationship between plasma drug concentration and concentration at the receptor site.

Mean residence time (MRT)—the average time for intact drug molecules to transit or reside in the body.

Model—a simplified mathematical simulation of physiologic processes used to predict the time course of drug concentrations or effect in the body.

Model-independent parameter—a pharmacokinetic parameter, such as clearance, that can be calculated without the use of a specific model.

Model-independent pharmacokinetics—pharmacokinetic calculations using parameters that do not require the use of specific compartmental models (e.g., one-compartment, two-compartment, etc.).

Pharmacodynamics—the relationship between drug concentrations at the site of action and the resulting effect, including the time course and intensity of therapeutic and adverse effects.

Pharmacokinetics—the relationship of drug dose to the time course of drug absorption, distribution, metabolism, and excretion.

Plasma—the fluid portion of blood (including soluble proteins but not formed elements).

Receptor—a structure on the surface of a cell to which a drug binds and causes an effect within the cell.

Serum—the fluid portion of blood that remains when the soluble protein fibrinogen is removed from plasma.

Steady state—the point at which, after multiple doses, the amount of drug administered over a dosing interval equals the amount of drug being eliminated over that same period.

Therapeutic drug monitoring—determination of plasma drug concentrations and clinical data to optimize a patient's drug therapy.

Therapeutic range—the plasma concentration range that is effective and safe in treating specific diseases.

Tolerance—decreased drug effectiveness with continued use.

Volume of distribution (V)—an important indicator of the extent of drug distribution into body fluids and tissues, V relates the amount of drug in the body to the measured concentration in the plasma. Thus, V is the volume required to account for all of the drug in the body if the concentration in all tissues is the same as the plasma concentration.

Volume of distribution at steady state (V_{ss})—a parameter that relates total amount of drug in the body to a particular plasma concentration under steady-state conditions.

Zero-order elimination—when the amount of drug eliminated for each time interval is constant, regardless of the amount of drug in the body.

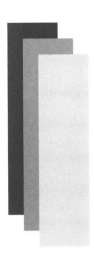

Index

Page numbers followed by *f* refer to figures; those followed by *t* indicate tables.